Medullary Thyroid Carcinoma

Cancer médullaire de la thyroïde

Colloques **INSERM**
ISSN 0768-3154

Other *Colloques* published as co-editions by John Libbey Eurotext and INSERM

133 Cardiovascular and Respiratory Physiology in the Fetus and Neonate. *Physiologie Cardiovasculaire et Respiratoire du Fœtus et du Nouveau-né.*
Scientific Committee : P. Karlberg,
A. Minkowski, W. Oh and L. Stern;
Managing Editor : M. Monset-Couchard.
ISBN : John Libbey Eurotext 0 86196 125 0
INSERM 2 85598 340 1

134 Porphyrins and Porphyrias. *Porphyrines et Porphyries.*
Edited by Y. Nordmann.
ISBN : John Libbey Eurotext 0 86196 087 4
INSERM 2 85598 281 2

137 Neo-Adjuvant Chemotherapy. *Chimiothérapie Néo-Adjuvante.*
Edited by C. Jacquillat, M. Weil and D. Khayat.
ISBN : John Libbey Eurotext 0 86196 125 0
INSERM 2 85598 340 1

139 Hormones and Cell Regulation (10th European Symposium). *Hormones et Régulation Cellulaire (10ᵉ Symposium Européen).*
Edited by J. Nunez, J.E. Dumont and R.J.B. King.
ISBN : John Libbey Eurotext 0 86196 125 0X
INSERM 2 85598 340 1

147 Modern Trends in Aging Research. *Nouvelles Perspectives de la Recherche sur le Vieillissement.*
Edited by Y. Courtois, B. Faucheux, B. Forette, D.L. Knook and J.A. Tréton.
ISBN : John Libbey Eurotext 0 86196 126 0X
INSERM 2 85598 340 1

149 Binding Proteins of Steroid Hormones. *Protéines de liaison des Hormones Stéroïdes.*
Edited by M.G. Forest and M. Pugeat.
ISBN : John Libbey Eurotext 0 86196 125 0
INSERM 2 85598 340 1X

151 Control and Management of Parturition. *La Maîtrise de la Parturition.*
Edited by C. Sureau, P. Blot, D. Cabrol, F. Cavaillé and G. Germain.
ISBN : John Libbey Eurotext 0 86196 125 0
INSERM 2 85598 340 1

Medullary Thyroid Carcinoma

Cancer médullaire de la thyroïde

Proceedings of the first European Congress on medullary thyroid carcinoma held in Paris (France), November 15-17, 1990

Initiated by the Groupe d'Étude des Tumeurs à Calcitonine (GETC) and sponsored by the Institut National de la Santé et de la Recherche Médicale (INSERM), the Centre National de la Recherche Scientifique (CNRS) and the Association pour la Recherche sur le Cancer (ARC)

Edited by

Claude Calmettes
Jean-Michel Guliana

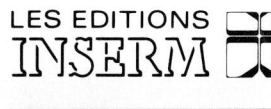

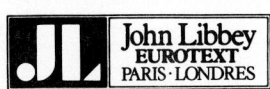

British Library Cataloguing in Publication Data

Medullary thyroid carcinoma
   Humans. Thyroid gland. Cancer
   I. Calmettes Claude. II. Guliana Jean-Michel
   616 44

ISBN 0 86196 287 7
ISSN 0768-3154

First published in 1991 by

Editions John Libbey Eurotext
6 rue Blanche, 92120 Montrouge, France. (1) 47 35 85 52
ISBN 0 86196 287 7

John Libbey and Company Ltd
13 Smiths Yard, Summerley Street, London SW18 4HR, England.
(1) 947 27 77

Institut National de la Santé et de la Recherche Médicale
101 rue de Tolbiac, 75654 Paris Cedex 13, France.
(1) 45 84 14 41
ISBN 2 85598 444 0

ISSN 0768-3154

© 1991 Colloques INSERM/John Libbey Eurotext Ltd,
All rights reserved
Unauthorized publication contravenes applicable laws

Preface

Thirty years have passed since the description by Hazard, Hawk and Crile of medullary cancer of the thyroid. Improvement in the knowledge of the disease has concerned all its aspects, such as malignancy, endocrinology, genetics and epidemiology. This is a time of exciting discoveries in basic research but also of European collaboration. So, the Groupe d'Etude des Tumeurs à Calcitonine has initiated a congress devoted to this tumor, in order to point out and transmit a statement of the question as full as possible and to open the way to a more collaborative approach of the disease.

Trente ans se sont écoulés depuis la description par Hazard, Hawk et Crile du cancer médullaire de la thyroïde. Les progrès réalisés depuis lors concernent tous les domaines dans lesquels se situe cette affection tumorale, endocrinienne, sporadique ou héréditaire à transmission autosomique dominante. Nous sommes dans une période fructueuse tant en recherche fondamentale que du fait d'une collaboration plus marquée au sein de l'Europe. Le Groupe d'Etude des Tumeurs à Calcitonine a pris l'initiative de ce congrès destiné tant à faire le point des connaissances actuelles sur cette maladie que d'en assurer la diffusion parmi les médecins et chercheurs de toutes spécialisations, mais aussi à permettre des rencontres et des échanges qui ouvrent la voie à une approche plus collective sur le continent.

C. Calmettes
J.M. Guliana

Honorary presidents / *Présidents d'honneur*
Pr Gérard Milhaud and Pr Maurice Tubiana

President
Dr Claude Calmettes

Organizing Committee / *Comité d'organisation*
C. Calmettes, M.J. Delisle, N. Feingold, B. Franc, P.J. Guillausseau, J.M. Guliana, E. Modigliani

Scientific Committee / *Conseil scientifique*

J.L. Baulieu (France)
B. Busnardo (Italy)
C. Calmettes (France)
P. Dor (Belgium)
N. Feingold (France)
J.A. Fischer (Switzerland)
B. Franc (France)
A. Garcia (Spain)
B.M. Goslings (The Netherlands)

P.J. Guillausseau (France)
J.M. Guliana (France)
C. Jaffiol (France)
G. Lenoir (France)
E. Modigliani (France)
M.S. Moukhtar (France)

C. Parmentier (France)
B.A.J. Ponder (UK)
Ch. Proye (France)
F. Raue (Germany)
M. Telenius-Berg (Sweden)
J. Tourniaire (France)
M. Weissel (Austria)

Acknowledgements

The First European Congress on Medullary Thyroid Carcinoma was held in Paris, from the 15th to 17th of November 1990, initiated by the French Medullary Study Group to review the substantial progress made since thirty years and define the fields of collaborative efforts for the next years. Participants to this meeting came from laboratories and hospitals in Europe, North America and North Africa.

We are greatly indebted to the Ministre de la Recherche et de la Technologie for allowing this Congress to take place in such a prestigious setting as the Amphithéâtre Poincaré in the Ministère de la Recherche et de la Technologie.

The meeting was sponsored by the Institut National de la Santé et de la Recherche Médicale (INSERM), the Centre National de la Recherche Scientifique (CNRS) and the Association pour la Recherche sur le Cancer (ARC). This book has been published by INSERM in co-edition with John Libbey Eurotext. We also would like to thank CIS bio international for its technical assistance in the organization of this Congress and I.C.I Pharma, Miles, Sandoz, Roucaire, Sophra, Unipath, Wild-Leitz for sponsoring the meeting.

Remerciements

Le Premier Congrès Européen sur le Cancer Médullaire de la Thyroïde s'est tenu à Paris, du 15 au 17 novembre 1990, à l'initiative du Groupe d'Etude des Tumeurs à Calcitonine (GETC) dans le but de présenter les progrès accomplis en trente ans et de définir les voies d'un effort commun pour les prochaines années. Les participants à ce congrès sont venus de laboratoires et d'hôpitaux d'Europe, d'Amérique du Nord et d'Afrique du Nord.

Nous sommes grandement redevables au Ministre de la Recherche et de la Technologie d'avoir permis que ce Congrès se tienne dans un lieu aussi prestigieux que l'Amphithéâtre Poincaré du Ministère de la Recherche et de la Technologie.

Le congrès a bénéficié du soutien de l'Institut National de la Santé et de la Recherche Médicale (INSERM), du Centre National de la Recherche Scientifique (CNRS) et de l'Association pour la Recherche sur le Cancer (ARC). La publication de cet ouvrage a été réalisée par l'INSERM en co-édition avec John Libbey Eurotext. Nous tenons à remercier également CIS bio international pour son aide technique à l'occasion de ce Congrès, ainsi que I.C.I Pharma, Miles, Sandoz, Roucaire, Sophra, Unipath, Wild-Leitz pour le soutien apporté.

List and addresses of participants
Liste et adresses des participants

Abs Roger, Université d'Anvers, Universiteits Plein, 2610 Wilrijk, Belgique

Alevizaki Maria, Alexandra Hospital, 80, Vassilissis Sofias Avenue, 11528 Athènes, Grèce

Allannic Hubert, Médecine F.B., Hôpital Sud, BP 129, 35056 Rennes, France

Amokrane Lounis, Secteur Pierre-et-Marie-Curie, Endocrinologie, Hôpital Mustapha, 16000 Alger, Algérie

Amparo Santos M., Lab. Endocrinologia, Instituto Francisco Gentil, R. Prof. Lima Basto, 1093 Lisbonne, Portugal

Andry Guy, Institut Jules Bordet, Rue Héger-Bordet, 1, 1000 Bruxelles, Belgique

Ardilouze Jean-Luc, 12, avenue Nord, CHUS, Jihici, Canada

Aubert Pierre, Service d'Endocrinologie-Diabétologie, Hôpital Saint-Antoine, 75571 Paris Cedex 12, France

Auersperg Marija, The Institute of Oncology, Zaloska 2, 61000 Ljubljana, Yougoslavie

Bacourt François, Hôpital Américain, 63, boulevard Victor-Hugo, 92200 Neuilly/Seine, France

Bailey Floyd, Department of Medicine (Endocrinology), Royal Postgraduate Medical School, Du Cane Road, Londres, W120NN, Royaume-Uni

Bailly Alain, CIS BIO-International, BP 32, 91192 Gif-sur-Yvette, France

Bakiri Faouzi, Secteur Pierre-et-Marie-Curie, Endocrinologie, Hôpital Mustapha, 16000 Alger, Algérie

Baldet Line, Service d'Endocrinologie, Hôpital Lapeyronie, 34059 Montpellier, France

Baulieu Jean-Louis, INSERM U.316 et Médecine Nucléaire, CHRU Bretonneau, 37044 Tours Cedex, France

Behmel Anne-Marie, Karl-Franzens-Universität Graz, Institut für Medizinische Biologie und Humangenetik, 8010 Graz, Autriche

Bellis G., Département d'Anthropologie et de Démographie Génétiques, INED, 27, rue du Commandeur, 75014 Paris, France

Bera Odile, CIS BIO-International, BP 32, 91192 Gif-sur-Yvette, France

Beressi Jean-Paul, INSERM U.30, Hôpital Necker-Enfants-Malades, 149, rue de Sèvres, 75743 Paris Cedex 15, France

Bergant Damjan, The Institute of Oncology, Zaloska 2, 61000 Ljubljana, Yougoslavie

Berger-Dutrieux Nicole, Laboratoire d'Anatomie Pathologique, Hôtel-Dieu, 1, place de l'Hôpital, 69288 Lyon Cedex, France

Bernard Anne-Marie, INSERM U.335, Centre Eugène-Marquis, CHR Pontchaillou, rue Henri-Le-Guilloux, 35033 Rennes Cedex, France

Bernard Marie-Hélène, Clinique Endocrinologique, Hôpital de l'Antiquaille, 1, rue de l'Antiquaille, 69005 Lyon, France

Berthelsen Anne, Copenhagen County Hospital Herlev, Oncology Department 54 C3, 2730 Herlev, Danemark

Bigorgne Jean-Claude, INSERM U.298, Centre Hospitalier Régional et Universitaire, 1, avenue de l'Hôtel-Dieu, 49033 Angers Cedex, France

Billaud Eliane, Service de Pharmacologie, Hôpital Broussais, 96, rue Didot, 75674 Paris Cedex 14, France

Blind Eberhard, Medizinische Universität Klinik Heidelberg, Abteilung Innere Medizin I, Bergheimer Strasse 58, 6900 Heidelberg, Allemagne

Body Jean-Jacques, Institut Jules-Bordet, 1, rue Héger-Bordet, 1000 Bruxelles, Belgique

Boiteau Valérie, Endocrinologie, Hôpital de Maison Blanche, 45, rue Cognacq-Jay, 51095 Reims, France

Bondeson Anne Greth, University of Lund, Malmö General Hospital, 21401 Malmö, Suède

Bondeson Lennart, University of Lund, Dept of Cytology, Malmö General Hospital, 21401 Malmö, Suède

Boneu Andrée, Centre Claudius Regaud, 20-24, rue du Pont-Saint-Pierre, 31052 Toulouse Cedex, France

Born Walter, Research Laboratory for Calcium Metabolism, Klinik Balgrist, Forchstrasse 340, 8008 Zurich, Suisse

Bornant-Rousselot Anne, 62, avenue du Général-Bizot, 75012 Paris, France

Bouizar Zhor, INSERM U.113, Faculté de Médecine Saint-Antoine, 27, rue Chaligny, 75571 Paris Cedex 12, France

Bouyge Nicole, Service de Médecine Nucléaire, Hôpital Saint-Antoine, 75571 Paris, France

Brambilla Sandrine, 20, rue Jouvenet, 75016 Paris, France

Broussoux B., CHRU, 37044 Tours Cedex, France

Brunaud-Liguory Marie-Dominique, Hôpital Américain, 63, boulevard Victor-Hugo, 92200 Neuilly/Seine, France

Bugalho Maria João, Instituto Português de Oncologia - Lisboa, Urbanizacau da Portels Lote 112 5 DTA, 2685 Sacavem, Portugal

Buhr H.J., Department of Surgery, University of Heidelberg, Im Neuenheimer Feld 110, 6900 Heidelberg, Allemagne

Busnardo Benedetto, Istituto di Semeiotica Medica, Universita di Padova, via Ospedale Civile, 105, 35128 Padoue, Italie

Cabezas Coppola Rosa, Serv. Endocrinologia, Hospital Santa Cruz y San Pablo, Avd. S. Antonio M. Claret, 167, 08025 Barcelone, Espagne

Caillou Bernard, INSERM U.66, Anatomie Pathologique, Institut Gustave-Roussy, 39, rue Camille-Desmoulins, 94805 Villejuif Cedex, France

Calmettes Claude, INSERM U.113, Faculté de Médecine Saint-Antoine, 27, rue Chaligny, 75571 Paris Cedex 12, France

Campos Béatrice, Instituto Português de Oncologia de Francisco Gentil, 1093 Lisbonne codex, Portugal

Carnaille Bruno, CHU de Lille, Clinique Chirurgicale de l'Est, 16, rue de la Meuse, 59155 Faches-Thumesnil, France

Caron Jean, Endocrinologie, Hôpital de Maison Blanche, 45, rue Cognacq-Jay, 51092 Reims Cedex, France

Caron Philippe, Service d'Endocrinologie, CHU de Rangueil, 1, avenue Pouilhet, 31054 Toulouse, France

Casanova Sylvie, Endocrinologie, Hôpital Avicenne, 93000 Bobigny, France.

Cassuto Dominique, Service de Médecine Générale et Nutrition, Hôtel-Dieu, Place du Parvis-Notre-Dame, 75181 Paris Cedex 04, France

Cerf Isabelle, 53, rue Gustave-Courbet, 49000 Angers, France

Chabre Olivier, Service d'Endocrinologie, CHU de Grenoble, BP 217 X, 38043 Grenoble Cedex, France

Chabrier Gérard, 24, place Kléber, 67000 Strasbourg, France

Chadenas Denis, Service d'Endocrinologie, CHR d'Orléans, Hôpital de la Source, Avenue de l'Hôpital, 45067 Orléans, France

Chapuis Yves, Service de Chirurgie Générale, Hôpital Cochin, 27, rue du Faubourg Saint-Jacques, 75674 Paris Cedex 14, France

Charpentier Guillaume, Service d'Endocrinologie-Diabétologie, Hôpital Henri-Dunant, 91100 Corbeil-Essonnes, France

Charrie Anne, Hôpital de l'Antiquaille, 69321 Lyon Cedex, 01, France

Chaventré André, Département d'Anthropologie et de Démographie Génétiques, INED, 27, rue du Commandeur, 75675 Paris Cedex 14, France

Chayvialle Jean-Alain, INSERM U.45, Hôpital Edouard-Herriot, Pavillon H bis, 69374 Lyon Cedex 02, France

Chesneau Anne-Marie, Centre Hospitalier René-Dubos, 95301 Pontoise, France

Chomant Jean, Centre Henri-Becquerel, 1, square d'Amiens, 76000 Rouen, France

Clarke Susan E.M., Dept of Nuclear Medicine, Guy's Hospital, St Thomas Street, Londres, SE 19 RT, Royaume-Uni

Clément Karine, Service d'Endocrinologie, Hôpital Saint-Antoine, 75571 Paris, France

Coequyt Serge, Service Central de Médecine Nucléaire, CHR de Lille, 1, place de Verdun, 59000 Lille, France

Cohen Régis, INSERM U.113 et Service d'Endocrinologie, Hôpital Avicennes, 93000 Bobigny, France

Coppe Pascal, 16, quai aux Bois, 59140 Dunkerque, France

Couette J.-Etienne, Centre F. Baclesse, Route de Lion, 14000 Caen, France

Cougard Patrick, Clinique chirurgicale, Hôpital du Bocage, CHU de Dijon, boulevard du Maréchal-de-Lattre-de-Tassigny, 21034 Dijon, France

Cressent Michèle, INSERM U.113, Faculté de Médecine Saint-Antoine, 27, rue Chaligny, 75571 Paris Cedex 12, France

Cubertafond Pierre, CHRU Dupuytren, 2, avenue Alexis-Carrel, 87042 Limoges, France

Cusumano Fabio, Istituto Nazionale Tumori, Via Foppa 9, 20133 Milan, Italie

Da Cruz Ferreira M. Teresa, Academisch Ziekenhuis Leiden, Isotopendiagnostiek, G1-C4Q, 2333 AA Leiden, Pays-Bas

Damian Alexandru, Str. Rafael Sanzio, 2, Sector II, Bucarest, Roumanie

David Jean-Marc, Centre Claudius-Regaud, 20-24, rue du Pont-Saint-Pierre, 31052 Toulouse, France

Dejax Catherine, Centre Jean-Perrin, Place Henri-Dunant, BP 392, 63011 Clermont-Ferrand, France

Delehaye Marie-Christine, INSERM U.113, Faculté de Médecine Saint-Antoine, 27, rue Chaligny, 75571 Paris Cedex 12, France

Delemer Brigitte, Endocrinologie, Hôpital de Maison-Blanche, 45, rue Cognacq-Jay, 51095 Reims, France

Delepine Nicole, Service d'Oncologie Pédiatrique, Hôpital Robert-Debré, 48, boulevard Sérurier, 75019 Paris, France

Delisle Marie-Joëlle, Service de Médecine Nucléaire, Institut Jean-Godinot, BP 171, 51056 Reims Cedex, France

Delprat C.C., Antoni van Leeuwenhoek, Ziekenhuis, Plesmanlaan 121, 1066 CX Amsterdam, Pays-Bas

De Micco Catherine, Laboratoire d'Anatomie-Pathologie, Faculté de Médecine, 27, boulevard Jean-Moulin, 13385 Marseille Cedex, France

De Rosa Giovina, Viale Colli Portuensi, 442, 00151 Rome, Italie

Desbois Jean-Claude, Service d'Oncologie Pédiatrique, Hôpital Robert-Debré, 48, boulevard Sérurier, 75019 Paris, France

Di Sacco G., Department of Endocrinology, Niguarda Hospital, 21100 Milan, Italie

Djemli Kheira, Secteur Pierre-et-Marie-Curie, Endocrinologie, Hôpital Mustapha, 16000 Alger, Algérie

Dor Pierre, Institut Jules-Bordet, Rue Héger-Bordet, 1, 1000 Bruxelles, Belgique

Dotto S., Istituto di Semeiotica Medica e Patologia Chirurgica, Universita di Padova, via Ospedale Civile, 105, 35128 Padoue, Italie

Dralle Henning, Medizinische Hochschule Hannover, Klinik für Abdominal und Transplantations chirurgie, 3000 61 Hanovre, Allemagne

Duhirel Raoul, Service d'Endocrinologie, Hôpital Saint-Antoine, 75571 Paris Cedex 12, France

Dupont Jean-Louis, Service de Médecine Interne, Hôpital Jean-Minjoz, 3, boulevard Fleming, 25000 Besançon, France

Duprey Jacques, Policlinique, Hôpital Ambroise-Paré, 9, avenue Charles-de-Gaulle, 92100 Boulogne, France

Durez Marianne, IMS Hornu, avenue Lefebvre, 7120 Haulchin, Belgique

Duron Françoise, Hôpital Saint-Antoine, 184, rue du Faubourg Saint-Antoine, 75571 Paris, France

Estour Bruno, Hôpital Bellevue, Pavillon 22, boulevard Pasteur, 42023 Saint-Etienne, France

Ettore Francette, Centre Antoine-Lacassagne, 36, voie Romaine, 06054 Nice, France

Farkas Diane, INSERM U.155, Université Paris 7, 2, place Jussieu, 75005 Paris, France

Fatourechi Vahab, Mayo Clinic, 200 First Street, Southwest, Rochester, MN 55905, États-Unis

Feingold Nicole, INSERM U.155, Université Paris VII, 2, place Jussieu, 75005 Paris, France

Fischer Jan, Klinik Balgrist, Forchstrasse 340, 8008 Zurich, Suisse

Fleury-Goyon Marie-Claude, Hôpital de l'Antiquaille, 1, rue de l'Antiquaille, 69321 Lyon Cedex 05, France

Flocquet Jean, Laboratoire d'Anatomie-Pathologie, Faculté de Médecine, Route de Maron, 54500 Vandœuvre-les-Nancy, France

Foidart Jacqueline, Service de Médecine Nucléaire, CHU de Liège, Sart-Tilman, 4000 Liège, Belgique

Foucart Annick, Rue Bosquet 47, bte 35, 1060 Bruxelles, Belgique

Fragu Philippe, INSERM U.66, Institut Gustave-Roussy, 39, rue Camille-Desmoulins, 94805 Villejuif Cedex, France

Franc Brigitte, Service d'Anatomie Pathologique, Hôpital Ambroise-Paré, 9, avenue Charles-de-Gaulle, 92100 Boulogne/Seine, France

Frank Hanna, Dept of Oncology and Radiotherapy, Norrebrogade 44, Aarhus Kommunehospital, DK 8000 Aarhus C, Danemark

Frank-Raue Karin, Department of Internal Medicine I, University of Heidelberg, Bergheimerstrasse 58, 6900 Heidelberg, Allemagne

Frantz Jacques, CHR de Metz-Bon-Secours, 1, place Philippe-de-Vigneulles, BP 1065, 57038 Metz Cedex 01, France

Franz Claudia, Service de Chirurgie Générale et Endocrinienne, CHR de Lille, 46, rue des Pyramides, 59000 Lille, France

Frilling A., Department of Surgery, Heinrich-Heine University, Moorenstrasse 5, 4000 Düsseldorf, Allemagne

Fritzsche Heinz, Department of Nuclear Medicine, Landeskrankenhaus, Carinagasse, 47, A-6800 Feldkirch, Autriche

Fulla Yvonne, Hôpital Cochin, Médecine Nucléaire, 27, rue du Faubourg Saint-Jacques, 75674 Paris, France

Galera-Davidson Hugo, Departamento de Anatomia Patologica, Hospital Universario "Virgen Macarena", Avda. Dr. Fedriani, s/n°, 41009 Séville, Espagne

Garcia-Almeijeiras Angela, 316 Maple Leaf D2, Toronto, Ontario M6L 1P6, Canada

Gardet Paule, Institut Gustave-Roussy, 39, rue Camille-Desmoulins, 94805 Villejuif Cedex, France

Gay Gérard, Service de Médecine Interne A, Hôpital Saint-Nicolas, 55100 Verdun, France

Geerdink R.A., University Hospital, Heidelberglaan 100, 3584 CS Utrecht, Pays-Bas

Genel Myron, Yale University School of Medicine, 333 Cedar Street, Box 3333, New Haven, CT 06510, USA

Gerard Jacques, Ulq, 396, rue du Sart-Tilman, B. 4900, Ansleur-Liese, Belgique

Gianello Pierre, Université Catholique de Louvain, Clinique Saint-Luc, Avenue Hippocrate 10, 1200 Bruxelles, Belgique

Giannasio Paolo, CHUV-Lausanne, Hôtel de l'Ours, Rue du Bugnon, 2 1011 Lausanne, Suisse

Giuffrida Dario, Istituto Endocrinologia, University of Catania, Via del Bosco 222, 95125 Catane, Italie

Glinoer Daniel, University Hospital Saint-Pierre, 322, rue Haute, 1000 Bruxelles, Belgique

Goellner John R., Mayo Clinic, 200 First Street, Southwest, Rochester, Minnesota 55905, États-Unis

Goslings Bernard, Stofwisselingsziekten en Endocrinologie, Gebouw 1, C4-R, Postbus 9600, 2300 RC Leiden, Pays-Bas

Grulet Henri, Service d'Endocrinologie, Hôpital Maison Blanche, 51100 Reims, France

Guillausseau Pierre-Jean, Service de Médecine Interne, Hôpital Lariboisière, 75475 Paris Cedex 10, France

Guillausseau-Scholer Claudine, Service de Médecine Nucléaire, Hôpital de la Pitié, 83, boulevard de l'Hôpital, 75013 Paris, France

Guilloteau Denis, INSERM U.316 et Laboratoire de Biophysique Médicale, CHRU Bretonneau, 2 bis, boulevard Tonnellé, 37032 Tours Cedex, France

Guliana Jean-Michel, INSERM U.113, Service d'Endocrinologie-Diabétologie, Hôpital Saint-Antoine, 75571 Paris Cedex 12, France

Guyot Martine, Médecine Nucléaire, Hôpital Pellegrin, Place Amélie Raba-Léon, 33076 Bordeaux, France

Hadden David R., Royal Victoria Hospital, Department of Medical Genetic, Queen's University of Belfast, Belfast, BT 126 BA, Royaume-Uni.

Hansen Hanne Sand, Onkologisk afd. Rigshospitalet afsnit 5072, Blegdamsvej 9, 2100 Copenhague, Danemark

Harach H. Reuben, Dept of Pathology, University Hospital of Wales, Heath Park, Cardiff, CF 44 XN, Royaume-Uni

Harmer, The Royal Marsden Hospital, Fulham Road, Londres, SW3, Royaume-Uni

Hay Ian D., Mayo Thryoid Group, Mayo Clinic, 200 First Street, Southwest, Rochester, Minnesota 55905, États-Unis

Hecart A.C., Endocrinologie, Hôpital de Maison Blanche, 45, rue Cognacq-Jay, 51095 Reims, France

Helal C. Badia, Hôpital de Bicêtre, Service de Médecine Nucléaire, 78, rue du Général-Leclerc, 94250 Le Kremlin-Bicêtre, France

Henry Jean-François, Unité de Chirurgie Endocrinienne, CHU de la Timone, boulevard Jean-Moulin, 13385 Marseille Cedex 05, France.

Hermans Jacques, Hôpital de Jolimont, rue Ferrier, 7161 Haine-Saint-Paul, Belgique

Herry Jean-Yves, C.R.L.C., CHR de Pontchaillou, 35033 Rennes, France

Hoch Michèle, Centre Antoine-Lacassagne, 36, voie Romaine, 06054 Nice, France

Hochberg-Parer Ghislaine, 276, boulevard Raspail, 75014 Paris, France

Hoefnagel C.A., Dept of Nuclear Medicine, The Netherlands Cancer Institute, Plesmanlaan 121, 1066 CX Amsterdam, Pays-Bas

Hoie Johan, The Norwegian Radium Hospital, O Montebello, 0310 Oslo 3, Norvège

Holm Ruth, Department of Pathology, The Norwegian Radium Hospital, Montebello, 0310 Oslo, Norvège

Houdent Chantal, Hôpital de Bois-Guillaume, CHU de Rouen, 147, avenue du Maréchal-Juin, 76230 Bois-Guillaume, France

Huschitt Niels, Endokrinologie Universität-Klinik Mainz, Langenbeckstrasse, 6500 Mayence, Allemagne

Hvid-Jacobsen Keld, Herlev Hospital, University of Copenhagen, Ulrikkenborg Alle 46, 2800 Lungby, Danemark

Iacconi Pietro, Via dei Colli, 29, 54100 Massa (ms), Italie

Icard Philippe, Clinique Chirurgicale, Hôpital Cochin, 75014 Paris, France

Ivanova Radina Stefanova, Institute of Endocrinology, bul. Christo Michailov 6, 1303 Sofia, Bulgarie

Jaffiol Claude, Hôpital Lapeyronie, 34000 Montpellier, France

James-Deidier Annick, Laboratoires Sandoz, 51, rue Louis-Blanc, 69006 Lyon, France

Janser Jean-Claude, Centre Régional de Lutte contre le Cancer Paul-Strauss, 3, rue Porte de l'Hôpital, 67000 Strasbourg, France

Jansson Svante, Department of Surgery, Sahlgrens Hospital, S-41345 Göteborg, Suède

Jarry Jean-Marc, Centre Hospitalier d'Aix-en-Provence, Avenue des Tamaris, 13616 Aix-en-Provence, France

Joannidis Sylvie, Service d'Endocrinologie, Hôpital Avicenne, 125, route de Stalingrad, 93000 Bobigny, France

Jorgensen Karsten E., Institute of Oto-Rhino-Laryngology, Odense University Hospital, Odense Sygehus, Sdr. Boulevard 29, 5000 Odense, Danemark

Joubert Isabelle, INSERM U.155, Université Paris VII, 2, place Jussieu, 75005 Paris, France

Jullienne Annick, INSERM U.113, CHU Saint-Antoine, 27, rue Chaligny, 75571 Paris Cedex 12, France

Kadi Anne-Marie, Laboratoire d'Anatomie Pathologique, CHD "Les Oudaines", 85025 La Roche-sur-Yon, France

Kainz Hans, 2 Medizinische Universität Klinik, Garnisongasse 13, A-1090 Vienne, Autriche

Kaloustian Edgar, Centre Hospitalier de Compiègne, Rue de Paris, 60200 Compiègne, France

Kauffmann Philippe, Centre Jean-Perrin, 30, place Henri-Dunant, 63011 Clermont-Ferrand, France

Koutras Demetrios, University of Athens, Dept of Clinical Therapeutics, 80, Vas. Sofia Avenue, 11528 Athènes, Grèce

Kraimps Jean-Louis, Hôpital Jean-Bernard, Service de Chirurgie B, BP 577, 86021 Poitiers Cedex, France

Labat-Moleur Françoise, CHRU de Grenoble, Laboratoire de Pathologie Cellulaire, BP 217 X, 38043 Grenoble Cedex, France

Lacroix André, Institut de Recherches Cliniques de Montréal, 110, avenue des Pins O., Montréal H2W 1R7, Canada

Landsvater Rudy M., Department of Pathology, University Hospital, Heidelberglaän 100, 3584 CX Utrecht, Pays-Bas

Lapicque Jean-Charles, Service de Chirurgie Générale, Hôpital Nord, Chemin de Bourrely, 13015 Marseille, France

Lasmoles Françoise, INSERM U.113, CHU Saint-Antoine, 27, rue Chaligny, 75571 Paris Cedex 12, France

Leclere Jacques, Service d'Endocrinologie, Hôpital de Brabois, 54511 Vandœuvre-les-Nancy, France

Lecomte Pierre, CHRU de Tours, 37044 Tours Cedex, France

Lecomte-Houcke Martine, Laboratoire d'Anatomie et Cytologie Pathologique A, CHU de Lille, Place de Verdun, 59045 Lille Cedex, France

Leenhardt Laurence, Service de Médecine Nucléaire, Hôpital de la Pitié, 83, boulevard de l'Hôpital, 75013 Paris, France

Lefebvre Jean, CHU de Lille, 25, avenue du Maréchal Leclerc, 59110 La Madeleine, France

Le Gall François, CHR Pontchaillou, 2, rue H. Le Guillou, 35000 Rennes, France

Léger Aubène, Service Central de Radio-Isotopes, Hôpital Necker, 149, rue de Sèvres, 75743 Paris, France

Leguillouzic Danièle, Hôpital de Bicêtre, Service de Médecine Nucléaire, 78, rue du Général-Leclerc, 94250 Le-Kremlin-Bicêtre, France

Le Moullec Nathalie, Hôpital Sud, boulevard de Bulgarie, 35000 Rennes, France

Lenoir Gilbert, CIRC, 150, cours Albert-Thomas, 69372 Lyon Cedex 08, France

Leopaldi Ennio, Clinica Chirurgica I, Via Cornodi Cavento, 19, 20148 Milan, Italie

Leroy Florence, 5, avenue Adeline, 92700 Colombes, France

Lescouarc'h J., Centre Eugène-Marquis, CHR de Pontchaillou, 35033 Rennes, France

Libroia Alfonso, Department of Endocrinology, Ospedale La Granda Niguarda, Piazza Ospedale Maggiore 3, 20162 Milan, Italie

Limbert Eduardo, Servico de Patologia Morphologica, Instituto Português de Oncologia de Francisco Gentil, 1093 Lisbonne Codex, Portugal

Lips C.J.M., University Hospital, Heidelberglaan 100, 3584 CX Utrecht, Pays-Bas

Lorcy Yannick, Médecine F, Hôpital Sud, 16, boulevard de Bulgarie, 35000 Rennes, France

Louvel Albert, 13, avenue Boudon, 75016 Paris, France

Machayekhi Jean-Pierre, Laboratoire d'Analyses Médicales, 7, boulevard de la Liberté, B.P. 87, 35002 Rennes Cedex, France

Maes Béatrice, Institut Jean-Godinot, 1, rue du Général-Koenig, BP 171, 51056 Reims, France

Mahler Charles, A.Z. Meddelheim Lindendreff 1, 2020 Anvers, Belgique

Manzl Monika, Institution of Nuclear Medicine and Endocrinology, Mullner-Hauptstrasse 48, 5020 Salzbourg, Autriche

Marchand Jean-Pierre, CHR d'Orléans, Hôpital de la Source, Avenue de l'Hôpital, BP 6709, 45067 Orléans Cedex 2, France

Marmousez Thierry, Clinique du Chapeau Rouge, 3, rue Saint-Sébastien, 59140 Dunkerque, France

Massart Catherine, Laboratoire d'Hormonologie-Enzymologie, CHU de Pontchaillou, 35043 Rennes, France

Massien Christine, 7, cours de Vincennes, 75020 Paris, France

Maubras Laurence, INSERM U.113, Faculté de Médecine Saint-Antoine, 27, rue Chaligny, 75571 Paris Cedex 12, France

Maunand Bernard, Service d'Endocrinologie, Centre Hospitalier Louise-Michel, 91014 Evry, France

M'Bemba Jocelyne, 3, rue Pierre-Mille, 75015 Paris, France

Mechelany Carine, Institut Gustave-Roussy, 94805 Villejuif Cedex, France

Meer Anne, Service de Médecine Générale et Nutrition, Hôtel-Dieu, 1, place du Parvis-Notre-Dame, 75181 Paris Cedex 04, France

Merchie Georges, Service de Médecine Nucléaire, CHU du Sart-Tilman, 4000 Liège, Belgique

Meurisse Michel, CHU, Domaine Universitaire du Sart-Tilman, B 35, 4080 Liège, Belgique

Mey Pascaline, Centre Paul-Papin, 2, rue Moll, 49100 Angers, France

Milhaud Gérard, INSERM U.113, CHU Saint-Antoine, 27, rue Chaligny, 75571 Paris Cedex 12, France

Minvielle Stéphane, INSERM U.113, CHU Saint-Antoine, 27, rue Chaligny, 75571 Paris Cedex 12, France

Mirkine Nelly, Service de Médecine, Hôpital Universitaire, 1020 Bruxelles, Belgique

Modigliani Elisabeth, Endocrinologie, Hôpital Avicenne, 125, rue de Stalingrad, 93000 Bobigny, France

Møller Pâl, Genetic Department, The Norwegian Radium Hospital, N-0315 Oslo, Norvège

Mornex René, INSERM U.197 et Hôpital Edouard-Herriot, Pavillon X, 69003 Lyon, France

Moukhtar M.S., INSERM U.113, CHU Saint-Antoine, 27, rue Chaligny, 75571 Paris Cedex 12, France

Mulligan Lois, Dept of Pathology, University of Cambridge, Tennis Court Road, Cambridge CB2 1QP, Royaume-Uni

Munck Anne, Service de Gastro-Entérologie, Hôpital Robert-Debré, 48, boulevard Sérurier, 75019 Paris, France

Mundschank Jochen, Endokrinologie, UniKlinik Mainz, Langenbeckstrasse, 6500 Mayence, Allemagne

Muratori Fabrizio, Dept of Endocrinology, Niguarda Hospital Milan, Via G.B. Vico 7, 21100 Varèse, Italie

Naoun Amar, Service de Médecine Nucléaire, CHRU, 18, rue Lionnois, 54000 Nancy, France

Nemry Claude, 38, rue Froissart, 1000 Bruxelles, Belgique

Neumann Hartmut P.H., Abteilung für Medizin, Klinikum der Albert-Ludwigs-Universität, Hugstetterstrasse 55, 7800 Fribourg, Allemagne

Niederle Bruno, 1st Department of Surgery, University of Vienna, Spitalgass 1, 1090 Vienne, Autriche

Noel Michèle, INSERM U.66, Institut Gustave-Roussy, 39, rue Camille-Desmoulins, 94805 Villejuif Cedex, France

Opocher G., Istituto di Semeiotica Medica, Universita di Padova, 35128 Padoue, Italie

Orefice Seriyo, Istituto Tumori Milano, 20100 Milan, Italie

Pacini Furio, Istituto di Endocrinologia, Metodologia Clinica E Medicina del Lavoro, Via del Terreno, 64, 56018 Terrenia / Pise, Italie

Pages André, Laboratoire d'Anatomopathologie, CHU Gui-de-Chauliac, 34059 Montpellier Cedex, France

Pantazi H., Second Endocrine Service, Alexandra Hospital, 11528 Athènes, Grèce

Papadodima-Lakker Elli, Endocrinology, 4, Trenulenudoni Str. Zografou, 15773 Athènes, Grèce

Papapetrou Peter D., Alexandra Hospital, Vas. Sofias and Lourou Street, 11528 Athènes, Grèce

Parmentier Claude, INSERM U.66, Institut Gustave-Roussy, 39, rue Camille-Desmoulins, 94805 Villejuif Cedex, France

Patey Martine, Laboratoire d'Anatomie Pathologique, CHU Robert-Debré, rue Alexis-Carrel, 51092 Reims Cedex, France

Pegg Christopher A.S., University Hospital, Queen's Medical Centre, Nottingham NG7 2UH, Royaume-Uni

Peix Jean-Louis, Hôpital de l'Antiquaille, 1, rue de l'Antiquaille, 69321 Lyon Cedex 5, France

Pelizzo M.R., Istituto di Chirurgica Patologica, Giustiniani 2, 35128 Padoue, Italie

Perichon Isabelle, 108, rue Didot, 75014 Paris, France

Perie Guy, Service d'Anatomie-Pathologie, Centre Hospitalier, 20, rue Armagis, 78105 Saint-Germain-en-Laye, France

Petit Sylvie, Service Central de Médecine Nucléaire, 1, place de Verdun, 59037 Lille Cedex, France

Pfragner Roswitha, Universitäts-Institut für Funktionelle Pathologie, Mozartgasse 14/II, 8010 Graz, Autriche

Pidoux Elisabeth, INSERM U.113, Faculté de Médecine Saint-Antoine, 27, rue Chaligny, 75571 Paris Cedex 12, France

Plouin Pierre-François, Département d'Hypertension, Hôpital Broussais, 96, rue Didot, 75674 Paris Cedex 14, France

Ponder Bruce A.J., Dept of Pathology, University of Cambridge, Tennis Court Road, Cambridge CB2 1QP, Royaume-Uni

Pons-Anicet Dominique, CIS-Bio-Industries, BP n° 6, 91192 Gif-sur-Yvette, France

Portman Luc, Division d'Endocrinologie, CHU Vaudois, Rue de Bugnon, 1011 Lausanne, Suisse

Probst Thomas, Endokrinologie Universität-Klinik Mainz, Langenbeckstrasse, 6500 Mayence, Allemagne

Proye Charles, Service de Chirurgie Générale et Endocrinienne, Hôpital Huriez, Place de Verdun, 59037 Lille Cedex, France

Pueyo E. Maria, Hôpital de Bicêtre, Service de Médecine Nucléaire, 78, rue du Général Leclerc, 94250 Le-Kremlin-Bicêtre, France

Pusel Jean, Centre Paul-Strauss, 3, rue de la Porte de l'Hôpital, 67085 Strasbourg, France

Putelat Roger, 17, rue d'Hauteville, 21121 Daix, France

Raue Friedhelm, Abteilung Innere Medizin-Endokrinologie und Stoffweichsel Klinikum der Universität Heidelberg, Luisenstrasse 5, 6900 Heidelberg 1, Allemagne

Rebattu Paul, Centre Léon-Bérard, 28, rue Laënnec, 69008 Lyon, France

Reubi Jean-Claude, Sandoz Laboratories, Montbijou Street, PO Box 2175, 3001 Berne, Suisse

Richard Alain, 6, boulevard de l'Hôpital, 75013 Paris, France

Rocco Bruno, CHUV Lausanne, Hôtel de l'Ours, Rue du Bugnon, 2, 1011 Lausanne, Suisse

Roger Patrick J.M., Service d'Endocrinologie, Hôpital du Haut-Lévêque, CHU de Bordeaux, 33600 Pessac, France

Rohmer Vincent, INSERM U.298, Médecine C, CHU d'Angers, 49033 Angers Cedex 01, France

Rolland Catherine, Service d'Endocrinologie, Hôpital Saint-Joseph, rue Pierre-Labrousse, 75014 Paris, France

Rosenberg-Bourgin Myriam, INSERM U.155, Université Paris VII, Tour 16, 3e étage, 2, place Jussieu, 75005 Paris, France

Ruszniewski Philippe, INSERM U.10, CHU Bichat, Service d'Hépato-Gastro-Entérologie, 46, rue Henri-Huchard, 75877 Paris Cedex 18, France

Saint-André Jean-Paul, Laboratoire d'Anatomie-Pathologie, CHRU, 49033 Angers Cedex, France

Sambade Clara, Laboratorio de Anatomia Patologica, Facultade de Medizina, 4200 Porto, Portugal

Sandrock Dirk, Department of Nuclear Medicine, Georg August University, Robert-Koch-Strasse 40, 3400 Göttingen, Allemagne

Santini José, Centre Antoine-Lacassagne, 36, avenue Voie Romaine, 06054 Nice, France

Sarrazin Roger, Vaulnaveys-Le-Haut, 38410 Uriage, France

Sassolas Geneviève, Hôpital Neuro-Cardiologique, 59, boulevard Pinel, 69394 Lyon-Montchat, France

Schaadt Bente, Dept of Oncology, Heplev University Hospital, Hjort Holms Alle 3 A street H2, 2400 Copenhague, Danemark

Scheumann G.F.W., Medizinische Hochshule Hannover, Klinik für Abdominal und Transplantationschirurgie, Postfach 61 01 80, 3000 Hanovre 81, Allemagne

Schlumberger Martin, INSERM U.66, Institut Gustave-Roussy, 39, rue Camille-Desmoulins, 94805 Villejuif Cedex, France

Scopsi Lucio, Anatomia Patologica, Istituto Nazionale per lo Studio e la Cura dei Tumori, via G. Venezian 1, 20133 Milan, Italie

Segond Nadine, INSERM U.113, Faculté de Médecine Saint-Antoine, 27, rue Chaligny, 75571 Paris Cedex 12, France

Siame-Mourot C., CHR de Lille, USNA, rue du Professeur Laguesse, 59800 Lille, France

Siemen Christine, Service d'Endocrinologie, Hôpital Sud, CHU de Rennes, 16, boulevard de Bulgarie, 35036 Rennes, France

Simioni Natalino, Ospedale di Cittadella, Via del Brenta 2/1, 35013 Cittadella, Italie

So Daniel, Hôpital Bel Air, CHR de Metz-Thionville, rue de Friseaty, 57100 Thionville, France

Soares Jorge, Servico de Patologia Morphologica, Instituto Português de Oncologia de Francisco Gentil, 1093 Lisbonne, Portugal

Sobol Hagay, Département d'Oncologie et de Génétique, Centre Léon-Bérard, 28, rue Laënnec, 69373 Lyon Cedex 08, France

Sobrinho-Simões Manuel, Laboratorio de Anatomia Patologica, Facultade de Medicina, 4200 Porto, Portugal

Spitz-Muller Maryline, Hôpital Necker, 75015 Paris, France

Squifflet Jean-Paul, Université Catholique de Louvain, Clinique Saint-Luc, Avenue Hippocrate 10, 1200 Bruxelles, Belgique

Szanto Janos, Rath György u. 7/9, H-1122 Budapest, Hongrie

Taboulet Jacqueline, INSERM U.113, Faculté de Médecine Saint-Antoine, 27, rue Chaligny, 75571 Paris Cedex 12, France

Teissier Marie-Pierre, Service de Médecine Interne B, Hôpital du Chezeau, 87042 Limoges, France

Telenius Häken, CRC Human Cancer Genetics Research Group, Department of Pathology, University of Cambridge, Tennis Court Road, Cambridge CB2 1QP, Royaume-Uni

Telenius-Berg Margareta, Björbang, Kristianstad, 529 185 Kristianstad, Suède

Tenenbaum Florence, Institut Gustave-Roussy, 39, rue Camille-Desmoulins, 94805 Villejuif, France

Tourniaire Jacques, Clinique Endocrinologique, Hôpital de l'Antiquaille, 69321 Lyon Cedex 05, France

Tran Ba Huy Patrice, Service O.R.L., Hôpital Lariboisière, 2, rue Ambroise-Paré, 75010 Paris, France

Treffot Marie-José, Centre Hospitalier Général, 33, avenue Rioudet, 83400 Hyères, France

Treilhou-Lahille Françoise, Université Paris-Sud, URA 11116 CNRS, Bât. 441, 91405 Orsay, France

Troncone Luigi, Istituto di Medicina Nucleare, Universita Cattolica Sacro Cuore, L. go A. Gemelli, 8, 00168 Rome, Italie

Trouillet Jacques, Service de Médecine Nucléaire, Hôpital Saint-Antoine, 75571 Paris, France

Tubiana Maurice, INSERM U.66, Institut Gustave-Roussy, 39, rue Camille-Desmoulins, 94805 Villejuif, France

Us-Krasovec Marija, The Institute of Oncology, Zaloska 2, 61000 Ljubljana, Yougoslavie

Vasen Hans, Foundation for the Detection of Hereditary Tumours, PO Box 12 009, 3501AA Utrecht, Pays-Bas

Vaudrey Colette, Service d'Endocrinologie, Hôpital de Maison-Blanche, 45, rue Cognacq-Jay, 51100 Reims, France

Veraldi Domenico, Institution Semeiotica Chirurgica, Universita di Verona, Via A. di Cambio, 16, 37138 Vérone, Italie

Verdy Maurice, Hôtel-Dieu de Montréal, 3840 Saint-Urbain, Montréal H2WIT8, Canada

Verga Uberta, Ospedale La Granda Niguarda, Via del Carmine 5, 20133 Milan, Italie

Verier-Mine Odile, Centre Hospitalier de Valenciennes, BP 479, 59322 Valenciennes Cedex, France

Vesco Lydia, 2, allée Royale, 64440 Villecresnes, France

Viennet Gabriel, CHU Jean-Minjoz, boulevard Fleming, 25030 Besançon, France

Vilde Françoise, Laboratoire d'Anatomie-Pathologie, Hôpital Boucicaut, 78, rue de la Convention, 75015 Paris, France

Vuillez Jean-Philippe, Médecine Nucléaire / LER URA CNRS 1287, CHU A. Michallon, BP 217 X, 38043 Grenoble Cedex, France

Waeber Catherine, FMH Médecine Interne, boulevard de Pérolles 12, 17000 Fribourg, Suisse

Weiss Peter, Department of Nuclear Medicine, Carinagasse, 47, A-6800 Feldkirch, Autriche

Weissel Michael, 2 Medizinische Universität Klinik, Garnisongasse, 13, A-1090 Vienne, Autriche

Wemeau Jean-Louis, Clinique médicale, USN A, CHU, 59037 Lille Cedex, France

Wheeler Malcom H., Department of Surgery, University Hospital of Wales, Heath Park, Cardiff CF44XN, Royaume-Uni

Williams Edwin D., Department of Pathology, The Welsh National School of Medicine, Heath Park, Cardiff CF44XN, Royaume-Uni

Wimalawansa Sunil J., Royal Postgraduate Medical School, Du Cane Road, Londres W12ONN, Royaume-Uni

Zimmer Adeline, Endokrinologie UniKlinik Mainz, Langenbeckstrasse, 6500 Mayence, Allemagne

Contents
Sommaire

- V   Preface
  Préface
- VIII Acknowledgements
- IX *Remerciements*
- XI List and addresses of participants
  Liste et adresses des participants

INTRODUCTION
INTRODUCTION

- 3 **M. Tubiana**
  Thyrocalcitonin - its discovery and development
  Thyrocalcitonine - découverte et développement

- 5 **G. Milhaud**
  Histoire du cancer médullaire de la thyroïde
  Medullary thyroid carcinoma story

- 9 **C. Calmettes**
  Medullary cancer of the thyroid : a general view
  Cancer médullaire de la thyroïde : aperçu général

I. CALCITONIN GENES, EXPRESSION AND BIOLOGICAL FUNCTIONS
I. LES GÈNES DE LA CALCITONINE, EXPRESSION ET FONCTIONS BIOLOGIQUES

- 19 **J.M. Guliana, A. Jullienne, F. Lasmoles, S. Minvielle, N. Segond, G. Milhaud, M.S. Moukhtar**
  Calcitonin gene family
  La famille des gènes de la calcitonine

- 31 **F. Raue, A. Zink, H. Scherübl**
  Regulation of calcitonin secretion
  Régulation de la sécrétion de calcitonine

39 **W. Born, J.A. Fischer**
Relevance of the amino-terminal cleavage peptide of procalcitonin (PAS-57), calcitonin and calcitonin gene-related peptide for the diagnosis of medullary thyroid carcinoma
Intérêt du peptide amino-terminal clivé de la procalcitonine (PAS-57), de la calcitonine et du "calcitonin gene-related peptide" pour le diagnostic de cancer médullaire de la thyroïde

II. FROM C-CELL TO MEDULLARY THYROID CARCINOMA
II. DE LA CELLULE C AU CANCER MÉDULLAIRE DE LA THYROIDE

45 **E.D. Williams**
Medullary carcinoma of the thyroid, thirty years after its discovery
Le cancer médullaire de la thyroïde, trente ans après sa découverte

53 **B. Caillou**
Histogenesis of medullary thyroid carcinoma
Histogenèse du cancer médullaire de la thyroïde

59 **C. Sambade, J.M. Nesland, R. Holm, M. Sobrinho-Simões**
Medullary carcinoma of the thyroid : a microfollicular carcinoma
Cancer médullaire de la thyroïde : un cancer microfolliculaire

65 **A. Pages, B. Franc**
De la cellule C au CMT. Les cancers thyroïdiens à sécrétions peptitiques
From C-cell to MTC. Peptidic secreting cancers of the thyroid

III. DIAGNOSTIC MEANS OF THE DISEASE
III. LES MÉTHODES DE DIAGNOSTIC DE LA MALADIE

Biochemical factors
Facteurs biochimiques

73 **D. Guilloteau, D. Bellet**
Calcitonine et ACE pour le dépistage et le suivi des CMT
Calcitonin and CEA for the diagnosis and the follow-up of MTC

81 **F. Pacini, F. Basolo, L. Fugazzola, A. Cola, A. Pinchera**
Somatostatin and other peptides in medullary thryoid cancer
Somatostatine et autres peptides dans le cancer médullaire de la thyroïde

85 **J.C. Reubi, E. Modigliani, C. Calmettes, L. Kvols, E.P. Krenning, S.W.J. Lamberts**
In vitro and in vivo identification of somatostatin receptors in medullary thyroid carcinomas, pheochromocytomas and paragangliomas
Identification des récepteurs de la somatostatine in vitro et in vivo dans les cancers médullaires de la thyroïde, les phéochromocytomes et les paragangliomes

89 **J.A. Chayvialle**
Bombesin/gastrin-releasing peptide in medullary thyroid carcinoma
Bombésine/"gastrin-releasing peptide" dans le cancer médullaire de la thyroïde

95 **L. Scopsi**
Peptide regulatory factors in the thyroid C cell system : an updating
Les facteurs peptidiques de régulation dans le système des cellules C de la thyroïde : une mise à jour

Cytology and imaging
Cytoponction et imagerie

101 **L. Bondeson**
Aspiration cytology of medullary thyroid carcinoma
Cytoponction du cancer médullaire de la thyroïde

103 **M.J. Delisle**
Les différentes modalités de l'imagerie dans le diagnostic, le traitement et la surveillance du cancer médullaire de la thyroïde (CMT)
Multimodality imaging in the management of the medullary cancer of the thyroid (MCT)

111 **S.E.M. Clarke**
Nuclear medicine techniques for imaging medullary thyroid carcinoma (MTC) (summary)
Techniques d'imagerie du cancer médullaire de la thyroïde en médecine nucléaire (résumé)

Pheochromocytoma detection
Dépistage du phéochromocytome

115 **P.F. Plouin, G. Chatellier, E. Billaud, E. Grouzmann, E. Comoy, P. Corvol**
Biochemical tests for phaeochromocytoma : diagnostic yield of the determination of urinary metanephrines, plasma catecholamines and plasma neuropeptide Y

Tests biochimiques dans le phéochromocytome : intérêt diagnostique de la mesure des métanéphrines urinaires, des catécholamines plasmatiques et du neuropeptide Y plasmatique

121 **H.P.H. Neumann, R.J. Hsiao, R.J. Parmer, J.A. Barbosa, D.T. O'Connor**
Chromogranin A in pheochromocytoma
Chromogranine A dans le phéochromocytome

125 **J.L. Baulieu**
Imagerie des phéochromocytomes
Imaging of pheochromocytomas

131 **Diagnostic means of the disease : discussion**
Les méthodes de diagnostic de la maladie : discussion

IV. EPIDEMIOLOGY AND GENETICS
IV. ÉPIDÉMIOLOGIE ET GÉNÉTIQUE

137 **L.M. Mulligan, E. Gardner, C. Jones, S.E. Mole, J. Moore, Y. Nakamura, I. Papi, H. Telenius, B.A.J. Ponder**
Clinical and molecular genetics of multiple endocrine neoplasia type 2A (MEN 2A)
La génétique clinique et moléculaire dans la néoplasie endocrinienne multiple de type 2A (NEM 2A)

145 **G.M. Lenoir, H. Sobol, I. Schuffenecker, S. Narod and the Groupe d'Etude des Tumeurs à Calcitonine (GETC)**
Linkage analysis for hereditary medullary thyroid carcinoma
Analyse de liaison des formes héréditaires de cancer médullaire de la thyroïde

149 **M. Rosenberg-Bourgin, D. Farkas, C. Calmettes, N. Feingold and the French GETC**
Epidemiologic and genetic analysis of medullary thyroid carcinoma in France
Analyses épidémiologique et génétique du cancer médullaire de la thyroïde en France

159 **B. Franc, A. Akrwight, B. Caillou, N. Dutrieux-Berger, J. Floquet, M. Houcke-Lecomte, E. Justrabo, F. Labat-Moleur, F. Lange, M.F. Le Bodic, A. Pages, M. Pluot, M. Patey, C. Rigaud, G. Viennet, F. Vildé, J.P. Saint-André, B. Auvert**
Expressions morphologiques des carcinomes médullaires de la thyroïde (CMT) dans les formes familiales
Pathologic expressions in the familial forms of medullary thyroid carcinomas

163 **A. Chaventré, C. Calmettes, C. Houdent, H. Sobol, C. Proye, G. Bellis, H. Allannic**
Rôle de l'anthropologie génétique (généalogie) dans le diagnostic de la forme familiale du cancer médullaire de la thyroïde
Relevance of genealogic studies for the diagnosis of familial forms of medullary thyroid carcinomas

V. MULTIPLE ENDOCRINE NEOPLASIA TYPE 2
V. NÉOPLASIE ENDOCRINIENNE MULTIPLE TYPE 2

169 **J. Caron, V. Boiteau, S. Casanova, D. Farkas, M. Rosenberg-Bourgin, N. Feingold, C. Calmettes, E. Modigliani and the GETC**
MEN 2A pheochromocytomas : GETC French multicentric retrospective study (1960 - 1988)
Les phéochromocytomes des NEM 2A : étude rétrospective multicentrique du GETC en France (1960 - 1988)

175 **P.J. Guillausseau, C. Guillausseau-Scholer, E. Sarfati, P. Chanson, M.E. Chauveau, J.L. Baulieu, G. Gay, J. Lubetzki and the GETC**
Hyperparathyroïdie et néoplasie endocrinienne multiple de type 2A. Aspects cliniques, biologiques et chirurgicaux
Hyperparathyroidism and multiple endocrine neoplasia type 2A. Clinical, biological and surgical aspects

183 **A. Meer, C. Calmettes, A. Munck and the GETC**
La néoplasie endocrinienne multiple de type 2B. Etude de 25 cas apparemment sporadiques. Recherche d'éléments de pronostic
Multiple endocrine neoplasia type 2B. Study of 25 apparently sporadic cases. Prognostic factors

187 **J.L. Baulieu, C. Calmettes, J. Caron, J.L. Dupont, J.F. Henry, R. Mornex, G. Opocher, P.J. Plouin, C. Proye, F. Raue**
Round table : screening diagnosis and treatment of pheochromocytomas associated with MTC
Table ronde : bilan, diagnostic et traitement des phéochromocytomes associés au CMT

VI. THERAPEUTIC MEANS
VI. MOYENS THÉRAPEUTIQUES

193 **C. Parmentier, P. Gardet, F. de Vathaire, J.P. Travagli, B. Caillou, M. Schlumberger**
Prognostic factors in medullary thyroid carcinoma (MTC) : a study based on 207 patients treated at the Institut Gustave Roussy

Facteurs pronostiques du cancer médullaire de la thyroïde : étude de 207 patients traités à l'Institut Gustave-Roussy

199 **C. Proye, T. Marmousez and the Association Française de Chirurgie Endocrinienne and the GETC**
Cancer médullaire de la thyroïde : moyens thérapeutiques, chirurgie de première intention
Medullary thyroid carcinoma : therapeutic means, surgery in first management

207 **G. Andry, P. Dor**
Medullary thyroid carcinoma : surgery for persistent disease
Cancer médullaire de la thyroïde : chirurgie de rattrapage

213 **M. Schlumberger, P. Gardet, F. de Vathaire, D. Sarrazin, J.P. Travagli, C. Parmentier**
External radiotherapy and chemotherapy in MTC patients
Radiothérapie externe et chimiothérapie chez les patients souffrant de cancer médullaire de la thyroïde

221 **C.A. Hoefnagel, R.A. Valdes Olmos, C.C. Delprat**
Therapy of medullary thyroid carcinoma using I-131 MIBG and radiolabelled monoclonal antibodies
Utilisation de la I-131 MIBG et des anticorps monoclonaux radioactifs dans le traitement du cancer médullaire de la thyroïde

VII. PHYSICIAN'S STRATEGY FOR THE MANAGEMENT OF MEDULLARY THYROID CARCINOMA
VII. STRATÉGIE DU CLINICIEN DEVANT UN CANCER MÉDULLAIRE DE LA THYROIDE

Strategy for the diagnosis and the follow-up
Stratégie de diagnostic et de suivi

229 **E. Modigliani, M. Weissel, B.M. Goslings, P.J. Guillausseau, B. Busnardo**
Round table : strategy of diagnosis and follow-up of medullary thyroid carcinoma
Table ronde : stratégie de diagnostic et de suivi dans le cancer médullaire de la thyroïde

Strategy in familial forms
Stratégie dans les formes familiales

237 **P. Gardet, M. Schlumberger, B. Caillou, J.P. Travagli, H. Sobol, D. Bellet, G. Lenoir, C. Parmentier**
Early detection of inherited MTC
Détection précoce des formes familiales de cancer médullaire de la thyroïde

241 **H.F.A. Vasen, C.J.M. Lips**
Strategy for an approach to familial medullary thyroid cancer. Practical, physiological and genetic aspects of screening
Stratégie en présence d'une forme familiale de cancer médullaire de la thyroïde. Aspects pratiques, psychologiques et génétiques de l'enquête

245 **H. Sobol, S. Narod, I. Schuffenecker, G.M. Lenoir and the Groupe d'Etude des Tumeurs à Calcitonine (GETC)**
Genetic screening for hereditary medullary thyroid carcinoma (MTC)
Enquête génétique dans les formes héréditaires de cancer médullaire de la thyroïde

VIII. EPIDEMIOLOGY OF MEDULLARY THYROID CARCINOMA IN EUROPE
VIII. ÉPIDÉMIOLOGIE DU CANCER MÉDULLAIRE DE LA THYROIDE EN EUROPE

255 **C. Calmettes, H. Hansen, E. Limbert, P. Moller, B. Ponder, F. Raue, H. Vasen, M. Weissel**
Epidemiology and genetics of medullary thyroid cancer. Preliminary of an European concerted action
Epidémiologie et génétique du cancer médullaire de la thyroïde. Résultats préliminaires de l'action concertée européenne

267 CONCLUSIONS
J. Tourniaire

269 **Author Index**
Index des auteurs

Introduction

Thyrocalcitonin, its discovery and development

Maurice Tubiana

Institut Gustave-Roussy and INSERM U.66, 39, rue Camille-Desmoulins, 94805 Villejuif Cedex, France

The discovery of thyrocalcitonin was due to cooperation between oncologists and biologists. In 1968 oncologists were puzzled and frustrated by the enigma of medullary thyroid cancers whose morphological appearance was that of a poorly differentiated cancer and whose natural history with its slow growth and progression evoked that of a well differentiated carcinoma. Biologists had found a hormone termed, calcitonin, and were searching for diseases releasing large amounts of this hormone. Over the past century most advances in endocrinology were related to the study of diseases in which there was either a hypersecretion of the hormone or a lack of secretion.

There was, therefore, a convergence between the aims of oncologists and biologists which materialized during a long conversation between Gérard Milhaud and myself and led to cooperation and the discovery of the synthesis of calcitonin in medullary cancers.

It is noteworthy that the subsequent development of studies on calcitonin was also related to collaboration between oncologists, pathologists, geneticists and biologists. The management of patients with medullary cancer greatly benefited from the use of calcitonin as a marker. After initial treatment, the serum calcitonin level was found to be a potent prognostic factor and when assayed in catheterized veins it can help to localize the source of secretion and therefore residual disease. Monoclonal antibodies directed against calcitonin make it a useful agent for tumor localization and metastasis detection.

Medullary carcinoma is one of the few hereditary cancers. When a cancer is diagnosed, one of the main uses of calcitonin is the search for medullary cancers in members of the same family. Its assay has played a crucial role in the early diagnosis of medullary cancer at a time when the tumor is barely palpable even during surgery. Currently the association of the calcitonin assay and the analysis of the karyotype has provided new technique for the screening of the disease and its cure.

The history of calcitonin is therefore a good illustration of the efficacy of a multidisciplinary approach. Further progress should result from such joint studies and a symposium like this one, which has been so well organised by C. Calmettes, should contribute to this endeavour.

Histoire du cancer médullaire de la thyroïde

Gérard Milhaud

INSERM U 113, Laboratoire Associé au CNRS 163, CHU Saint-Antoine, 27, rue Chaligny, 75571 Paris Cedex 12, France

Le premier congrès européen consacré au cancer médullaire de la thyroïde réunit 300 participants représentant 20 pays. Certains sont venus des Etats-Unis d'Amérique et du Canada. Organisé sous l'égide de l'INSERM, du CNRS et de l'Association pour la Recherche sur le Cancer, ce congrès permet de mettre en commun nos connaissances les plus récentes sur tous les aspects du cancer médullaire, en particulier dans la dimension diagnostique, thérapeutique et pronostique.

Ce congrès a la légitime ambition de programmer les études de demain. Faisons un bref rappel historique. C'est en 1965 que nous décrivons l'existence de la calcitonine chez l'Homme et que nous démontrons que la calcitonine porcine est capable de faire baisser la calcémie du sujet normal.

C. R. Acad. Sc. Paris, t. 261, p. 4513-4516 (22 novembre 1965).   Groupe 12.

ENDOCRINOLOGIE. — *Existence et activité de la thyrocalcitonine chez l'Homme.* Note (*) de MM. Gérard Milhaud, Mohsen S. Moukhtar, Jacques Bourichon et Mlle Anne-Marie Perault, présentée par M. Jacques Tréfouël.

Cette découverte fut accueillie avec beaucoup du septicisme. La communauté scientifique avançait qu'il s'agissait d'une hormone vestigiale, qui avait perdu sa fonction au cours de l'évolution, lorsque des vertébrés quittèrent le milieu marin pour vivre à l'air libre.

On déniait tout rôle de la calcitonine en pathologie humaine, puisque l'on n'a décrit aucun nanisme ou gigantisme provoqué par un trouble de production de la calcitonine : dans toute l'histoire de l'endocrinologie, la description du tableau clinique n'a-t-elle pas toujours précédé la reconnaissance du désordre endocrinien causal et l'identification de l'hormone responsable du trouble incriminé ?

Le doute n'était pas de notre fait et nous étions convaincu qu'il nous revenait le découvrir les entités anatomo-cliniques associées aux troubles de la sécrétion de la calcitonine chez l'Homme. Je demande au Professeur TUBIANA s'il connaissait un cancer thyroïdien susceptible de dériver des cellules parafolliculaires - les cellules C - sécrétrices de calcitonine.

Très rapidement, Maurice TUBIANA nous fait parvenir des échantillons de sang et des prélèvements de tissu tumoral provenant de deux malades atteints de cancer médullaire de la thyroïde, entité anatomopathologique décrite par HAZARD, HAWK et CRILE quelques années auparavant.

A l'aide du dosage biologique, pourtant peu sensible, nous mettons en évidence la calcitonine présente en quantités très élevées en mettant à profit les effets hypocalcémiant et hypophosphatémiant de l'hormone.

C. R. Acad. Sc. Paris, t. 266, p. 608-610 (5 février 1968)   Série D

ENDOCRINOLOGIE. — *Epithélioma de la thyroïde sécrétant de la thyrocalcitonine.* Note (*) de MM. **Gérard Milhaud, Maurice Tubiana, Claude Parmentier** et **Gérard Coutris,** présentée par M. Maurice Fontaine.

Rappelons qu'à l'époque la structure chimique de la calcitonine humaine était encore inconnue. Le cancer médullaire de la thyroïde produisait donc de la calcitonine, qui est sécrétée dans le sang. Cette observation, qui s'accordait avec une hypothèse émise par le Professeur WILLIAMS que nous avons le plaisir d'avoir parmi nous aujourd'hui, ouvrait le chapitre des hypercalcitonies.
Nous décrivons ensuite un cancer trabéculaire particulier producteur de grandes quantités de calcitonine.

Separatum EXPERIENTIA 26, 1381 (1970)
Birkhäuser Verlag, Basel (Schweiz)

An Unusual Trabecular Thyroid Cancer Producing Calcitonin

G. Milhaud, C. Calmettes, G. Dreyfuss
and M. S. Moukhtar

Il convenait aussi de rechercher les sécrétions ectopiques ou inapropriées de calcitonine. Les carcinoïdes bronchiques et intestinaux sont identifiés et de nombreuses entités productrices de calcitonine sont rapidement dénombrées

C. R. Acad. Sc. Paris, t. 270, p. 2195-2198 (4 mai 1970)   Série D

ENDOCRINOLOGIE. — *Carcinoïde sécrétant de la thyrocalcitonine.* Note (*) de M. **Gérard Milhaud**, Mme **Claude Calmettes**, MM. **Jean-Paul Raymond, Jean Bignon** et **Mohsen S. Moukhtar**, présentée par M. Maurice Fontaine.

En 1971 au congrès de Chapel Hill (Caroline du Nord) sur les hormones régulatrices du calcium nous présentons le rapport sur ce nouveau chapitre de pathologie humaine, celui des troubles de sécrétion de la calcitonine.

Reprinted from
International Congress Series No. 243 (ISBN 90 219 0153 6)
CALCIUM, PARATHYROID HORMONE AND THE CALCITONINS
Proceedings of the Fourth Parathyroid Conference, Chapel Hill, N.C., March 15-19, 1971.
Excerpta Medica, Amsterdam

A NEW CHAPTER IN HUMAN PATHOLOGY:
CALCITONIN DISORDERS AND THERAPEUTIC USE

G. MILHAUD, C. CALMETTES, A. JULLIENNE, D. THARAUD,
H. BLOCH-MICHEL, J. P. CAVAILLON, R. COLIN and M. S. MOUKHTAR

En fait la calcitonine deviendra le marqueur tumoral des années 1970.

Les conséquences de ces travaux allaient être nombreuses. Citons :

- L'isolement de la calcitonine humaine et l'élucidation de sa structure, rendus possibles du fait de la très forte teneur en hormone de la tumeur primitive et des métastase du cancer médullaire. La thyroïde tumorale contient jusqu'à mille fois plus de calcitonine que la glande normale.

- La mise au point du dosage de l'hormone par voie radioimmunologique, grâce aux anticorps obtenus par immunisation des animaux avec des extraits de cancer médullaire de la thyroïde. Désormais quelques gouttes de sang suffisent pour poser le diagnostic de cancer médullaire de la thyroïde, pour vérifier le résultat du traitement, pour déceler la formation de métastases bien avant toute traduction clinique.

Le cancer médullaire de la thyroïde est un des très rares cancers héréditaires à produire son propre marqueur. Il devrait nous apporter la réponse à la question du mécanisme génétique selon lequel s'opère la transmission héréditaire d'un cancer.

- Les processus qui président à l'association du cancer médullaire de la thyroïde à d'autres affections dans le cadre de neuroendocrinopathies de type II sont discutés.

- L'élucidation des étapes de la biosynthèse de la calcitonine est réalisée. A. JULLIENNE et M.S. MOUKHTAR donnent la séquence complète, comprise entre le codon signal et le codon terminal.

The complete sequence of human preprocalcitonin

J.M. Le Moullec*, A. Jullienne⁺, J. Chenais, F. Lasmoles, J.M. Guliana, G. Milhaud and M.S. Moukhtar

Etait-il prévisible que la découverte du cancer médullaire de la thyroïde permette d'aborder la régulation de l'expression génétique, le même gène conduisant à la production soit de calcitonine soit du peptide apparenté au gène de la calcitonine ?

- D'un point de la santé publique, l'initiative du Dr. C. CALMETTES a conduit à la création du groupe de travail interdisciplinaire intitulé le "Groupe d'Etudes des Tumeurs à Calcitonine" (G.E.T.C.), qui réunit plus d'une centaine de spécialistes français. Il jouera un rôle déterminant dans la transformation du pronostic du cancer médullaire de la thyroïde, qui est très sombre s'il est laissé à son évolution naturelle. Si le diagnostic est posé au stade préclinique, l'ablation de la ou des tumeurs de taille microscopique entraîne une normalisation de tous les paramètres tumoraux dans près de 100 % des cas : il faudra cinq années de recul pour affirmer la guérison.

En conclusion, les études concernant le cancer médullaire de la thryoïde illustrent les apports réciproques de la recherche fondamentale et de l'investigation clinique, dans l'enchaînement extra-ordinairement rapide des découvertes et de leurs applications. Les tumeurs à calcitonine contribueront à l'élucidation des mécanismes de transformation de la cellule normale en cellule maligne.

Medullary cancer of the thyroid : a general view

Claude Calmettes

INSERM U 113, CHU Saint-Antoine, 27, rue Chaligny, 75571 Paris Cedex 12, France

Medullary thyroid carcinoma (MTC) is a disease particularly interesting from multiple points of view, - oncology, but this malignant tumor can be associated with usually benign disorders of neuroendocrine cells derived from the neural crest -in the clinical syndromes of multiple endocrine neoplasia (MEN)- :
- biology, chiefly as it secretes its own marker, calcitonin (CT) ;
- endocrinology, with the production of different hormones and peptides ;
- pathology, presenting various forms essential to be known ;
- genetics and epidemiology, as it exists in sporadic and familial forms, a model of hereditary cancer.

All these aspects are inseparable and must o be taken into account in the study of the disease.

Three principal forms of MTC can be summarized on scheme (fig.1): briefly, it appears as sporadic or familial, isolated(MTC only) or associated with other diseases developed from cells of neural crest origin, but sporadic MENs as well as familial MTC only seem to be seldom on the view of extensive familial screening including genealogical research and must be proved : so, it is preferable to speak about apparently sporadic MEN or familial MTC only until the gene responsible for the MTC is identified.

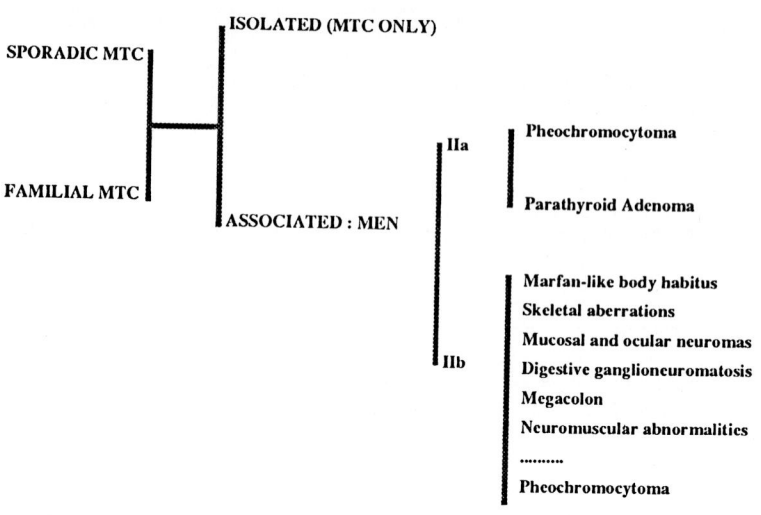

Fig. 1

HISTORY

The history of the disease underlines the progress in our knowledge of it ; it can be divided in three large periods:
The clear cell thyroid cancer had been described by Pagès (1955) but the identification of medullary cancer with amyloid stroma is due to Hazard, Hawk and Crile in 1959 (Hazard et al.1959) and was rapidly followed by the description of the main forms of the disease
1961 - Sipple : association of thyroid cancer and pheochromocytoma
1965 - Williams : medullary thyroid cancer is characteristic of Sipple's syndrome
Schimke and Hartman: Sipple's syndrome is a distinct genetic entity
1966 - Williams : histogenesis
1968 - Gorlin: The hereditary form is linked with autosomal transmission
The discovery of the secretion of calcitonin -identified by Hirsch in1963 (Hirsch et al 1963)- by MCTs successively by Milhaud, Tubiana et al (Milhaud et al. 1968), Meyer and Abdel Bari (1968) is the key event opening the way to MCT biology, allowing preoperative diagnosis and survey of the disease and discovery of atypical histological MTC (Milhaud et al. 1970).
1973 - Wolfe et al.: Description of the C-cell hyperplasia in familial medullary thyroid cancer
1974 - Hennessy et al.: stimulation of calcitonin by secretagogues
1975 - Chong et al: Classification of multiple endocrine neoplasia in MEN II a and b.

The progress in the last ten years are due to molecular biology and cooperative works:
1983 - Amara et al: production of different polypeptides by the CT gene
- Founding of the French and English Study Groups for Calcitonin Tumors
1984 - Moukhtar et al : Identification of the sequence of human preprocalcitonin
1987 - Mathew et al, Simpson et al : Assignement of MEN II to chromosome 10 by linkage.
Motte et al.: Mature CT assay.

CLINICAL PICTURE

Sporadic MTC as the index case of the familial form appears usually as a cold thyroid nodule, bilateral when familial or in case of MEN ; it can be painful on palpation and accompanied by diarrhea and/or flushes. Lymph node metastases are precocious ; they can even reveal the cancer. Distant metastases occur in lungs, bones,and, characteristically, liver. The cancer can also be diagnosed prior to tangible thyroid nodule by CT assay when suspected on clinical signs, an extrathyroidal association or in family screening.
In MEN IIa, pheochromocytoma generally occurs bilaterally and multicentrically; malignant degeneration is very rare.Clinical manifestations of parathyroid adenomas rarely constitute the first sign of the disease.
Extrathyroidal manifestations other than pheochromocytoma, associated in various ways to MTC, constitute MEN IIb syndromes, of bad prognosis. The Hirschsprung's pseudosyndrome is often diagnosed in the first days of life and MTC appears early ; other clinical features of MEN IIb, obvious later, include musculoskeletal abnormalities, marfanoid appearance, abnormal, corneal and cutaneous innervation, mucosal neuromas, digestive ganglioneuromatosis...

DIAGNOSIS

MTC is characterized by CT secretion ; successive advances in the sensivity and specificity of the assay of the hormone have been realized from biological quantitation to successive radioimmunological (Calmettes et Moukhtar 1982) and, recently, radioimmunometric methods. Plasmatic CT assay allows the diagnosis of the tumor, especially after stimulation for the early detection of the familial form. In situ CT detection must authenticate the diagnosis in surgically removed tissues, particularly in atypical forms.
The carcinoembryonic antigen level has essentially a prognostic value.
Multiple hormones and peptides are also secreted by MTC, among them bioactive ACTH can be responsible for a Cushing syndrome.

Imaging techniques are essential in search of preoperative tumoral extension, for the detection of metastases and for pheochromocytoma diagnosis.

The diagnosis of the hereditary form is made by recognition of a second case in the family. A third to a quarter of the cases are familial. Diagnosis of gene carriers can already be supported by linkage studies in some large MEN families ; nethertheless the early detection of the disease relies on an abnormal CT level obtained after stimulation of the hormone and, when negative, it is necessary to repeat provocative tests. Advances in familial screening have been progressive since the clinical detection of the first cases, with the following steps :
- elevated circulating CT level assay
- abnormal increase of CT level after stimulation
- improvement of pathological diagnosis : recognition of atypical MTC forms
- systematic familial screening using CT provocative tests
- national registers allowing to link apparently sporadic cases
- genealogic studies defining branches of families affected with the hereditary form (Houdent et al. 1990)
- assay of mature calcitonin earlier detecting an increase of the hormone.

PATHOLOGY
We will only mention that besides the classical medullary form with amyloidosis, many atypical types of MTC have been described, i.e. trabecular, papillary, follicular, possibly producing thyroglobulin besides CT (Franc 1990).

TREATMENT
MTC can only be cured by surgery : total thyroidectomy with central neck dissection remains essential. Other therapies do not lead to a complete remission of the disease.

PROGNOSIS
It depends on the precocity of the diagnosis and clinically obvious MTC are in most of the cases accompanied by lymph nodes metastases, the surgical cure of which is often uncomplete; nethertheless, the evolution is usually long, even in the presence of tumoral spread. That is to say that early detected familial forms are of good prognosis and it is possible to formulate the following equations :
sporadic and familial index cases = bad prognosis
early detected and surgically cured familial forms = good prognosis
This is confirmed by recent studies : Marmousez et al. (1990) report 68 per cent and 73 per cent of lymph nodes metastases respectively in 168 sporadic and 41 obvious familial MTC and only 8 per cent of metastases in occult familial cancers- 2 per cent macroscopic and 6 per cent microscopic-. If the diagnosis of occult cancer is made by means of provocative test and assay of mature CT, no lymph node extension was observed in 21 cases with basal normal CT level, i.e. under 10 pg/ml (data unpublished).

MTC UNSOLVED PROBLEMS

Though step-by-step substantial progress in the knowledge and treatment of MTC has been achieved, many problems are still unsolved; among the chief questions remaining to be solved, I will mention some :

Directly concerning the patients, methods, age, rhythm... of familial screening are difficult to establish ; there is no agreement on the choice of imaging methods ; do "clinically and biologically healthy transmitters" exist ?

Specific markers for C-cells implied in MTC, for pretumoral C-cell hyperplasia and for C-cells carcinogenesis are lacking.

The biology of the C-cells is not really known.

Discrimination between sporadic and familial forms is not always possible.

The significance of its various secreted hormones and peptides is not clear

No adjuvant therapy is up to now efficient.

The genes implied in tumorigenesis and the determination of the mutation(s) on chromosome 10 will have to be identified ; the process implied in carcinogenesis must be discovered ; these are preliminary steps to establish the existence of mutations de novo and possible gene therapy.

All substantial progress has been and will be achieved thanks to collaboration between specialists, practitioners, nurses and patients. Both a bilateral relationship, patient-practitioner, and a triple one, limited to patient-practionner-family, are out dated. The management of a patient must now take into account many points of view which are summarized on the scheme presented here (fig. 2) and established with the help of M. Rosenberg ; moreover, it must often be considered not only at a local but at a national or even international level for which scientific meetings are the best way to become acquainted and to plan projects.

RESUME

Le cancer médullaire de la thyroïde, sporadique ou familial, isolé ou élément d'une polyendocrinopathie de type II, est intéressant à de multiples points de vue. Son histoire peut être divisée en trois grandes périodes, descriptive, puis biologique - avec la découverte de la sécrétion tumorale de calcitonine qui permettait diagnostic et suivi de la maladie, détection précoce des formes familiales - et récente, bénéficiant des progrès de la biologie moléculaire et des dosages hormonaux par anticorps monoclonaux, avec l'apport d'études de groupe.

Néanmoins, malgré de substantiels progrès, de nombreuses questions restent en suspens, qui ne peuvent être résolues que par une collaboration entre praticiens et spécialistes; leurs compétences sont nécessaires pour traiter un malade et explorer sa famille à la recherche d'une forme héréditaire de la maladie.

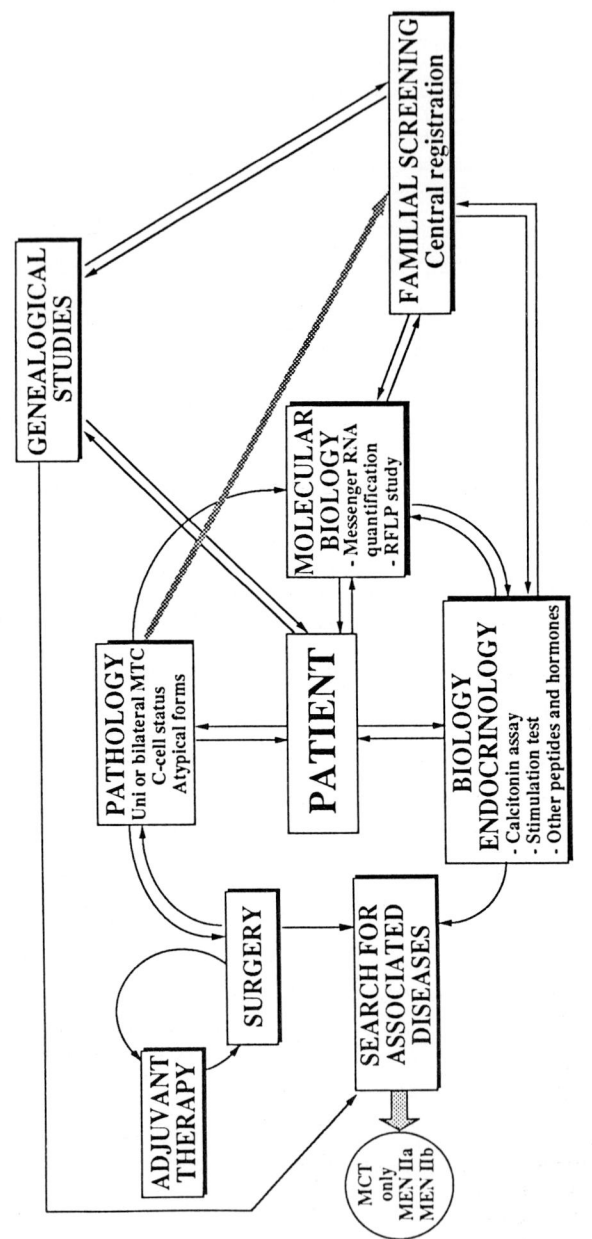

Fig. 2

Amara S.G. et al. (1982): Alternative RNA processing in calcitonin gene expression generates mRNAs encoding different polypeptide products. Nature 298 : 240-244.

Calmettes C. and Moukhtar M.S. (1982): Calcitonin in health and disease. Endocrinology of Calcium Metabolism, J.A. Parsons ed., pp 211-233, New york, Raven Press.

Chong G.C. et al. (1975) : Medullary carcinoma of the thyroid gland. Cancer 35, 2173-2183.

Franc B. (1990) : Le cancer médullaire de la thyroïde : acquisitions récentes. Sem. Hôp. Paris 66 : 111-117.

Gorlin A. et al. (1968) : Multiple mucosal neuromas, phéochromocytoma and medullary carcinoma of the thyroid - a syndrome. Cancer 2 : 293-299.

Hazard J.B. et al. (1959) : Medullary (solid) carcinoma of the thyroid: a clinicopathologic entity. J. Clin. Endocrinol. Metab.19 : 152-161.

Hennessy J.F. et al. (1973) : Stimulation of thyrocalcitonin secretion by pentagastrin and calcium in two patients with medullary carcinoma of the thyroid. J.Clin. Endocrinol. Metab. 36 : 200-203.

Hirsch P.F.et al. (1964): Thyrocalcitonin : hypocalcemic hypophosphatemic principle of the thyroid gland. Science 146 : 412-413.

Houdent Ch. et al. (1990): Cancer médullaire familial de la thyroïde. Apport de la généalogie et de la génétique à l'étude de deux familles. Presse Méd. 19 : 549-552.

Marmousez T. et al. (1990): Actualisation de la prise en charge chirurgicale des cancers médullaires de la thyroïde (tumeurs thyroïdiennes à calcitonine). Lyon Chir.86: 104-107.

Mathew C.G.P. et al. (1987): A linked genetic marker for multiple endocrine neoplasia type 2A on chromosome 10. Nature 328 : 527-528.

Meyer J.S. et Abdel Bari W. (1968) : Granules and thyrocalcitonin activity in medullary carcinoma of the thyroid gland. N. Eng. J. Med. 278 : 523-529

Milhaud G. et al. (1968): Epithélioma de la thyroide sécrétant de la thyrocalcitonine. C.R.Acad. Sci.(D), Paris, 266: 608-610.

Milhaud G. et al. (1970): An unusual trabecular thyroid cancer producing calcitonin. Experentia (Basel) 26: 1381-1383.

Motte P. et al. (1988):Construction and clinical validation of sensitive and specific assay for serum mature calcitonin using monoclonal anti-peptide antibodies. Clin. Chim. Acta 174 : 35-54.

Pagès A.- Essai sue le système des cellules claires de Feyrter. Thèse de doctorat en médecine, Montpellier, 1955.

Schimke R.N. et HARTMAN W.H. (1965) : Familial amyloid-producing mdullary thyroid carcinoma and pheochromocytoma - a distinct genetic entity. Am. J. Int.Med 63, 1027-1039.

Simpson N.E. et al. (1987): Assignment of multiple endocrine neoplasia type 2A to chromosome 10 by linkage. Nature 328 : 528-530.

Sipple J.H. (1961): The association of pheochromocytoma with carcinoma of the thyroid gland. Am. J. Med.,31: 163-166.

Williams E.D. (1965): A review of 17 cases of carcinoma of the thyroid and pheochromocytoma. J. Clin. Path., 18 : 288-292.
Williams E.D. (1966): Histogenesis of medullary carcinoma of the thyroid. J. Clin. Path.19,: 114-118.
Wolfe H.J.et al. (1973) : C-cell hyperplasia preceeding medullary thyroid carcinoma. N. Eng. J. Med.,289 : 437-441.

I. Calcitonin genes, expression and biological functions

I. Les gènes de la calcitonine, expression et fonctions biologiques

Calcitonin gene family

J.M. Guliana[1][2], A. Jullienne[1], F. Lasmoles[1], S. Minvielle[1], N. Segond[1], G. Milhaud[1] and M.S. Moukhtar[1]

(1) INSERM U 113, Faculté de Médecine Saint-Antoine, 75571 Paris Cedex 12, and
(2) Service d'Endocrinologie Diabétologique, Hôpital Saint-Antoine, 75571 Paris Cedex 12, France

ABSTRACT

The concept of calcitonin (CT) gene includes several genes with common structural particularities encoding for different peptides which have some homologies in their structure. These gene constitute the Calc Gene Family. Two genes are well identified, Calc I gene encoding for CT and calcitonin gene-related peptide I (CGRP I) and Calc II gene encoding for CGRP II only. At least, three considerations determine the importance of Calc I gene: the alternative splicing mechanism, a model for studying relationships between genomic expression and cellular differentiation, particularly in neuronal and endocrine tissue functions; the modifications of its expression with tumoral development of C-cells and with ectopic production of CT; the potential relations between the expression of this gene and the familial determinism of medullary thyroid carcinoma (MTC). The relative importance of physiological role of Calc II gene and the relations between the 2 genes remain to be clarified. On the basis of species evolution of CT and CGRP and structural similarities between peptides, the presence of other genes is postulated in the Calc gene family: a non-mammalian vertebrate apparented gene and the gene of amylin, a recently discovered peptide with 50 % of homology with CGRP I and II.

I. INTRODUCTION

The importance of CT secretion studies in normal and pathologic situations results from the role of this hormone as the main tumoral marker (Milhaud et al. 1968) of a cancer: medullary thyroid carcinoma (MTC) which exists in 2 forms, sporadic or familial. CT secretion appears without relation in discriminating the both forms of this disease. However, biochemical studies of CT production shown the presence of several molecular forms of the hormone, particularly the presence in human serum (Tobler et al. 1983) and thyroid gland (Fischer et al. 1983) of CT molecular forms specifically recognized by antibodies raised against salmon CT. Thus, the existence in the human genome of at least 2 different genes could be postulated. In 1982, the report by Amara et al. that the first identified CT gene (Calc I gene) in the rat encodes for two peptides, CT and calcitonin gene-related peptide

(CGRP), raises the interest of studies concerning CT production and CT/CGRP (Calc) gene expression.

From the C-cells activity to the development of MTC, several physiologic and pathologic aspects may justify the great interest to extend studies concerning Calc genes. 1- CGRP is widely synthetized and distributed in the central and peripheral nervous system. Thus, Calc I gene appears as a model for studying alternative splicing, and so, the relations between genomic expression and tissular differentiation. 2- The role of the CT and newly identified related peptides as tumoral markers of MTC have to be respectively defined again. 3- The regulating factors of these genes have to be identified in order to appreciate their role in normal and pathologic C-cells activities.

II. HUMAN CALC GENES

The two identified Calc genes of the human genome are located in the short arm of chromosome 11: Calc I gene is in the p13-p15 region, between catalase and PTH genes loci (Höppener et coll. 1984, Kittur et coll. 1985); Calc II gene locus has been first situated to the q12-pTer region (Höppener et coll. 1985). Calc I gene is composed of 6 exons. This gene encodes for CT (exon 4) and CGRP I (exons 5). The 3 first exons are common to the 2 peptides, exon 6 is associated to the maturation of CGRP I mRNA. Calc II gene has 5 exons (Steenberg et al. 1984). It only encodes for CGRP II (Steenberg et al. 1985). This gene is a pseudo-gene for CT (Alevizaki et al. 1986) (Figure 1). The comparison of the nucleotidic sequence of these genes shows a strong homology (95%) for the CGRP coding-exons and only 60% sequence identity between the CGRP non-coding exons and between exon 4 of Calc I gene and the corresponding region of Calc II gene.

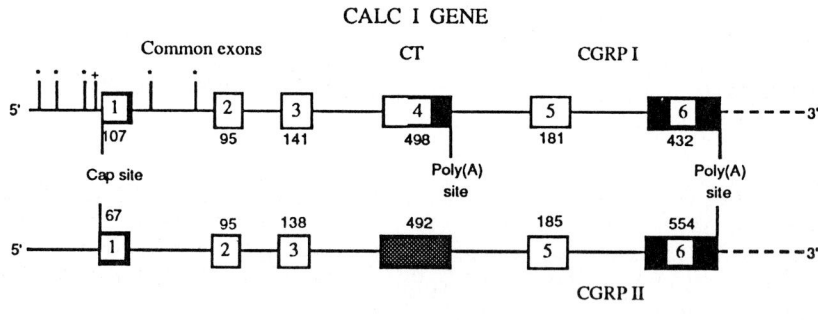

Figure 1: Schematic representation of the 2 Calc gene structure indicating: exon size (number), non-coding exon (black boxes), CT-like sequence of Calc II gene (grey box), 5 of the Msp I and Hpa II restriction sites (*), TATA box (+). See text for references and further explanations.

On the basis of these similarities, it is postulated that the 2 genes identified in human and rat are more probably due to a duplication from a common gene in mammalian species than to different evolution from an ancestral Calc gene.

The organisation of Calc I gene is similar in rat (Amara et al. 1982), human (Jonas et coll. 1985), and chicken (Minvielle et al. 1987). The nucleotidic structure of this gene is known on approximatively 5 kb from exon 1 to 3' end and on 1.5 kb of the 5' flanking region. In 1981, Rosenfeld et al. show the presence in rat transplantable MTC of a new mRNA, hybridizable with specific cDNA for CT mRNA, longer than the CT specific messenger, appearing in some low-producer CT tumours. These authors first characterize the existence of two distinct mRNAs produced by the expression of the same gene, implicating an alternative splicing mechanism during the transcription. The same group of co-workers then identified the structure of rat Calc I gene (Amara et al. 1982) and demonstrated the tissue-specific alternative splicing between thyroid C-cells, predominantly producing CT mRNA, and neural tissue, producing large amounts of CGRP mRNA (Rosenfeld et al. 1983). This model of gene expression implicates common regions in the structure of specific mRNA for CT and CGRP I and of their respective precursor peptide (figure 2): the 5' end of mRNAs and a 75 amino-acid N-terminal peptidic sequence. The 21 amino-acid C-terminal related peptide of CT precursor is called katacalcine or PDN-21 in human (PDN-18 in rat CT precursor). This peptide is interesting for its equimolar secretion with CT.

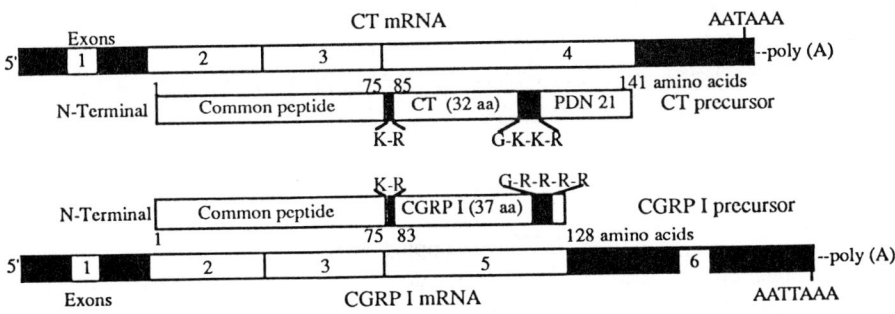

Figure 2: Schematic representation of the structure of hCT and hCGRP I specific mRNA and precursor polyproteins, illustrating the size of respective precursors, non-coding nucleotidic sequences (black), common regions of mRNAs and precursors, polyadenylation activating sites (AATAAA for CT mRNA, ATTAAA for CGRP I mRNA), C-terminal related-peptide of CT precursor (katacalcine or PDN 21 in human).

III. STRUCTURES POTENTIALLY IMPLICATED IN THE REGULATION OF CALC GENE EXPRESSION.

The respective expression of Calc I gene for both peptides is variable according to the tissue. CGRP appears the major product of Calc gene expression as the result of neuronal activity, including the large role of this peptide in several regulation system (for review see Breimer et al. 1988). CGRP mRNA represents 98% of Calc I gene expression in neural tissue, and less than 3% in adult thyroid C-cells (Sabate et al. 1985). Thus, it is of great interest to identify the regulating structures of the 5' flanking region of this gene, the factors implicated in tissue specific gene expression and the mechanisms determinating alternative splicing.

THE 5' FLANKING REGION OF CALC I GENE.

The 5' flanking region of rat and human Calc I gene have been sequenced for around 1.5 kb. The analysis of the nucleotidic chain shows the presence of some concensus sequences for potentially regulating factors (Figure 3). The initializing transcription sequence, TATA box (AATAA), has been identified 27 bases upstream cap site in murin and human species. The cAMP responsive element binding site (TGACGTCA) is located around to position -250 from cap site. In human Calc I gene, Cote et al. (1990) have recently identified 8 sequences compatible with activator protein-1 (AP-1) binding sites and 5 sequences for activator protein-2 (AP-2) binding sites. Using Msp 1 and Hpa II restriction enzymes, Baylin et al. (1986) have mapped 3 potentially methylated CCGG sites in the 5' flanking region and 3 others between exons 1 to 3 of human Calc I gene. The importance of these elements results from their potential implications in the regulation of Calc I gene expression.

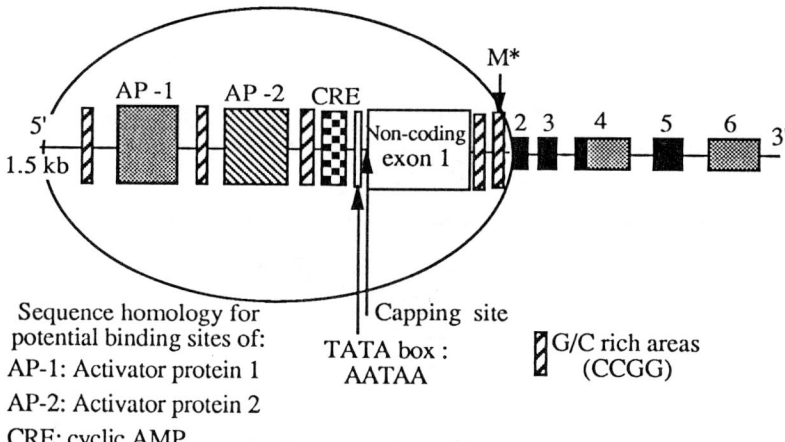

Figure 3: Schematic representation of the 5' flanking region of Calc I gene showing the concensus sequences for potential binding sites of AP-1 (n=8), AP-2 (n=5), the cAMP responsive element (CRE) and the potential methylated CG sites with mention of the normally methylated site 5 in normal thyroid (M*). See text for references.

DNA methylation of C-G rich areas of 5' flanking region of genes plays a role in gene expression (Feinberg et Vogelstein, 1983). High degree of methylation is associated with a low genomic expression of some genes in normal tissue as in neoplastic conditions. The DNA methylation pattern of CCGG sites of Calc I gene have been studied in normal tissues and some tumours, including MTC (Baylin and al. 1986). An hypomethylation pattern of Calc I gene in MTC has been found as a result of a lack of the normally methylated site 5 (between exons 1 and 2) in normal tissue. In contrast, other aggressive tumours as lymphomas and several types of lung tumours, including small-cell lung carcinoma (SCLC), have a high proportion of methylated sites for this gene. However, no references to the level of CT or CGRP production by the studied tumours are mentionned, essentially in MTC and in SCLC (which often is a CT secreting cancer). Moreover, the methylation pattern of DNA appears identical for several studied genes located in the short arm of chromosome 11 (catalase, Calc I gene, HRAS and the pADJ 762 region) but not for genes of other chromosomes in different forms of neoplasms (De Bustros and al. 1988).The authors suggest that the short arm of chromosome 11 is a "hot spot" for hypermethylation in human neoplasia.

The potential role of concensus sequences in Calc I gene expression. A number of factors has been studied for their role in the production of CT by normal or pathologic C-cells. Some of them probably interact with Calc I gene transcriptional unit: phorbol esters (De Bustros et al. 1985, 1986), cAMP (De Bustros et al. 1986), glucocorticoid (Muszinski et al. 1983, Cote et Gagel. 1986, Russo et al. 1988), 1-25 dihydroxyvitamin D3 (Segond et al. 1985). Phorbol esters increase Calc gene expression in human medullary carcinoma cell lines (De Bustros et al. 1985). The mechanism of action of these factors includes the activation of protein kinase C (Imagawa et al. 1987). Cis-concensus sequences for a trans-acting factor AP-1 had been previously identified in different TPA-inducible genes as collagenase, stromelysin, human metallothionein IIa gene (Angel et al.1987, Lee et al. 1987). The presence of such sequences, associated to the protein kinase C pathway, suggest possible relations between Calc gene expression and some proto-oncogenes. The introduction of v-Ha-ras oncogene into cultured human medullary carcinoma cells induces a cellular differentiation with an increase of Calc gene expression (Nakagawa et al. 1987) and an increase of c-jun protein and c-jun mRNA levels (Nelkin et al. 1990). Cyclic AMP, the protein kinase A activator, also increases Calc I gene expression (De Bustros et al. 1986). A cAMP responsive element binding (CREB) site, described above in the Calc I gene, has also been identified as a regulatory element of the somatostatin gene (Montminy et Bilezikjian, 1987).

In order to demonstrate the implication of the 5' flanking region of Calc gene in the regulation of gene expression, Cote et al. (1990) have transfected a human medullary carcinoma cell line, the TT cells, with 2 plasmid constructs associating the mouse metallothionein promoter and the human growth hormone (GH) mRNA with addition into the 5' end of one plasmid of the 5' flanking region of Calc I gene (HindIII/BamH1 fragment). These authors show an increase of GH production by TT cells transfected with the plasmid containing the 5' flanking Calc I gene fragment and an enhanced production of GH when they add phorbol ester PMA or forskolin (cAMP analog) into the medium. They conclude on the presence of promoter elements in the 5' flanking region of Calc I gene without direct evidence of a relation with the described concensus sequences. They don't observe the same in the fibroblast derived cell line NIH 3T3, suggesting the presence of a tissue specific enhancer factor in the TT cell line. Similar conclusions have been obtained using different fragments of the 5' flanking region of rat Calc I gene. Stolarski-Fredman et al. (1990) suggest the presence of a tissue specific enhancer in the 5' region of rat Calc I gene which is only active in neuroectodermic derived cells, neural cell line (B103) and the CA77 cell line (a rat medullary carcinoma cell line), but not in cell lines of other origin as monkey kidney (CV-1), fibroblast (NIH 3T3), human epithelial (HeLa) pancreatic islet (HIT) and pituitary (AtT20) derived cell lines.

THE ALTERNATIVE SPLICE-SITES IN CALC I GENE

At the moment where Calc I gene expression was demonstrated to produce 2 distinct mRNAs, this gene became one of the models for studying not only the alternative splicing transcription of the primary transcript but also the tissue specific mechanisms which determinate different ways of the gene expression. In a first time, alternative splicing of Calc I gene expression was suggested as tissue-specific (Rosenfeld et al. 1983), resulting from the demonstration that CGRP mRNA is the predominant product of the expression of this gene in neural tissue, as CT mRNA predominates in thyroid C-cells (figure 4). However, the co-localization of the both peptides and of their respective mRNAs in the same cells, rat thyroid C cells (Sabate et al. 1985), human pituitary (Jonas et al. 1985), human MTC (Jonas et al. 1985, Zajac et al. 1986) and human MTC cell line (Gkonos et al. 1986) suggest that the production of CT and CGRP mRNA is not mutually exclusive. Different mechanisms of alternative splicing have been demonstrated for many genes in eukaryotic cells (for review see Breitbard et al. 1987).

In order to evaluate the mechanisms of alternative splicing in Calc I gene expression, 3 successive steps have been accomplished by now. In a first time, the existence of 2 different polyadenylation sites for the selective processing of mature CT and CGRP mRNA has been demonstrated in rat (Rosenfeld et coll. 1983, Amara et coll. 1984) and human (Jonas et al., 1985) Calc I genes. Then, transgenic mice transfected with the rat Calc I gene associated to the mouse metallothionein promoter were demonstrated to produce rat CT mRNA in non-neuronal tissues while CGRP transcripts were selectively expressed in a wide variety of neurones (Crenshaw et al. 1987).Thus, the presence of neuronal selective factor(s) was suggested. Two potential mechanisms have been proposed for the regulation of alternative splicing in the Calc I gene: the regulating action of factors at the polyadenylation signal sites or at the 3' acceptor splice-sites of CT or CGRP exons. In order to evaluate the implication of polyadenylate activator sites at the 3' end of exon 4 and exon 6, lymphocyte A20 and teratocarcinoma F9 cell lines have been transfected using different rat Calc I mutated genes with either an inactive exon 4 polyadenylation site, or a Pst I deletion of the third intron, or a Bgl II deletion of exon 4 (Leff et al. 1987). The Bgl II fragment of the gene, including exon 4 polyadenylation site, was found to be implicated by containing an acceptor site for factor(s) predominantly expressed in neuronal derived cells which might modify the secondary structure of the transcript in order to drive the splice between exons 3 and 5. More recently, in order to evaluate the role of splice acceptor sites, human epithelial (HeLa) and mouse teratocarcinoma (F9) cell lines have been transfected with different constructed Calc I gene: deletions of the third intron, exon 4 and exon 5 splice acceptor deletions, substitution of exon 4 splice acceptor region with a heterologous splice acceptor (Emeson et al. 1989). The authors show that tissue-specific processing of the Calc I primary transcript is the result of alternative splice-site selection primarily regulated by cis-active sequences at the CT-specific 3'-splice junction. Using in vitro studies, Bovenberg et al. (1988) and Adema et al. (1988) describe the presence of a distinct branch point for lariat formation upstream the splice site of exon 4 and exon 5. The presence of uridine, in position -23 from the cleavage site of exon 4, slows down the splicing between exons 3 and 4, which can constitute the first cis-factor for the predominant production of CGRP mRNA (Adema et al.1990).

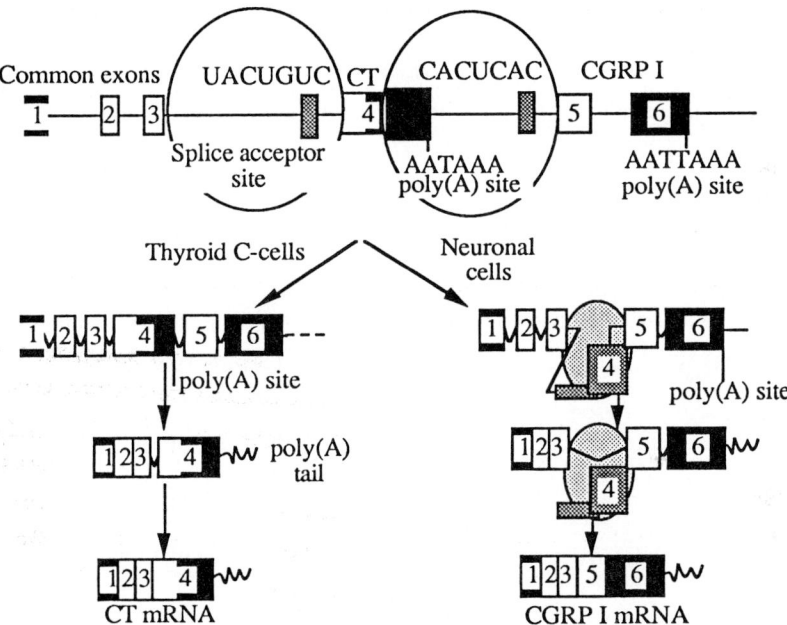

Figure 4: schematic representation of transcription steps from primary transcript of Calc I gene with reference to the alternative splicing mechanisms for maturation of specific CT or CGRP I mRNA. See text for references.

These studies show that the alternative splicing of Calc I primary transcript is directly linked to regulating sequences around CT exon. The polyadenylation signal at the 5' end of exon 4, activated or not inhibited, turns the transcription into the maturation of CT mRNA. However, the respective role of cis-regulating sequences, splice acceptor and polyadenylation sites of exon 4, and the trans-regulating factors remains to be evaluated. In these experiments, the role of an hypothetic "machinery" modifying the secondary structure of transcripts appears dependant of a first event which implicates the splice acceptor site of exon 4. This hypothesis results from the following facts:

lymphocyte cell lines transfected with Bgl II deletion construct, suppressing the splice acceptor region of exon 4, turn the transcription in part into the maturation of CGRP mRNA and not CT mRNA (Leff et al. 1987); F9 cells transfected with a heterologous splice acceptor sequence before exon 4 lost their ability to mature CGRP mRNA and product mature CT mRNA (Emeson et al. 1989).

IV. THE PRESENCE OF OTHER GENES

THE CALC III GENE: Alevisaki et al. (1987) have described a genome sequence with 90% homology with exons 2 and 3 of Calc I gene. Specific probes for CT and CGRP do not hybridize with this genomic structure.

HYPOTHESIS OF AN ANCESTRAL CALC GENE IN THE HUMAN GENOME. A lot of works suggest the presence in human genome of an ancestral Calc gene, relative to a non-mammalian Calc gene. Lasmoles et al. (1985), using a chicken cDNA probe for CT, detect in a human medullary thyroid carcinoma the presence of a specific CT mRNA, distinct from the CT mRNA produced by Calc I gene expression.

THE AMYLIN GENE: A MEMBER OF CALC GENE FAMILY ?. The amylin, first called Islet Amyloid Polypeptide (IAPP), has been identified in pancreatic islets of Langherans in human insulinoma, diabetic patients and diabetic cats (Westermark et al. 1987a, 1987b). Human IAPP shows 46% amino-acid sequence homology with CGRP II. Specific mRNAs for amylin have been identified, and the precursor structure deduced, in human (Mosselman et al. 1988) and in rat (Leffert et coll. 1989). The human amylin gene is assigned to chromosome 12 (Mosselman et al. 1988) and its structure is composed of 3 exons (for review and references see Nishi et al. 1990). This gene remains to be studied in order to determine the evolutionary relations with Calc genes.

V. CONCLUSIONS

Calcitonin genes product CT and other related peptides (CGRP I and II, PDN) which are used for the diagnosis and the follow-up of MTC. From studies concerning the structure and the activity of Calc genes, we can expect to understand the potential relations between these genes and the tumoral development of C cells, the role of their products as tumoral markers, the importance of Cis and Trans regulating factors implicated in normal or pathologic gene expression. Moreover, because medullary thyroid carcinoma has a familial form, the relations between the hereditary pattern and the tumoral development of C cells implicate directly or not the expression of Calc gene.

Thus, further studies will probably show the respective physiologic place of genes of the Calc gene family, their role in the development of MTC, and their relation with other genomic events.

REFERENCES

Adema, G.J., R.A.L. Bovenberg, H.S. Jansz and P.D. Baas (1988): Unusual branch point involved in splicing of the alternatively processed Calcitonin/CGRP I pre-mRNA. Nucleic Acids Res., 16, 9513-9526.

Adema, G.J., K.L. van Hulst and P.D. Baas (1990): Uridine branch acceptor is a cis-acting element involved in regulation of the alternative processing of calcitonin/CGRP I pre-mRNA. Nucleic Acids Res., 18, 5365-5373.

Alevizaki, M., A. Shiraiszhi, F.V. Rassool, G.J.M. Ferrier, I. MacIntyre and S. Legon (1986): The calcitonin-like sequence of the beta CGRP gene. FEBS Lett., 206, 47-52.

Alevizaki, M., F.V. Rassool, K.L.S. Collyear, I. MacIntyre and S. Legon (1987): A third calcitonin related sequence in the human genome. Calcified Tissues, 41 (suppl.2), abstract.

Amara, S.G., V. Jonas, M.G. Rosenfeld, E.S. Ong and R.M. Evans (1982) Alternative RNA processing in calcitonin gene expression generates mRNAs encoding different polypeptide products. Nature, 298, 240-244.

Amara, S.G., R.M. Evans and M.G. Rosenfeld (1984): Calcitonin/calcitonin gene-related peptide transcription unit: tissue-specific expression involves selective use of alternative polyadenylation sites. Mol. Cell. Biol., 4, 2151-2160.

Angel, P., M. Imagawa, R. Chiu, B. Stein, R.J. Imbra, H.J. Rahmsdorf, C. Jonat, P. Herrlich and M. Karin (1987): Phorbol ester-inducible genes contain a common Cis element recognized by a TPA-modulated Trans-acting factor. Cell, 49, 729-739.

Baylin, S.B., J.W.M. Höppener, A. de Bustros, P.H. Steenbergh, C.J.M. Lips and B.D. Nelkin (1986): DNA methylation patterns of calcitonin gene in human lung cancers and lymphomas. Cancer Res., 46, 2917-2922.

Bovenberg, R.A.L., G.J. Adema and P.D. Baas (1988): Model for tissue specific Calcitonin/CGRP I RNA processing in vitro experiments. Nucleic Acids Res., 16, 7867-7883.

Breimer, L.H., I. MacIntyre and M. Zaidi (1988): Peptides from the calcitonin genes: molecular genetics, structure and function. Biochem. J., 255, 377-390.

Breitbard, R.E., A. Andreadis and B. Nadal-Ginard (1987): Alternative splicing: a ubiquitous mechanism for the generation of multiple protein isoforms from single genes. Ann. Res. Biochem., 56, 467-495.

de Bustros, A., S.B. Baylin, C.L. Berger, B.A. Roos, S.S. Leong and B.D. Nelkin (1985): Phorbol esters increase calcitonin gene transcription and decrease c-myc mRNA levels in cultured human medullary thyroid carcinoma. J. Biol. Chem., 260, 98-104.

de Bustros, A., S.B. Baylin, M.A. Levine and B.D. Nelkin (1986): Cyclic AMP and phorbol esters separately induce growth inhibition, calcitonin secretion and calcitonin gene transcription in cultured human medullary thyroid carcinoma. J. Biol. Chem., 261, 8036-8041.

de Bustros, A., B.D. Nelkin, A. Silverman, G. Ehrlich, B. Poiesz and S.B. Baylin (1988): The short arm of chromosome 11 is a "hot spot" for hypermethylation in human neoplasia. Proc. Natl. Acad. Sci. (USA), 85, 5693-5697.

Cote, G.J. and R.F. Gagel (1986): Dexamethasone differentially affects the levels of calcitonin and calcitonin gene-related peptide mRNAs expressed in a human medullary thyroid carcinoma cell line. J. Biol. Chem., 261, 15524-15528.

Cote, G.J., R.V. Abruzzese, C.J.E. Lips and R.F. Gagel (1990): Transfection of calcitonin gene regulatory elements into a cell culture model of the C cell. J. Bone Mineral Res., 5, 165-171.

Crenshaw, III E.B., A.F. Russo, L.W. Swanson and M.G. Rosenfeld (1987): Neuron-specific alternative RNA processing in transgenic mice expressing a metallothionein calcitonin fusion gene. Cell, 49, 389-398.

Emeson, R.B., F. Hedjran, J.M. Yeakley, J.W. Guise and M.G. Rosenfeld (1989): Alternative production of calcitonin and CGRP mRNA is regulated at the calcitonin-specific splice acceptor. Nature, 341, 76-80.

Feinberg, A.P., and B. Vogelstein (1983): Hypomethylation distinguishes genes of some human cancers from their normal counterparts. Nature, 301, 89-92.

Fischer, J.A., P.H. Tobler, H. Henke and P.A. Tshopp (1983): Salmon and human calcitonin-like peptides coexist in the human thyroid and brain. J. Clin. Endocrinol. Metab., 57, 1314-1316.

Gkonos, P.J., W. Born, B.N. Jones, J.B. Peterman, H.T. Keutmann, R.S. Birnbaum, J.A. Fischer and B.A. Roos (1986): Biosynthesis of calcitonin gene-related peptide and calcitonin by a human medullary thyroid carcinoma cell line. J. Biol. Chem., 261, 14386-14391.

Höppener, J.W.N., P.H. Steenbergh, J. Zandberg, E. Bakker, P.L. Pearson, A.H.M. Geurts Van Kessel, H.S. Jansz and C.J.M. Lips (1984): Localization of the polymorphic human calcitonin gene on chromosome 11. Hum. Genet., 66, 309-312.

Höppener, J.W.N., P.H. Steenbergh, J. Zandberg, A.H.M. Geurts Van Kessel, S.B. Baylin, D.B. Nelkin, H.S. Jansz and C.J.M. Lips (1985): The second human calcitonin/CGRP gene is located on chromosome 11. Hum. Genet., 70, 259-263.

Imagawa, M., R. Chiu and M. Karin (1987): Transcription factor AP-2 mediates induction by two different signal-transduction pathways: protein kinase C and cAMP. Cell, 51, 251-260.

Jonas V., C.R. Lin, E. Kawashina, D. Semon, L.W. Swanson, J.J. Mermod, R.M. Evans and M.G. Rosenfeld (1985): Alternative RNA processing events in human calcitonin/calcitonin gene-related peptide gene expression. Proc. Natl. Acad. Sci. (USA), 82, 1994-1998.

Kittur, S.D., W.M. Hoppener, S.E. Antonarakis, J.D.J. Daniels, D.A. Meyers, N.E. Maestri, M. Jansen, R.G. Korneluk, B.D. Nelkin and H.H. Kazazian Jr. (1985) Linkage map of the short arm of human chromosome 11: location of the genes for catalase, calcitonin, and insulin-like growth factor II. Proc. Natl. Acad. Sci. (USA), 82, 5064-5067.

Lasmoles F., A. Jullienne, F. Day, S. Minvielle, G. Milhaud and M.S. Moukhtar (1985): Elucidation of the nucleotique sequence of chicken calcitonin mRNA: direct evidence for the expression of a lower vertebrate calcitonin-like gene in man and rat. EMBO J., 4, 2603-2607.

Lee, W., P. Mitchell and R. Tjian (1987): Purified transcription factor AP-1 interacts with TPA-inducible enhancer elements. Cell, 49, 741-752.

Leff, S.E., R.M. Evans and M.G. Rosenfeld (1987): Splice commitment dictates neuron-specific alternative RNA processing in calcitonin/CGRP gene expression. Cell, 48, 517-524.

Leffert, J.D., C.B. Newgard, H. Okamoto, J.L. Milburn and K.L. Luskey (1989) Rat amylin: cloning and tissue specific expression in pancreatic islets. Proc. Natl. Acad. Sci. (USA), 86, 3127-3130.

Milhaud, G., M. Tubiana, C. Parmentier et G. Coutris (1968): Epithélioma de la thyroïde secrétant de la thyrocalcitonine. C.R. Acad. Sci. (D), Paris, 266, 608-610.

Minvielle, S., M. Cressent, M.C. Delehaye, N. Segond, G. Milhaud, A. Jullienne, M.S. Moukhtar and F. Lasmoles (1987): Sequence and expression of the chicken calcitonin gene. FEBS Lett., 223, 63-68.

Montminy, M.R. and L.M. Bilezikjian (1987): Binding of a nuclear protein to the cyclic AMP response element of the somatostatin gene. Nature, 328, 175-178.

Mosselman, S., J.W.M. Höppener, J. Zandberg, A.D.M. van Mansfeld, A.H.M. Geurts van Kessel, C.J.M. Lips and H.S. Jansz (1988): Islet amyloid polypeptide: identification and chromosomal localization of the human gene. FEBS Lett., 239, 227-232.

Muszinski, M., R.S. Birnbaum and B.A. Roos (1983): Glucocorticoids stimulate the production of preprocalcitonin-derived secretory peptides by a rat medullary thyroid carcinoma cell line. J. Biol. Chem., 258, 11678-11683.

Nakagawa, T., M. Mabry, A. de Bustros, J.N. Ihle, B.D. Nelkin and S.B. Baylin (1987): Introduction of v-Ha-ras oncogene induces differentiation of cultured human medullary thyroid carcinoma. Proc. natl. Acad. Sci. (USA), 84, 5923-5927.

Nelkin, B.D., M. Borges, M. Mabry and .S.B. Baylin (1990): Transcription factor levels in medullary thyroid carcinoma cells differentiated by Harvey ras oncogene: c-jun is increased. Biochem. Biophys. Res. Comm., 170, 140-146.

Nishi, M., T. Sanke, S. Nagamatsu, G.I. Bell and D.F. Steiner (1990): Islet amyloid polypeptide: a new ß cell secretory product related to islet amyloid deposit. J. Biol. Chem., 265, 4173-4175.

Rosenfeld M.G., S.G. Amara, B.A. Roos, E.S. Ong and R.M. Evans (1981): Altered expression of the calcitonin gene associated with RNA polymorphism. Nature, 290, 63-65.

Rosenfeld, M.G., J.J. Mermod, S.G. Amara, L.W. Swanson, P.E. Sawchenko, J. Rivier, W.W. Vale and R.M. Evans (1983): Production of a novel neuropeptide encoded by the calcitonin gene via tissue-specific RNA processing. Nature, 304, 129-135.

Russo, A.F., C. Nelson, B.A. Roos and M.G. Rosenfeld (1988): Differential regulation of the coexpressed calcitonin/α-CGRP and β-CGRP neuroendocrine genes. J. Biol. Chem., 263, 5-8.

Sabate M.I., L.S. Stolarsky, J.M. Polak, S.R. Bloom, I.M. Varndell, M.A. Ghatei, R.M. Evans and M.G. Rosenfeld (1985): Regulation of neuroendocrine gene expression by alternative RNA processing: colocalization of calcitonin and calcitonin gene-related peptide in thyroid C-cells. J. Biol. Chem., 260, 2589-2592.

Segond, N., B. Legendre, E.H. Tahri, P. Besnard, A. Julienne, M.S. Moukhtar and J.M. Garel (1985): Increased level of calcitonin mRNA after 1,25-dihydroxyvitamin D3 injection in the rat. FEBS lett., 184, 268-272.

Steenbergh, P.H., J.W.M. Höppener, J. Zandberg J.M. Van De Ven, H.S. Jansz and C.J.M. Lips (1984): Calcitonin gene related peptide coding sequence is conserved in the human genome and is expressed in medullary thyroid carcinoma. J. Clin. Endocrinol. Metab., 59, 358-360.

Steenbergh, P.H., J.W.M. Höppner, J. Zandberg, C.J.M. Lips and H.S. Jansz (1985): A second human calcitonin/CGRP gene. FEBS Lett., 183, 403-407.

Stolarsky-Fredman, L., S.E. Leff, E.S. Klein, E.B. Crenshaw, J. Yeakley and M.G. Rosenfeld (1990): A tissue-specific enhancer in the rat-calcitonin/CGRP gene is active in both neural and endocrine cell types. Molecul. Endocrinol., 4, 497-504.

Tobler P.H., A. Tschoppf, M.A. Dambacher, W. Born and J.A. Fischer ; 1983; Identification and characterization of calcitonin forms in plasma and urine of normal subjects and medullary carcinoma patients ; J. Clin. Endocrinol. Metab.; 57; 749-754.

Westermark, P., C. Wernstedt, T.O. O'Brien, D.W. Hayden and K.H. Johnson (1987a): Islet amyloid in type 2 human diabetes mellitus and adult diabetic cats contains a novel putative polypeptide hormone. Am. J. Pathol., 127, 414-417.

Westermark, P., C. Wernstedt, E. Wilander, D.W. Hayden, T.O. O'Brien and K.H. Johnson (1987b): Amyloid fibrils in human insulinoma and islets of Langherans of the diabetic cat are derived from a neuropeptide-like protein also present in normal islet cells. Proc. Natl. Acad. Sci. (USA), 84, 3881-3885.

Zajac, J.D., J. Penschow, T. Mason, G. Tregear, J. Coghlan and T.J. Martin (1986): Identification of calcitonin and calcitonin gene-related peptide messenger ribonucleic acid in medullary thyroid carcinomas by hybridization histochemistry. J. Clin. Endocrinol. Metab., 62, 1037-1043.

RESUME

La famille des gènes de la CT constitue un modèle d'étude de la production de la CT et du CGRP I par un même gène (Calc I) impliquant des mécanismes d'épissage alterné et de différenciation fonctionnelle cellulaire, des modifications d'expression des gènes au cours des processus de tumorisation, des relations potentielles entre l'expression du gène d'un marqueur tumoral et le déterminisme génomique des formes familiales de cancer médullaire de la thyroïde. D'autres gènes devraient s'inclure dans cette famille de gènes de la CT, principalement un gène proche du gène CT/CGRP des vertébrés inférieurs.

Regulation of calcitonin secretion

Friedhelm Raue[1], Angela Zink[1] and Hans Scherübl[2]

(1) Department of Internal Medicine I, Endocrinology and Metabolism, University of Heidelberg, Bergheimerstrasse 58, 6900 Heidelberg, Germany
(2) Department of Pharmacology, Free University of Berlin, Thielallee 69-73, 1000 Berlin 33, Germany

Summary

The concentration of extracellular calcium tightly regulates calcitonin secretion. This seems to be mediated via calcium influx through voltage dependent calcium channels leading to an increase in intracellular calcium concentration. The role of dehydropyridine-sensitive calcium channels for stimulus-secretion-coupling could be confirmed in experiments using the calcium channel agonist Bay K 8644 and the calcium channel blocker nifedipine. A rise in extracellular calcium evokes an increase of intracellular calcium after 5-8 seconds. There also exists a cAMP-dependent-pathway of calcitonin release activated by glucagon, epinephrine or rat growth hormone releasing factor. Dual regulation of the adenylate cyclase, mediated by Gi or Gs-proteins takes place: the cAMP production stimulated by the rat growth hormone releasing factor can be inhibited by somatostatin or the A1 receptor analogue PIA. This inhibitory pathway is partially neutralized by pertussis toxin. There is a complex interaction between the two second messenger systems, cAMP and intracellular calcium. In C-cells pretreated with glucagon intracellular calcium starts to oscillate when extracellular calcium is raised. An additive rather than a synergistic stimulatory effect of the calcium- and cAMP-dependent pathway on calcitonin secetion is observed.

Control of calcitonin secretion in vivo

Calcitonin (CT) secretion from the C-cells is clearly regulated by plasma calcium (Ca) levels. When plasma Ca rises acutely, there is a propotional increase in plasma CT. This is the basis for using calcium infusion as a provocative test for CT release in patients with medullary thyroid carcinoma (MTC). In contrast, the effect of chronic hypercalcemia and hypocalcemia are controversal and contradictory results have been reported. Normal, elevated, as well as decreased basal levels of CT have been observed in hyperparathyroidism, whereas CT reserve can be normal or decreased (Tiegs et al. 1986; Tørring, et al. 1985). During chronic hypercalcemia a reversible exhaustion of CT content was observed in rats, while basal serum CT levels remained unchanged (Raue et al. 1984). In contrast, chronic hypocalcemia enhanced CT storage and secretion in the rat. The serum Ca levels showed an inverse relationship to CT storage and CT response to acute stimuli (Raue et al., 1988).

The most important CT secretagogues apart from calcium probably are the gastrointestinal hormones, gastrin, cholecystokinin, glucagon, and secretin. Gastrin is the most effective and the gastrin analog, pentagastrin is also used as provocative test in patients with MTC. However, the physiological significance of the regulation of CT secretion by these hormones is unclear, since large doses have been used in most studies. An increase in plasma CT after meals and/or an oral

Ca load could be demonstrated in only a few clinical and experimental studies (Deftos & Roos, 1989).

Both sex and age appear to influence CT secretion in humans. Higher than normal plasma levels for adults have been reported in pregnant women, children and newborn infants. CT levels appear to decrease with age in humans, in contrast to rats. Women have been shown to have lower basal plasma CT levels and reduced responses to i.v. Ca or pentagastrin compared to men. These findings have led many to postulate, that lower CT levels in women might contribute to the higher female prevalence of symptomatic osteoporosis (McDermott & Kidd, 1987). When evaluating the relationship of CT secretion to osteoporosis variable findings have been reported: lower (Reginster et al.,1989), unchanged or even elevated basal CT levels with normal (Body et al., 1989) or impaired CT response. Replacement of estrogen resulted in increased or unchanged basal CT levels and in augmented CT response to Ca stimulation. The discrepancies presumably reflect the use of different estrogens, different treatment periods and different CT assays. The role of CT in pathogenesis of osteoporosis is still questionable.

Other steroid hormones like glucocorticoids or 1,25 $(OH)_2D_3$ are also involved in CT secretion and synthesis. Dexamethasone increases CT mRNA in adrenalectomized rats within 5 days (Besnard et al., 1989) while 1,25 $(OH)_2D_3$ decreases CT mRNA in rats (Naveh-Many & Silver, 1988) within 6 h. 1-2 hours after injection of 1,25 $(OH)_2D_3$ CT serum levels increased (Raue et al., 1983) and a transient rise in translatable CT mRNA activity was observed (Segond et al., 1985).

Control of calcitonin secretion in vitro

As in vivo, the extracellular calcium $[Ca^{2+}]_{ex}$ concentration tightly regulates CT secretion in vitro. Various gastrointestinal and hypothalamic peptide hormones trigger CT release by acting via different intracellular signalling systems like cAMP, IP3 or Ca. Steroid hormones exert their effects on CT secretion and storage by binding to specific nuclear receptors thereby directly regulating CT gen transcription.

Calcium dependent calcitonin secretion

An acute elevation of $[Ca^{2+}]_{ex}$ evokes a prompt release of preformed CT in C-cell of the carcinoma cell-line e.g. rMTC 6-23 or rMTC 44-2. There is a strong positive relationship between $[Ca^{2+}]_{ex}$ and CT secretion. Even a small acute decrease of $[Ca^{2+}]_{ex}$ cause a decrease of CT release in rat thyroid explants. It is an essential function of C-cells to monitor $[Ca^{2+}]_{ex}$ and to respond to changes in $[Ca^{2+}]_{ex}$ by regulating CT secretion, which in turn regulates serum Ca. This tight linkage between $[Ca^{2+}]_{ex}$ and CT secretion is mediated by changes in intracellular cytosolic free calcium $[Ca^{2+}]_i$ (Fried & Tashjian, 1986). A small increase of $[Ca^{2+}]_{ex}$ causes a distinct rapid elevation in $[Ca^{2+}]_i$ via Ca influx through dihydropyridine-sensitive Ca channels. The essential role of these voltage-dependent Ca channels could be confirmed by applying Ca channel activators (BAY K 8644), Ca channel blockers (nifedipine, verapamil) or by depolarisation of the plasma membrane by high external potassium. BAY K 8644 stimulates CT secretion, which is completely inhibited by equimolar concentration of nifedipine and by chelating $[Ca^{2+}]_{ex}$ (Hishikawa et al.,1985; Raue et al., 1989). In the human MTC cell line (TT), a rise of $[Ca^{2+}]_{ex}$ does not affect $[Ca^{2+}]_i$ and the secretion of CT, indicating a defect in Ca^{2+} signal transduction (Haller-Brem et al., 1987). These findings have suggested a prominent role of dihydropyridine-sensitive Ca channels for the Ca sensitivity of C-cells.

Electrophysiological studies on rMTC-cells now provide direct evidence for a voltage dependent long lasting Ca^{2+} current with a steady state conductivity for Ca^{2+} even at the normal resting membrane potential (Scherübl et al., 1990). While rMTC cells showed this slowly decaying Ca^{2+} inward current, C-cells of the "defective" TT cell-line exhibited only a transient Ca^{2+} current. Thus, the steady state conductivity for Ca^{2+} is a prerequisite for C-cells to be able to monitor $[Ca^{2+}]_{ex}$.

The anticonvulsant agent phenytoin which can inhibit the calcium channel activity and also inhibits calmodulin, and thereby inhibits CT release (Cooper et al., 1988). Similar actions are described by other more or less specific calmodulin inhibitors as W7, trifluoperazine, chlorpromazine and haloperidol (Cooper & Borosky, 1986). Other agents, which increase $[Ca^{2+}]_i$ by enhancing Ca influx or by mobilization of intracellular Ca, enhance CT release. This could be done with Ca ionophores

(ionomycin, A23187; Haller-Brem et al., 1988; Seitz & Cooper, 1989). These findings again indicate that changes in $[Ca^{2+}]_i$ play a functional role in CT secretion in C-cells.
Similar to the in vivo findings, the long term effect of high $[Ca^{2+}]_{ex}$ led to a decline of CT release to unstimulated levels within 4 hours in vitro. This decline proved to be reversible by lowering the high $[Ca^{2+}]_{ex}$ concentration to basal for 2 hours and than increasing Ca^{2+} again (Scherübl et al., 1989a). Thus, the Ca induced desensitization of CT release was not due to an exhaustion of the secretory reserve in the observation period. These results suggest, that a reversible modification of Ca channels of the C-cells may cause the desensitization of CT release to repetitive Ca stimulation. Also long term exposure to BAY K 8644 over 4 days results in a decrease of CT secretion and CT content in rMTC 6-23 cells, while short term experiments with BAY K 8644 caused a stimulation effect over 6 hours (Mekonnen et al., 1990). The different time course of desensitization by BAY K 8644 and $[Ca^{2+}]_{ex}$ might be explained by different modifications of the voltage dependent Ca channels.
The increase of $[Ca^{2+}]_i$ is the important step in activation the Ca dependent metabolic process e.g. activation of regulatory enzymes by Ca dependent protein kinase. Activators of protein kinase C like phorbol esters are highly effective in acute releasing CT within minutes (de Bustros et al., 1985). In addition, a CT specific cytoplasmic mRNA increases within hours. An acute effect of the Ca mediated pathway by depolarizing potassium concentration on CT mRNA has been observed within 30 min., probably by a post transcription effect (Jousset et al., 1988). In contrast to the acute effect, incubation with a high ionized Ca concentration (4mM) for 72-96 hours causes a decrease in CT secretion and also a decrease in specific CT mRNA (Zeytin et al., 1987). This demonstrates that the Ca dependent pathway controls secretion and possibly the transcription of CT in a time dependent fashion in the C-cell: Acutely affecting exocytosis of stored proteins and chronicaly affecting transcription as well as synthesis of CT and perhaps sustained secretory response. A prolongation of ionomycin-stimulated secretion of CT by TPA , a phorbol ester, could be demonstrated in the TT-cell-line (Haller-Brem et al., 1988). The various agents used suggest, that the Ca-dependent secretory pathways, involve plasma membrane Ca channels, $[Ca^{2+}]_i$, calmodulin and protein kinase C.

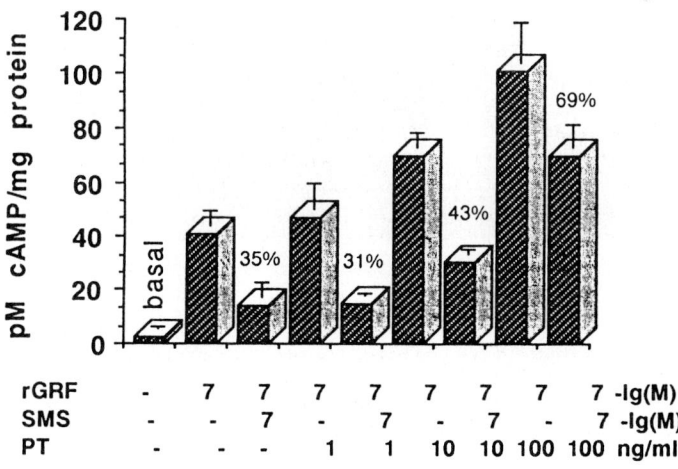

Fig.1 Effect of increasing doses of pertussis toxin (PT) on somatostatin (SMS) inhibited rat growth hormone releasing factor (rGRF) stimulated cAMP secretion in rMTC 6-23 cells.

cAMP dependent calcitonin secretion

Glucagon is one of the classical peptide hormones which acts upon the cell surface to stimulate the formation of cAMP by activation of the adenylate cyclase (AC). The effect of cAMP on cellular metabolism is mediated by protein kinase A which in turn stimulates hormon secretion (CT in rMTC-cells). This cAMP dependent CT secretion could be imitated by cAMP analogues (8-Br-cAMP, DB-cAMP) or substances like forskolin, a diterpene which enhances protein kinase A activity by stimulating the catalytic subunit of adenylate cyclase. Other protein kinase A activating substances are cholera toxin which stimulates ADP ribose transfer to the G-protein with consequent inhibition of its GTP-ase activity and prolonged activation of AC or theophyllin (or IBMX) which inhibits phosphodiesterase and the endogenous degradation of cAMP. AC and thereby CT secretion is also stimulated by catecholamines (epinephrin, norepinephrin) and other peptide hormones like GRF, VIP, gastrin, and CCK in C-cells. Hormones can exert inhibitory as well as stimulatory effect on AC. This dual control of hormone sensitive AC is mediated by specific guanyl nucleotide-binding regulatory proteins (G-proteins) in the plasma membrane, stimulatory Gs and inhibitory Gi proteins. cAMP production in rMTC cells stimulated by glucagon or rat growth hormone releasing factor (rGRF) could be dose dependently inhibited by somatostatin (SMS) and PIA, an analogue of the adenosine A1 receptor. This inhibition of AC could be partly neutralized by pertussis toxin (PT). Thus, the AC of the C-cells is controlled by a dual regulation and the inhibitory pathway involves a PT sensitive G protein (Höflich et al., 1990) (Fig.1). In parallel to inhibition or stimulation of cAMP CT secretion is inhibited or stimulated (Fig.2). SMS appears to inhibit CT release by a second, cAMP independent mechanism, as it reduces Ca stimulated CT secretion (Endo et al., 1988).

Not only secretion but also synthesis of CT is regulated by cAMP. cAMP binding to the regulatory unit of protein kinase A appears to be neccessary for activation of both secretion and synthesis. A cAMP regulatory element binding (CREB) protein as a trans-regulatoring factor has been identified (Cote et al., 1990), as well as a cis cAMP regulatory element (CRE) at the 5'flanking DNA of the CT gene. Phosphorylation of CREB protein by protein kinase A and interaction with specific cis elements 5'to the CT gene results in enhanced transcription.

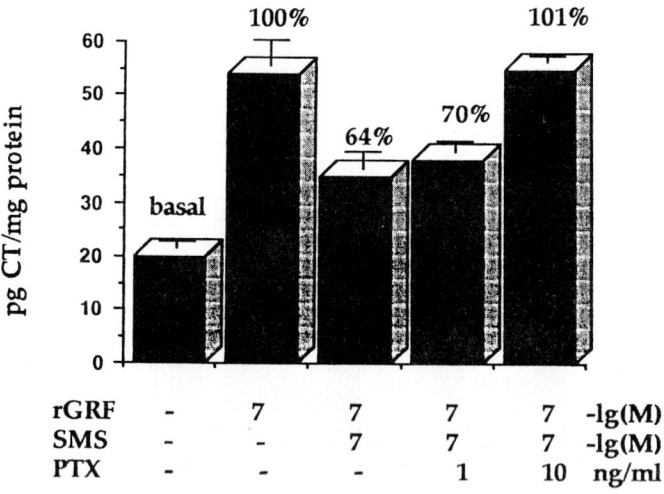

Fig.2 Effect of increasing doses of pertussis toxin (PT) on somatostatin (SMS) inhibited rat growth hormone releasing factor (rGRF) stimulated CT secretion in rMTC 6-23 cells

Interaction between calcium- und cAMP-dependent pathways

There are lots of interactions and "cross talkings" between to two main intracellular messenger systems at the different cellular levels. These interactions of effector systems are responsible for the spectrum of indiviudual target cell responses. Many hormones interact with both intracellular pathways and exert a rapid and a slow action that exerts both, acute secretion and long term growth effect via transcription. Epinephrine, for instance, acts simultaneously on cAMP and Ca dependent pathway (Fried & Tashjian, 1987). $[Ca^{2+}]_i$ has an important effect on AC activity (Scherübl et al., 1989b) and phosphorylation and controversely, the cAMP pathway acts by modulation of $[Ca^{2+}]_i$. Interaction of both pathways can result in a new signal, the oscillation: after activating the cAMP pathway by glucagon or Br-cAMP $[Ca^{2+}]_i$ started to oscillate when $[Ca^{2+}]_{ex}$ was raised in C-cells (Fig.3). These fluctuations in $[Ca^{2+}]_i$ could be stopped by chelating the $[Ca^{2+}]_{ex}$ with EGTA or by adding Ca channel blockers (Eckert et al., 1989). This points to a major role of voltage dependent Ca channels in maintaining the oscillations of $[Ca^{2+}]_i$ in C-cells. A cAMP and $[Ca^{2+}]_{ex}$ dependent mechanism at the site of the Ca channels in the plasma membrane has to be proposed. It is possible that some of the Ca-mediated responses may infact be frequency-modulated rather than amplitude-modulated.

The combination of the two secretagogues Ca and glucagon has been reported to result in higher CT release than would be expected from the sum of the effects of each stimulant alone (Aron et al., 1981). A synergistic effect of both intracellular pathways on CT secretion could be confirmed in other C-cell systems, while in rMTC 6-23 only an additive stimulatory effect was observed (Scherübl et al., 1989b). It appears that different regulatory pathways may be involved in primarily affecting exocytosis of stored proteins, whereas others may have a direct effect on exocytosis and transcription. Phorbolester, activator of protein kinase C, and cAMP have been demonstrated to increase the transcriptional rate of the CT gene by cis-regulatory elements in the 5`flanking DNA. There seemed to be several potential regulatory sequences which enhances the transcription efficiency and it is likely that cAMP transcription enhancement may occur through protein kinase C regulatory element. (Murray et al., 1988).

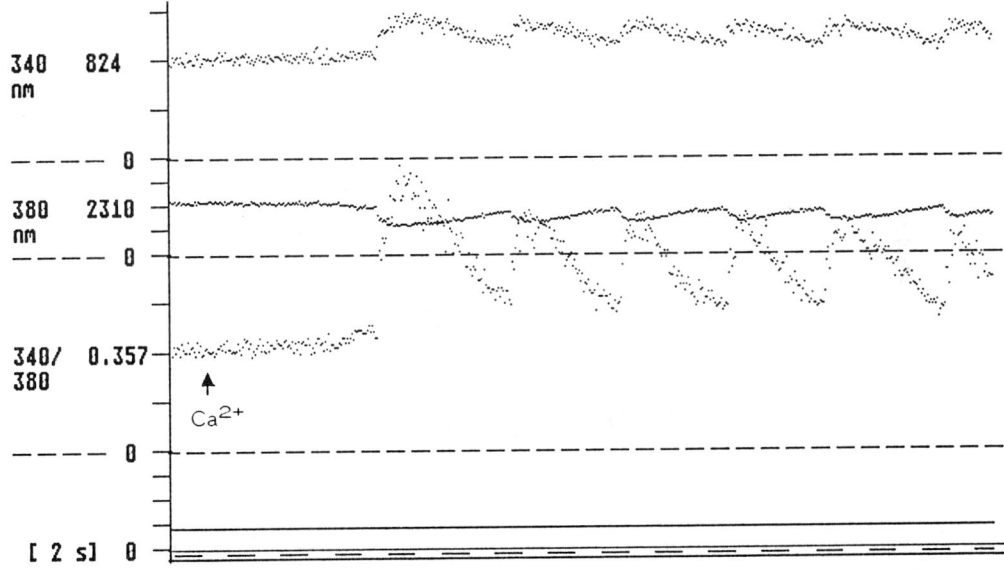

Fig.3 Action of 3 mM $[Ca^{2+}]_{ex}$ (arrow) on $[Ca^{2+}]_i$ in a single rMTC cell pretreated with glucagon. A single cell was loaded with with fura 2. The traces show relative changes in fluorescence intensity for wavelengths 340nm, 380 nm and the 340/380 ratio (Eckert et al.,1989)

Steroid hormone regulation of calcitonin synthesis and secretion

In their target tissue steroid hormones elicit specific cell responses by stimulating the expression of genes. The first step is binding to specific receptors that are present in the target cell followed by an activation of the hormone receptor complex that increases the affinity of the complex for nuclear binding sites. Estrogen and 1,25 (OH)$_2$D$_3$ receptors are well documented in C-cells (Yang et al., 1988; Freake et al., 1982). 1,25 dihydroxyvitamin D$_3$ has a negative effect on CT gene transcription: CT mRNA decreases and consequently CT content and CT secretion is reduced (Cote et al., 1987). This inhibition of transcription is specific, as the inactive analog 24, 25 (OH)$_2$D$_3$ has no effect on CT content and secretion. Dexamethasone, a synthetic glucocorticoid, has a stimulatory effect on CT gene transcription, CT content and secretion in different MTC cell lines (Cote & Gagel, 1986). It seems to be a direct regulation of CT gene expression since dexamethasone does not alter the stability of CT mRNA in the TT-cell line. Combining the agonistic effect of dexamethasone and the antagonistic effect of 1,25 (OH)$_2$D$_3$ surprisingly the stimulatory activity of dexamethasone could be abolished by 1,25 (OH)$_2$D$_3$. The explanation of this interaction might be a modulation of 1,25 (OH)$_2$D$_3$ receptor levels by glucocorticoids or interference with the action of transcriptional factors on the levels of the DNA binding sites (Lazaretti-Castro et al., 1990).

There is no direct stimulatory effect of estrogen on CT secretion in the C-cell carcinoma cell line in vitro, neither after short term (within 3 hours) nor after long term (up to 6 days) exposure. But there is a significant dose dependent increase on total cellular protein content. In contrast, a dose dependent transient inhibition of CT secretion and content with a nadir at 24 hours could be demonstrated (Raue et al., 1990). This discrepancy to the in vivo studies, which demonstrate a stimulatory effect of estrogen on CT secretion, might be best explained by the more complex environment with interfering factors due to the presence of other cell types.

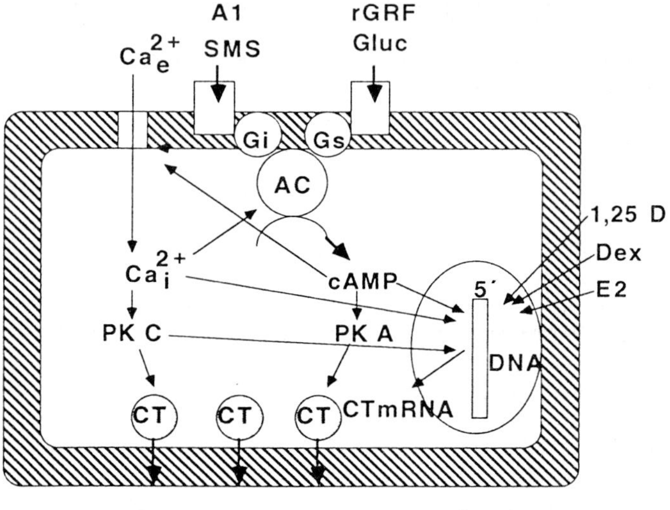

Fig. 4 Mechanism of calcitonin (CT) secretion and synthesis in C-cells.

Conclusion

Serum Ca seems to be the most important regulator of CT secretion. A very sensitive and specific system at the cell membrane is able to monitor $[Ca^{2+}]_{ex}$. A slowly inactivating Ca current appears to work as a Ca sensor by allowing transmembranous Ca influx even at normal resting potenital. Acute changes in $[Ca^{2+}]_{ex}$ are reflected in changes of cytosolic free Ca, mediating CT secretion and other cell processes. Beside this Ca dependent intracellular pathway, the cAMP mediated pathway, activated by intestinal and hypothalamic hormones and inhibited by adenosine (A1) or somatostatin, is involved in regulation of secretion and gene transcription. Interaction between the two pathways on every cellular level occurs modifying the response. 1,25 (OH)$_2$D$_3$ acts directly on gene transcription and has a negative effect on CT secretion. Two feedback relationships between the C-cells and the whole organism could be postulated: an acute rise in serum Ca is the adequate stimulus for secretion of CT which in turn normalizes serum Ca and a more prolonged interrelationship, whereby 1,25 (OH)$_2$D$_3$ inhibits CT synthesis and secretion, while CT stimulates 1,25 (OH)$_2$D$_3$ synthesis in the kidney (Jaeger et al., 1986).

References

Aron, D.C., Muszynski, M., Birnbaum, R.S., Sabo, S.W. & Roos, B.A. (1981): Somatostatin elaboration by monolayer cell cultures derived from transplantable rat medullary thyroid carcinoma synergistic stimulatory effects of glucagon and calcium. Endocrinology 109, 1830-1834.

Besnard, P., Jousset, V. & Garel, J.M. (1989): Additive effects of dexamethasone and calcium on the calcitonin mRNA level in adrenalectomized rats. FEBS Letters 258, 293-296.

Body, J.J., Struelens, M., Borkowski, A. & Mandrat, G. (1989): Effects of estrogens and calcium on calcitonin secretion in postmenopausal women. J.Clin.Endocrinol.Metab. 68, 223-226.

Cooper, C.W. & Borsky, S.A. (1986): Inhibition of secretion of rat calcitonin by calmodulin inhibitors. Calcif.Tissue Int. 38, 103-108.

Cooper, C.W., Yi, S.J. & Seitz, P.K. (1988): Inhibition by phenytoin of in vitro secretion of calcitonin from rat thyroid glands and cultured rat C-cells. J.Bone Mineral Res. 3, 219-223.

Cote, G.J., Abruzze, R.V., Lips, C.J.M. & Gagel, R.F. (1990): Transfection of calcitonin gene regulatory elements into a cell culture model of the C-Cell. J. Bone Mineral Res. 5, 165-171.

Cote, G.J. & Gagel, R.F. (1986): Dexamethasone differentially affects the levels of calcitonin and calcitonin gene-related peptide mRNA`s expressed in a human medullary thyroid carcinoma cell line. J.Biol.Chem. 261, 15524-15528.

Cote, G.J., Rodgers, D.G., Huang, E.S.C. & Gagel, R.F. (1987): The effect of 1,25-dihydroxyvitamin D_3 treatment on calcitonin and calcitonin gene-related peptide mRNA levels in cultured human thyroid C-cells. Biochem.Biophys.Res.Commun. 149, 239-243.

de Bustros, A., Baylin, S.B., Berger, C.L., Roos, A., Leony, S.S. & Nelkin, B.D. (1985): Phorbol ester increase calcitonin gene transcription and decrease c-myc mRNA levels in cultured human medullary thyroid carcinoma. J.Biol.Chem. 260, 98-104.

Deftos, L.J. & Roos, B.A. (1989): Medullary thyroid carcinoma and calcitonin gene expression. In Bone and Mineral Research 6, ed. W.A. Peck, pp. 267-316, Amsterdam: Elsevier Sci.Publ. B.V..

Eckert, R.W., Scherübl, H., Petzelt, Ch., Raue, F. & Ziegler, R. (1989): Rhythmic oscillations of cytosolic free calcium in rat C-cells. Molec.Cell.Endocrinol. 64, 267-270.

Endo, T., Saito, Uchida, T. & Onaga, T. (1988): Effects of somatostatin and serotonin on calcitonin secretion from cultured rat and parafollicular cells. Acta Endocrinol. 117, 214-218.

Freake, H.C. & McIntyre, I. (1982): Specific binding of 1,25 dihydroxycholecalciferol in human medullary thyroid carcinoma. Biochem.J. 206, 181-184.

Fried, R.M. & Tashjian, A.H. (1986): Unusual sensitivity of cytosolic free Ca^{2+} to changes in extracellular Ca^{2+} in rat C-cells. J.Biol.Chem. 261, 7669-7674.

Fried, R.M. & Tashjian, A.H. (1987): Action of rat growth hormone-releasing factor and norephinephrine on cytosolic free calcium and ionsitol trisphosphate in rat C-cells. J.Bone Mineral Res. 2, 579-585.

Haller, S., Muff, R. & Fischer, J.A. (1988): Calcitonin gene-related peptide and calcitonin secretion from a human medullary thyroid carcinoma cell line: effects of ionomycin, phorbol ester and forskolin. J.Endocr. 119, 147-152..

Haller-Brem, S., Muff, R., Petermann, J.B., Born, W., Roos, B.A. & Fischer, J.A. (1987): Role of cytosolic free calcium concentration in the secretion of calcitonin gene-related peptide and calcitonin from medullary thyroid carcinoma cells. Endocrinology 121, 1272-1277.

Hishikawa, R., Fukase, M., Takenaka, M. & Fujita, T. (1985): Effect of calcium channel agonist BAY K 8644 on calcitonin secretion from a rat C-cell line. Biochem.Biophys.Res.Com. 130: 454-459.

Höflich, M., Scherübl, H., Raue, F., Hoffmann, J. & Ziegler, R. (1990): Regulation of adenylate cyclase in rat C-cells. Acta Endocr. 122, Suppl. 1, Abstract 35.

Jaeger, P., Jones, W., Clemens, T.L. & Haystett, J.P. (1986): Evidence that calcitonin stimulates 1,25-dihydroxyvitamin D production and intestinal absorption of calcium in vivo. J.Clin.Invest. 78, 456-461.

Jousset, U., Besnard, P., Segond, N., Julliene, A. & Garel, J.M. (1988): Potassium administration and calcitonin mRNA levels in the rat. Molec.Cell.Endocr. 59, 65-169.

Lazaretti-Castro, M., Grauer, A., Raue, F. & Ziegler, R. (1990): 1,25-dihydroxyvitamin D_3 suppresses dexamethasone effects on calcitonin secretion. Molec.Cell.Endocrin. 71, R13-R18.

McDermott, M.T. & Kidd, G.S. (1987): The role of calcitonin in the development and treatment of osteoporosis. Endocrine Reviews 8, 377-390.

Mekonnen, Y., Lazaretti-Castro, M., Raue, F. & Ziegler, R. (1990): Long term exposure to the calcium channel agonist BAY K 8644 inhibits calcitonin secretion and content in a rat C-cell carcinoma cell line. J.Endocrinol.Invest. 13, Suppl. 2, Abstract P 316.

Murray, S.S., Burton, D.W. & Deftos, L.J. (1988): The effects of forskolin and calcium ionophore A 23187 on secretion and cytoplasmic RNA levels of chromogranin-A and calcitonin. J.Bone Mineral Res. 3, 447-452.

Naveh-Many, T. & Silver, J. (1988): Regulation of calcitonin gene transcription by vitamin D metabolites in vivo in the rat. J.Clin.Invest. 81, 270-273.

Raue, F., Deutschle, I., Küntzel, Ch. & Ziegler, R. (1984): Reversible diminished calcitonin secretion in the rat during chronic hypercalcemia. Endocrinology 115, 2362-2367.

Raue, F., Deutschle, I. & Ziegler, R. (1983): Acute effect of 1,25-dihydroxyvitamin D_3 on calcitonin secretion in rats. Horm.Metabol.Res. 15, 208-209.

Raue, F., Lazaretti-Castro, M., Grauer, A. & Ziegler, R. (1990): Effect of estradiol on calcitonin secretion and storage in a human C-cell carcinoma cell line. Endocrine Society, 72nd Meeting, Abstract 1432.

Raue, F., Serve, H., Grauer, A., Scherübl, H., Schneider, H.G. & Ziegler, R. (1989): Role of voltage-dependent calcium channels in secretion of calcitonin from human medullary thyroid carcinoma cells. Klin.Woschr. 67, 635-639.

Raue, F., Wieland, U., Weiler, Ch. & Ziegler, R. (1988): Enhanced calcitonin secretion in the rat after parathyroidectomy and during chronic calcium deprivation. Europ.J.Clin.Invest. 18, 284-289.

Reginster, J.Y., Deroisy, R., Albert, A., Denis, D., Lecart, M.P., Collette, J. & Franchimont, P. (1989): Relationship between whole plasma calcitonin levels, calcitonin secretory capacity, and plasma levels in estrone in healthy women and postmenopausal osteoporotics. J.Clin.Invest. 83, 1073-1077.

Scherübl, H., Raue, F., Zopf, G., Hoffmann, J. & Ziegler, R. (1989): Reversible desensitization of calcitonin secretion by repetitive stimulation with calcium. Mol.Cell.Endocrinol. 63, 263-266.

Scherübl, H., Raue, F., Zopf, G. & Ziegler, R. (1989): Calcitonin secretion and cAMP-efflux from C-cells, stimulated by glucagon and either calcium or BAY K 8644. Horm.Metab.Res., Suppl. 21, 18-21.

Scherübl, H., Schultz, G. & Hescheler, J. (1990): A slowly inactivating calcium current works as a calcium sensor in calcitonin-secreting cells. FEBS Letters, in press.

Segond, N., Legendre, B., Tahri, E.H., Besnard, P., Jullienne, A., Moukhtar, M.S. & Garel, J.M. (1985): Increased level of calcitonin mRNA after 1,25-dihydroxyvitamin D_3 injection in the rat. FEBS Letters 184, 268-272.

Seitz, P.K. & Cooper, C.W. (1989): Cosecretion of calcitonin and calcitonin gene-related peptide from cultured rat medullary thyroid C-Cells. J.Bone Mineral Res. 4, 129-134.

Tiegs, R.D., Body, J.J., Barta, J.M. & Heath III, H. (1986): Plasma calcitonin in primary hyperparathyroidism: failure of C-cell response to sustained hypercalcemia. J.Clin.Endocrinol.Metab. 63, 785-788.

Tørring, O., Bucht, E. & Sjöberg, H.E. (1985): Decreased plasma calcitonin response to a calcium clamp in primary hyperparathyroidism. Acta Endocrinol. 108, 372-376.

Yang, K., Pearson, C.E. & Samaan, N.A. (1988): Estrogen receptor and hormone responsiveness of medullary thyroid carcinoma cells in continous culture. Cancer Research 48, 2760-2763.

Zeytin, F.N., Rusk, S. & Leff, S.E. (1987): Calcium, dexamethasone, and the anticorticoid RU-486 differentially regulate neuropeptide synthesis in a rat C-cell line. Endocrinology 121, 361-370.

Relevance of the amino-terminal cleavage peptide of procalcitonin (PAS-57), calcitonin and calcitonin gene-related peptide for the diagnosis of medullary thyroid carcinoma

Walter Born and Jan A. Fischer

Research Laboratory for Calcium Metabolism, Departments of Orthopaedic Surgery and Medicine, University of Zürich, 8008 Zurich, Switzerland
Correspondence : Dr. W. Born, Research Laboratory for Calcium Metabolism, Klinik Balgrist, Forchstrasse 340, 8008 Zurich, Switzerland

INTRODUCTION

Tissue specific expression of the human calcitonin (CT)/CT gene-related peptide (CGRP) genes results in the production of CT predominantly in thyroid C-cell and of CGRP in the central and peripheral nervous system (Jonas et al., 1985; Steenbergh et al., 1986). The human CT precursor protein predicted from the CT/CGRP gene structure consists of CT, and N- and C-terminal flanking peptides abbreviated PAS-57 and PDN-21 according to Tatemoto and Mutt (1981). Similarly, the human CGRP precursor protein includes a nonidentified N-terminal flanking peptide, PAQ-55 with the amino acid sequence of PAS-57 up to residue 50, and CGRP. CT and PDN-21 have been identified in the circulation of normal subjects and of medullary thyroid carcinoma (MTC) patients where they are recognized in equimolar concentrations (Hillyard et al., 1983; Ittner et al., 1985; Roos et al., 1983) The isolation of PAS-57 from MTC tissue has confirmed the DNA-predicted amino acid sequence (Westermark et al., 1986). According to Burns et al. (1989) PAS-57 appears to be a growth factor with mitogenic activity in osteoblasts.

Normal plasma levels of CT which reaches its target organs through the circulation, have been recognized to range from 5 to 40 pgeq/ml (Body et al., 1983; Parthemore et al., 1975; Torring et al., 1985). Reported plasma concentrations of CGRP, widely accepted as a neuropeptide with a local mode of action, varied between 1 and 1000 pgeq/ml (Girgis et al., 1985; Kim et al., 1989; Mason et al., 1986; Saggese et al., 1989; Schifter et al., 1986; 1989). To this end, PAS-57 values were abnormally high in unextracted plasma of normal subjects due to nonspecific inhibition of the immunological reaction by plasma proteins (unpublished observation). Immunextraction methodology with specific antibodies to synthetic human PAS-57, CT and CGRP coupled to Affigel-10 (BioRad Laboratories, Richmond, California) was used to quantitate PAS-57, CT and CGRP in plasma of normal subjects, and to discriminate the values obtained from the raised levels measured in unextracted plasma of MTC patients.

The present study reveals that PAS-57 and CT are co-secreted in calcium dependent manner from normal thyroid C-cells, and from tumor tissue in MTC patients (Born et al., 1990).

RESULTS AND DISCUSSION

The levels of PAS-57, CT and CGRP measured after immunoextraction of serum from normal subjects before and 1.5 min after intravenous calcium infusions, are summarized in Table I. Mean plasma levels of PAS-57, CT and of CGRP were higher in normal male than female subjects, and PAS-57 and CT were increased in response to intravenous calcium. Plasma levels of PAS-57 immunoreactivity were one order of magnitude higher than those of CT. CT levels observed in the present study were similar to those reported by Parthemore et al. (1975) and Torring et al. (1985). The levels were higher than those obtained by Body and Heath (1983) using a silica-based extraction procedure.

In all 57 patients with surgically verified MTC and raised circulating CT (0.5 to 540 ngeq/ml; normal <0.05 ngeq/ml) plasma levels of PAS-57 were also increased (5 to 14'800 ngeq/ml; normal <0.7 ngeq/ml). In one MTC patient surgical removal of the MTC tumor tissue resulted in parallel falls of plasma PAS-57 and CT levels with a half life of disappearance of approximately 30 min (Raue and Blind, unpublished observation). This indicated that the circulating PAS-57 was of tumoural origin.

Interestingly, the ratio between PAS-57 and CT was 21 and 26 in male and female MTC patients, and even 1.7-fold higher than in normal subjects ($P<0.01$). PAQ-55 has not been identified so far. Due to its close structural homology with PAS-57, PAQ-55 is probably recognized by the antibodies raised to PAS-57. In view of the relatively low levels of CGRP in the circulation of normal subjects and of MTC patients it seems unlikely that large amounts of PAQ-55 derived from the CGRP precursor protein affect our PAS-57 measurements obtained in the serum of normal subjects and of MTC patients. It remains to be shown if the rate of secretion of PAS-57 is higher than that of CT and PDN-21 and/or the metabolism of PAS-57 slower than that of the other two peptides. Correlation analysis revealed that the values of PAS-57 and CT were related in MTC patients ($r=0.91$, $P<0.001$).

TABLE I. Plasma levels of PAS-57, calcitonin and CGRP in normal subjects before and 1.5 min after intravenous calcium infusions (2 mg per kilogram body weight)

	MEN (n=10)	WOMEN (n=8)
	pgeq/ml	
PAS-57		
Before	290 ± 50[*,†]	126 ± 14[†]
After iv calcium	1100 ± 240[†,‡]	325 ± 56[†,‡]
Calcitonin		
Before	27 ± 8[†]	17 ± 3.0[†]
After iv calcium	85 ± 14[†,‡]	31 ± 5.0[†,‡]
CGRP		
Before	8.4 ± 0.8[†]	5.5 ± 0.9[†]
After iv calcium	9.3 ± 1.0[†]	5.0 ± 0.8[†]

[*] Data are mean values ± SEM
[†] $P<0.05$ men vs. women
[‡] $P<0.001$, before and after intravenous calcium

CGRP was undetectable in the large majority of MTC patients when examined in unextracted plasma, and therefore presumably within the normal range (not shown). In contrast to PAS-57 and CT which was raised in response to intravenous calcium in normal sujects, CGRP levels remained unchanged. Controversial results have been obtained with respect to CGRP as a tumor marker in the plasma of MTC patients (Girgis et al., 1985; Kim et al., 1989; Mansson et al., 1990; Mason et al., 1986; Saggese et al., 1989; Schifter et al., 1986; 1989). Normal values have been reported to range between 1 pg/ml to over 1000 pg/ml, and to be elevated in some or the majority of MTC patients. The lowest concentrations in plasma of intravenously administered CGRP required to evoke cardiovascular, renal and gastrointestinal effects were approximately 40-fold higher than those recognized in the present study in normal subjects (Beglinger et al., 1988; Gnädinger et al., 1989). It seems therefore that under physiological conditions a paracrine mode of action accounts for the pronounced biological effects of CGRP, and that circulating CGRP largely represents a spillover from the nervous system. To this end, CGRP was increased 15-fold in rats after treatment with capsaicin which releases neuropeptides from sensory nerve fibres (Diez Guerra et al., 1988). The use of CGRP, however, as a tumor marker in the plasma of MTC patients appears to be rather limited.

In conclusion, the amino-terminal flanking peptide, PAS-57, is the most abundant CT/CGRP gene product in the plasma of normal subjects and of MTC patients. Much like CT, the concentrations are higher in normal male than female subjects, and the secretion is stimulated by raised extracellular calcium concentrations. PAS-57 is therefore a new sensitive marker of thyroid C cell hyperplasia and relapsing MTC.

REFERENCES

Beglinger, C., Born, W., Hildebrand, P., Ensink, J.W., Burckhardt, F. and Fischer, J.A. (1988): Calcitonin gene-related peptide I and -II and calcitonin: Distinct effects on gastric acid secretion in humans. Gastroenterology 95, 958-965.
Body, J.-J. and Heath, H. (1983): Estimates of circulating monomeric calcitonin: physiological studies in normal and thyroidectomized man. J. Clin. Endocrinol. Metab. 57, 897-903.
Born, W., Beglinger C. and Fischer J.A. (1990): Diagnostic relevance of the amino-terminal cleavage peptide of procalcitonin (PAS-57), calcitonin and calcitonin gene-related peptide in medullary thyroid carcinoma patients. Submitted for pulication.
Burns, D.M., Forstrom, J.M., Friday, K.E., Howard, G.A. and Roos, B.A. (1989): Procalcitonin's amino-terminal cleavage peptide (N-procalcitonin) is a bone cell mitogen. Proc. Natl. Acad. Sci. U S A 86, 9519-9523.
Diez Guerra, F.J., Zaidi, M., Bevis, P., MacIntyre, I. and Emson, P.C. (1988): Evidence for release of calcitonin gene-related peptide and neurokinin A from sensory nerve endings in vivo. Neurosci. 25, 839-846.
Girgis, S.I., Stevenson, J.C., Lynch, C., Self, C.H., MacDonald, D.W.R., Bevis, P.J.R., Wimalawansa, S.J. and Morris, H.R. (1985): Calcitonin gene-related peptide: potent vasodilator and major product of the calcitonin gene. Lancet ii, 14-16.
Gnädinger, M.P., Uehlinger, D.E., Weidmann, P., Sha, S.G., Muff, R., Born, W., Rascher W. and Fischer, J.A. (1989): Distinct hemodynamic and renal effects of calcitonin gene-related peptide and calcitonin in men. Amer. J. Physiol. 257, E848-E854.
Hillyard, C.J., Aberyasekera, G., Craig, R.K., Myers, C., Stevenson, J.C. and MacIntyre, I. (1983): Katacalcin: a new plasma calcium-lowering hormone. Lancet i, 846-848.

Ittner, J., Dambacher, M.A., Born, W., Ketelslegers, J.-M., Buysschaert, M., Albert, P.M., Lambert, A.E. and Fischer, J.A. (1985): Diagnostic evaluation of measurements of carboxyl-terminal flanking peptide (PDN-21) of the human calcitonin gene in human serum. J. Clin. Endocrinol. Metab. 61, 1133-1137.

Jonas, V., Lin, C.R., Kawashima, E., Semon, D., Swanson, L.W., Mermod, J.-J., Evans, R.M. and Rosenfeld, M.G. (1985): Alternative RNA processing events in human calcitonin/calcitonin gene-related peptide gene expression. Proc. Natl. Acad. Sci. U S A 82, 1994-1998.

Kim, S.H. and Morimoto, S.H. (1989): Circulating levels of calcitonin gene-related peptide in patients with medullary thyroid carcinoma. J. Clin. Chem. Clin. Biochem. 27, 423-427.

Mansson, B., Ahren, B., Nobin, A., Böttcher, G. and Sundler, F. (1990): Calcitonin, calcitonin gene-related peptide, and gastrin releasing peptide in familial thyroid medullary thyroid carcinoma. Surgery 107, 182-186.

Mason, R.T., Shulkes, A., Zajac, J.D., Fletcher, A.E., Hardy, K.J. and Martin, T.J. (1986): Basal and stimulated release of calcitonin gene-related peptide (CGRP) in patients with medullary thyroid carcinoma. Clin. Endocrinol. 25, 675-685.

Parthemore, J.G., Bronzert, D. and Deftos, L.J. (1975): The regulation of calcitonin in normal human plasma as assessed by immunoprecipitation and immuno-extraction. J. Clin. Invest. 56, 835-841.

Roos, B.A., Huber, M.B., Birnbaum, B.S., Aron, D.C., Lindall, A.W., Lips, K. and Baylin, S.B. (1983): Medullary thyroid carcinoma secrete a non-calcitonin peptide corresponding to the carboxyl-terminal region of preprocalcitonin. J. Clin. Endocrinol. Metab. 56, 802-807.

Saggese, G., Bertelloni, S., Baroncelli, G.I., Buggiani, B. and Biver, P. (1989) Variations of circulating calcitonin gene-related peptide levels during pregnancy and perinatal period, Neuroendocrinol. Lett., (1989) 103-108.

Schifter, S., Williams, E.D., Craig, R.K. and Hansen, H.H. (1986): Calcitonin gene-related peptide and calcitonin in medullary thyroid carcinoma. Clin. Endocrinol. 25, 703-710.

Schifter, S. (1989): Calcitonin gene-related peptide and calcitonin as tumor markers in MEN 2 family screening. Clin. Endocrinol. 30, 263-270.

Steenbergh, P.H., Höppener, J.W.M., Zandberg, J., Lips, C.J.M. and Jansz, H.S. (1986): Structure and expression of the human calcitonin/CGRP genes. FEBS Lett. 209, 97-103.

Tatemoto, K. and Mutt, V. (1981): Isolation and characterization of the intestinal peptide porcine PHI (PHI-27), a new member of the glucagon-secretin family. Proc. Natl. Acad. Sci. U S A 78, 6603-6607.

Torring, O., Bucht, E. and Sjoberg, H.E. (1985): Plasma calcitonin response to a calcium clamp. Influence of sex and age. Horm. metabol. Res. 17, 536-539.

Westermark, P., Wernstedt, C., Wilander, E. and Sletten, K. (1986): A novel peptide in the calcitonin gene-related peptide family as an amyloid fibril protein in the endocrine pancreas. Biochem. Biophys. Res. Commun. 140, 827-831.

ACKNOWLEDGEMENTS

This work was supported in part by the Swiss National Science Foundation by grant 3.924-0.87 and the Kanton of Zürich.

II. From C-cell to medullary thyroid carcinoma

II. De la cellule C au cancer médullaire de la thyroïde

Medullary carcinoma of the thyroid, thirty years after its discovery

Edwin D. Williams

Department of Pathology, University of Wales College of Medicine, Heath Park, Cardiff, CF4 4XN S. Wales, United Kingdom

In the 30 years since medullary carcinoma of the thyroid was established as a histopathological entity by Hazard, Hawk, Crile (1959) there have been major advances in our understanding of the pathology, the origin and the genetics of this tumour. Hazard was not the first to describe epithelial thyroid tumours which were solid, lacking papillary or follicular differentiation and which did not behave like anaplastic carcinomas. Indeed the history of recognition goes back nearly 100 years, starting with individual case reports (Burk 1901, Jacquet 1906, Stoffel,1910, Wegelin 1926). Shortly before Hazard's paper small series were reported by Horne (1951) and Laskowski (1957) who both clearly recognised some of the important pathological features of this tumour although neither recognised the frequent presence of amyloid. The delineation in 1959 of the histological appearances of the tumour, the correlation with survival, and the recognition of the amyloid occurred at about the same time as two other developments, at that time apparently unrelated.

The existence of a second type of epithelial cell in the thyroid had been a subject of argument since 1876 when Baber described "parafollicular cells" in the dog. Nonidez (1932) used silver impregnation to separate these cells from follicular cells and Getzowa (1907) and Godwin (1937) suggested that these cells were derived from the ultimo-branchial contribution to the thyroid. Interest in these cells was renewed in the early 1960s, when they were called 'light cells' by Stux et al (l961). Although some regarded them as degenerative follicular cells (Sarkar and Isler 1963, Young & Leblond 1963) most accepted that they were probably a separate cell type.

Recognition of the existence of a hypocalcaemic hormone came much later - and was at first complicated by uncertainty as to its source, with Copp (1962) initially suggesting that it was derived from the parathyroid while Hirsch et al (1963), finding activity in the thyroid, wished to introduce the name "thyrocalcitonin".

My own involvement and interest stemmed from recognising an example of this entity in man shortly after reading Hazard's paper and also from work in experimental thyroid tumours in the rat. The rat shows many cells with a clear cytoplasm in a parafollicular location which some authors suggested were degenerate follicular cells. However they appeared a distinct second cell type on routine histology and therefore a potential source of the recently discovered second thyroid hormone. It seemed likely from simple observation that the rat thyroid solid tumour - the so called gamma nodule - was derived from the para-follicular cells. It was therefore not difficult to recognise that it was likely that the human thyroid solid tumour, medullary carcinoma was derived from C cells and that it would be shown to secrete calcitonin (Williams 1966). If this tumour was derived from a different cell from other thyroid tumours it could well be linked to very different clinical features; in particular there might be a clinical syndrome associated with calcitonin over-production. I therefore set out to collect as many cases of medullary carcinoma as possible from the files of several London hospitals, to study the pathology and the clinical records. This of course required a review of the pathology of all cases of thyroid carcinoma recorded in these hospitals as medullary carcinoma had not been recognised in the past. The resulting study (Williams et al 1965, 1966), confirmed and extended Hazard's description of the tumour and its relative frequency, it also led to several new observations including the first recognition that medullary carcinoma could be inherited and that it was associated with diarrhoea (Williams 1966). The realisation that medullary carcinoma had a separate origin, and showed distinct clinical associations as well as a distinct pathological appearance and that it had commonly been mis-diagnosed in the past led to a review of some of the unusual associations of thyroid carcinoma. Sipple (1961) had drawn attention to the occurrence of a number of case reports of the coincidence of phaeochromocytoma and thyroid carcinoma without recognising that there was a genetic basis to the association, or that there was a link to a specific type of thyroid tumour. Re-reading the original case reports led to the realisation that some at least of the tumours described as follicular carcinoma might well be medullary carcinoma. The authors of the reported cases were asked to allow review of the histology, and all cases reviewed were found to be indisputably medullary carcinoma. The review together with our own study also showed that medullary carcinoma and phaeochromocytoma could be inherited together. The association of thyroid carcinoma and phaeochromocytoma was therefore re-defined as a specific association of phaeochromocytoma and medullary carcinoma which could be inherited (Williams, 1965); similar studies were carried out by Schimke and Hartmann (1965). A review of the few published cases of thyroid carcinoma and Cushing's syndrome again showed that this association was specifically with medullary carcinoma (Williams 1968). At about the same time a case reported as malignant phaeochromocytoma metastatic to the thyroid associated with so-called neurofibromatosis (Russell and Rubenstein 1963) was reviewed and found to be an example of phaeochromocytoma and medullary carcinoma of the thyroid with widespread metastases, together with facial neuromas and intestinal ganglioneuromatosis. Tracing the family of this old case showed that the father had had the same facial appearance as his daughter and had also had a thyroid carcinoma. Finding another unrelated case with exactly the same combination of neuromas of the eyelids, lips and tongue and with medullary carcinoma and bilateral phaeochromocytoma led to the recognition that this was a previously undescribed genetically determined syndrome, separate from the association of medullary carcinoma and phaeochromocytoma and separate from classical neurofibromatosis (Williams and Pollock 1966).

The recognition that MCT was an inherited tumour and that it was inherited together with phaeochromocytoma as an autosomal dominant (Williams 1967) but that the tumour did not become clinically apparent in many cases until well into adult life raised the question of what was the biological effect of the inherited gene and what further steps took place that led to tumour formation. Ljungberg (1972) and Wolff et al (1973) found that C cell hyperplasia preceded and accompanied inherited medullary carcinoma. The observation is important for the recognition of inherited cases, but is also very relevant to the pathogenesis of the tumour. Long-standing hyperplasia in endocrine glands not uncommonly leads to the development of tumours even when the cause of the hyperplasia has no direct link to the growth control of the gland concerned. This progression from hyperplasia to neoplasia in man can be clearly seen in acquired conditions such as chronic renal failure which may be associated with parathyroid hyperplasia and adenomas, and in genetically determined conditions where the defect is not directly concerned with growth control such as dyshormonogenesis of the thyroid or adrenal virilism. By analogy the genetic defect leading to hyperplasia of C cells is therefore not necessarily directly related to the subsequent tumour development, this could be the consequence of severe, prolonged hyperplasia of C cells whatever its cause.

The early pathological recognition of medullary carcinoma was based on the microscopic architecture and cytology and especially the presence of amyloid, indeed the early Mayo Clinic review referred to the tumour as "solid carcinoma with amyloid stroma" (Woolner et al 1961). It was not long before it was realised that tumours of similar morphology and behaviour might lack the amyloid. The introduction of calcitonin immunocytochemistry helped greatly in a more precise definition of the tumour and in particular led to the recognition that C cell tumours in man could on occasions show quite a wide range of histological patterns. The range may indeed be so wide that medullary carcinoma should be considered in the differential diagnosis of almost any architectural type of thyroid tumour. C cell tumours have been described as showing a papillary (Kakudo 1979) or a glandular structure (Harach & Williams 1983), other variants have been recorded including mucinous tumours (Fernandes et al 1982) and melanin containing tumours (Marcus et al 1982). An anaplastic variant has also been described (Mendelsohn et al 1980) but care must be taken to ensure that the giant cell response to amyloid is not mistaken for tumour pleomorphism.

The use of immunocytochemistry has also led to the recognition that a very small number of tumours show both C and follicular cell patterns of differentiation together with positive immunolocalisation for both calcitonin and thyroglobulin. A number of these mixed medullary/follicular carcinomas have been described, including metastatic tumours (Pfaltz et al 1983). The origin of these tumours is discussed elsewhere but it is of interest that when the thyroid gland is undescended cystic structures containing both C cells and thyroid follicles may be found adjacent to the upper parathyroid glands (Toyn et al 1989).

A 30 year perspective of the growth of our knowledge of the pathology of medullary carcinoma shows how a perceptive morphological observation in 1959 that established a new type of thyroid carcinoma (Hazard et al 1959) opened a new file for investigation that has led to the situation today, where we define the tumour by its specific peptide content, recognise a broad spectrum of pathological patterns that may mimic any other type of thyroid tumour and recognise its association with a wide range of humorally mediated and of genetically mediated syndromes. The location of the gene for the inherited medullary carcinoma syndromes has been identified (Simpson et al 1987, Matthew et al 1987) and the technique of restriction fragment length polymorphism is being used to supplement calcitonin provocation tests in the recognition of children at risk of developing medullary carcinoma..

The next 30 years will see equally significant advances in the pathology and pathogenesis of medullary carcinoma. Already in situ hybridisation is being used as a new differentiation marker; its use may extend the spectrum of medullary carcinoma still further. The recognition of the complexity of the calcitonin gene, with post translational modifications giving rise either to calcitonin gene related peptide or to calcitonin and the recognition of the presence of two calcitonin gene related peptides will give other markers for the normal, hyperplastic, and neoplastic C cell. The identification of the oncogenes involved in the transition from hyperplasia to neoplasia will coincidentally also give possible additional markers for malignancy. While there will doubtless be many other advances that cannot be foreseen, the identification of the gene that is defective in inherited medullary carcinoma, the characterisation of the mutation, the mechanism by which the mutation leads to hyperplasia and the role, if any, that the gene defect plays in the transition from hyperplasia to neoplasia in inherited cases are likely to be the major advances in the near future. These will be advances of great importance for clinical management and for our understanding of the pathology and pathogenesis of this uniquely fascinating tumour.

REFERENCES

Baber, E.C. 9 (1876) Contributions to the minute anatomy of the thyroid gland of the dog. Proc. R. Soc. Lond. (Biol) 24,240-241.

Burk,W. (1901): Uber einen Amyloidtumor mit Metastasen. Dissertation.Franz Pietzcker, Tubingen.

Copp, D.H., Cameron, E.C., Cheney, B., Davidson, A.G.F., Henze, K.G. (1962): Evidence for calcitonin: A new hormone from the parathyroid that lowers blood calcium. Endocrinology 70, 638-649.

Fernandes, B.J., Bedard Y.C., Rosen, I. (1982): Mucus-producing Medullary Cell Carcinoma of the Thyroid Gland. Am.J. Clinic. Path. 78,(4), 536-540.

Getzowa, S. (1907): Uber die Glandula parathyroidea, intrathyroideale Zell-haufen derselben und Reste des postbranchialen Korpers. Virchows Arch. Path.Anat. 188,181.

Godwin, M.C.(1937): Complex IV in the dog with special emphasis on the relation of the ultimobranchial body to interfolllicular cells in the postnatal thyroid gland. Am.J. Anat. 60, 299.

Harach, H.R., Williams, E.D. (1983): Glandular (tubular and follicular) variants of medullary carcinoma of the thyroid. Histopathology 7,83-97.

Hazard, J.B., Hawk, W.A., Crile, G.Jr. (1959): Medullary (solid) carcinoma of the thyroid: A clinicopathologic entity. J. Clin Endocrinol.Metab. 19, 152-161.

Hirsch,P.F., Gauthier, G.F., Munson, P.L. (1963): Thyroid hypocalcemic principle and recurrent laryngeal nerve injury as factors affecting the response to parathyroidectomy. Endocrinology 73, 244-252.

Horn,R.C.Jr (1951): Carcinoma of the thyroid: Description of a distinctive morphologic variant and a report of seven cases. Cancer 4,697-707.

Jacquet, J. (1906): Ein Fall von metastasierenden Amyloid-tumoren (Lymphosarcoma). Virchows Arch.Path.Anat. 185, 251-267.

Kakudo, K., Miyauchi, A., Takai, S., Katayama, S., Kuma,K., Kitamura, H. (1979): C Cell Carcinoma of the Thyroid. Acta. Path. Jap. 29, 653-659.

Laskowski, J. (1957):Carcinoma hyalinicum thyroideae. Nowotowory 7, 23-28.

Ljungberg, O. (1972): On medullary carcinoma of the thyroid: Acta. Pathol. Microbiol. Scand. (A) (Suppl) 231,1-57.

Ljungberg, O., Dymling, J.F.(1972) Pathogenesis of C-cell neoplasia in thyroid gland. C-cell proliferation in a case of chronic hypercalcaemia. Acta. Path. Microbiol. Scand. (A)80,577-588

Marcus, J.N. , Dise, C.A., Livolsi, V.A. (1982): Melanin Production in a Medullary Thyroid Carcinoma. Cancer 49, 2518-2526.

Mathew, C.G.P., Chin, K.S., Easton, D.F., et al (1987): A linked genetic marker for multiple endocrine neoplasia type 2A on chromosome 10. Nature 328,527-528.

Mendelsohn, G., Bigner, SH., Eggleston, J.C., Baylin S.B., Wells, S.A.Jr. (1980):Anaplastic variants of medullary thyroid carcinoma. Am.J.Surg.Path.4,333-341.

Nonidez, J.F. (1932): The origin of the "parafollicular" cell, a second epithelial component of the thyroid gland of the dog. Am. J. Anat. 49, 479-505.

Pfaltz, M., Hedinger, Chr.E., Muhlethaler, J.P. (1983): Mixed Medullary and Follicular Carcinoma of the Thyroid. Virchows Arch. (Pathol.Anat) 400, 53-59

Russell, D.S., Rubenstein, L.J. (1963): Pathology of tumours of the nervous system. Second Edition, London, Edward Arnold

Sarkar,SK. and Isler, H. (1963): Origin of the "Light Cells": of the Thyroid Gland. Endocrinology 73,199-204.

Schimke, R.N., Hartmann, W.H. (1965): Familial amyloid-producing medullary thyroid carcinoma and pheochromocytoma: A distinct genetic entity. Ann.Intern. Med. 63, 1027-1039.

Simpson, N.E., Kidd, K.K., Goodfellow, et al (1987): Assignment of multiple endocrine neoplasia type 2A to chromosome 10 by linkage. Nature. 328,528-530.

Sipple, J.H. (1961): The association of pheochromocytoma with carcinoma of the thyroid. Am. J. Med. 31, 163-166.

Stoffel, E. (1910): Lokales Amyloid der Schilddruse. Virchows Arch.Path. Anat. 201,245-252.

Stux, M., Thompson B, Isler H, Leblond, C.P.(1961):The "light cell" of the thyroid gland in the rat. Endocrinology 68,292-308.

Wegelin, C. (1926): "Im Handbuch der speziellen pathologischen Anatomie und Histologie", Bd.8, S.1 Berlin:Springer-Verlag.

Williams, E.D. (1965): A review of 17 cases of carcinoma of the thyroid and pheochromocytoma. J. Clin. Pathol. 18, 288-292.

Williams, E.D. (1966): Histogenesis of medullary carcinoma of the thyroid. J. Clin. Pathol. 19, 114.

Williams, E.D. (1967): Medullary Carcinoma of the Thyroid. J. Clin. Pathol. 20, 395-398.

Williams, E.D., Brown, C.L., Doniach, I. (1965): Familial Syndromes Associated with Medullary Carcinoma of the Thyroid. In:"Current Topics in Thyroid Research". Proc. 5th Int.Thy.Conf, Acad.Press. Inc. New York,1020-1022.

Williams, E.D., Brown, C.L., Doniach, I (1966): Pathological and clinical findings in a series of 67 cases of medullary carcinoma of the thyroid. J. Clin.Pathol. 19, 103-113.

Williams, E.D., Morales, A.M., Horn, R.C. (1968) Thyroid carcinoma and Cushing's syndrome. J. Clin. Pathol. 21, 129-135.

Williams, E.D., Pollock, D.J. (1966): Multiple mucosal neuromata with endocrine tumors: A syndrome allied to von Reckinghausen;s disease. J. Pathol. Bacteriol., 91, 71-80.

Williams, E.D., Toyn, C.E., Harach, H.R.(1989): The ultimobranchial gland and congential thyroid abnormalities in man. J. Path. 159,135-141.

Wolfe, H.J., Melvin, K.E.W., Cervi-Skinner, H.J, Al Saadi, A.A., Juliar, J.F., Jackson, C.E., Tashijian, A.H.Jr.(1973):"C" cell hyperplasia preceding medullary thyroid carcinoma. N. Eng. J. Med. 289,437-441.

Woolner, L.B., Beahrs, O.H., Black, B.M., McConahey, W.M., Keating, F.R. (1961): Classification and prognosis of thyroid carcinoma. Am. J. Surg. 102, 354-387.

Young, B.A. and Leblond, C.P. (1963):The Light Cell as Compared to the Follicular Cell in the Thyroid Gland of the Rat 73,669-686.

Histogenesis of medullary thyroid carcinoma

Bernard Caillou

INSERM U 66, Département d'anatomie pathologique, Institut Gustave-Roussy, 39, rue Camille-Desmoulins, 94805 Villejuif Cedex, France

The pathological entity termed "medullary thyroid carcinoma" was primarily defined on histological ground. In 1951, Horn reported seven cases. In 1959, Hazard, Hawks and Crile labelled the entity and described precisely the main morphological features of medullary carcinoma with amyloid stroma. In 1966, E.D. Williams proposed that this tumour develops from the parafollicular C cells which produce calcitonin. In the synopsis of his article E.D.Williams wrote :"It is suggested* that medullary carcinoma is derived from a parafollicular cell.....It is also concluded that the whole spectrum of clinical and pathological features of medullary carcinoma makes more sense* if it is considered as a parafollicular cell tumour". Thus, the key concept of medullary carcinoma was obtained not from experimental data but by an inductive process from a certain number of clinical and pathological facts which suggested a generic relationship between medullary carcinoma and calcitonin producing cells. The validity of such an approach was not challenged and indeed appeared obvious when, a little later, clinicians demonstrated the presence of an elevated level of calcitonin in the blood of patients suffering from medullary carcinoma (Tubiana et al.,1968)

At the same time, the C cell was at the origin of one of the most fruitful and provocative histogenetic concepts of the last decades: the APUD concept proposed by A.G.E. Pearse (1966). A little later, in a classical experimental study, Nicole Le Douarin (1970) showed, that calcitonin producing cells of neuroectodermal origin penetrate into the ultimobranchial body (UB) of the chicken. In humans, lateral UBs fuse with the median thyroid anlage. Thus, at this time and according to these views, there were two entirely different types of cells in the human thyroid gland : the epithelial follicular cell of endodermal origin and the C cell of neuroectodermal origin

At the beginning of the eighties, it was difficult to explain several findings using this theory which upheld the existence of two types of cells with a different origin.

---

* we underlined.

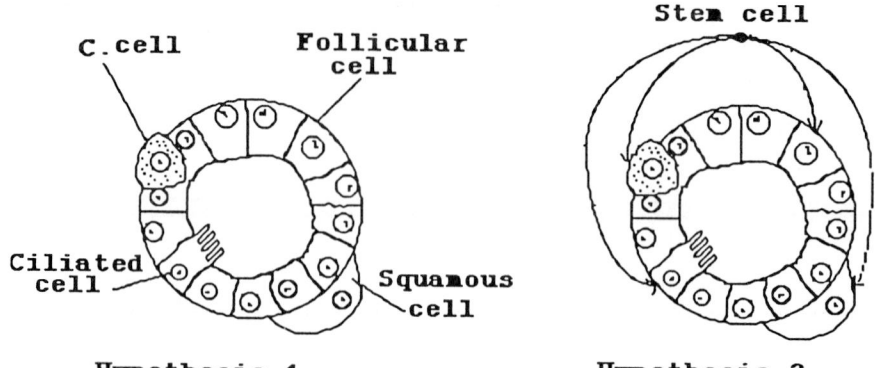

Fig. 1.

The main problem encounterd by several authors (Caillou, 1981; Hales, 1982; Ljungberg, 1983; Platz, 1983) was that of describing a tumour which associated both follicular and C cells . Moreover, neoplastic follicular and C cells were arranged according to their normal physiological pattern. Indeed, the tumour contained characteristic thyroglobulin positive thyroid follicles with calcitonin positive C cells located between two follicular cells, in the external part of the follicle, not directly in contact with the follicular lumen. These findings suggest that parafollicular and follicular proliferating cells may have a common stem cell.
In 1981, we described a thyroid carcinoma displaying a complex follicular structure associating follicular cells, C cells, ciliated cells, and squamous cells. All these cells are arranged in a similar manner to a second type of follicle in the mouse described by Wollman et al. (1969, 1971) and considered by the authors to be ultimobranchial in origin. This type of architecture was found both in the primary and metastases. To explain how all these cells originated in the same tumour we envisaged two hypotheses: i) each cell type was considered to have a different origin ; ii) all cells were thought to have a common stem cell (fig. 1). The latter hypothesis appeared to be far more satisfying and prompted us to seriously consider follicular and C cells as arising from a common stem cell.
We extended this concept to both, neoplastic and normal cells. We justified this further step by our constant attempt to choose the simplest explanation. We found it highly unlikely that the above-described differentiations could simply be explained by chance or by some kind of ectopic process resulting from malignancy. Moreover, it was possible to obtain similar conclusions from studies on non neoplastic or normal tissue (See the article of Harach in this issue).
Furthermore, it was necessary to clearly distinguish between the ultimobranchial and the germ layer origin of the follicular cell and the C cell. The ultimobranchial body is a poorly understood anatomical structure which originates from the endoderm.

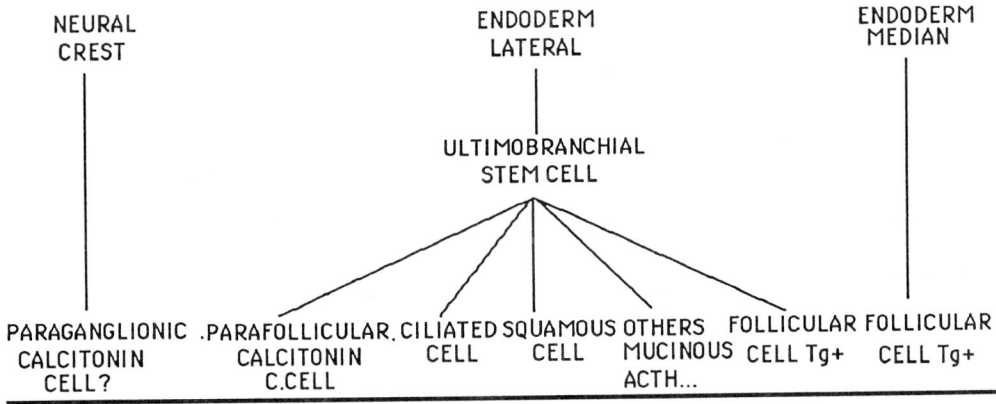

Table 1

To date, the only well recognized cells in this structure are the C cells. In fact, for a long time, some authors have stated that U.B has the capacity to form thyroid tissue with true follicular structures (Godwin,1937). From these data and from our own findings we suggested the following sequence (Caillou,1983,1984) : The endoderm is induced to form the ultimobranchial body which differentiates into follicular cells, C cells, mucinous cells, ciliated cells and squamous cells (Table 1).

There is an obvious homology of structure between the C cells in the thyroid and the enterochromaffin cell in the gut and today, there is a general consensus that enterochromaffin cells have the same endodermal stem cells as their neighbouring cells. This homology is clearly demonstrated in the primitive vertebrate, the lamprey. The corresponding thyroid follicle is opened in the mouth of its larvae whereas it.is entirely closed in the adult. If the histology of the main types of cells in the neck is compared to that of the same cell types in the abdomen (fig.2) we can see a symmetry between the neck and the abdomen provided one accepts the endodermal origin of C cells.

The paraganglionic cell has its origin in the neural crest origin (Böck 1982) and is only well recognized in certain sites as, in the abdomen, the Zuckerkandl's organ or in the neck, the carotid body. This type of cells is however far more represented than it appears to be but in a diffuse and isolated manner : the neuroendocrine complexes. The quantitative and qualitative importance of these structures have only been recently appreciated (Rode et al.,1982 Schmidt et al.,1986).In the abdomen, some neurones or paraganglonic cells synthesize the same peptides (e.g. vasointestinal peptide) as epithelial enterochromaffin cells. We suggest that some neurones or paraganglionic cells in the neck are able to synthesize calcitonin like parafollicular cells. This view is reinforced by the recent description of calcitonin producing cells located inside nervous structures in a "paraganglionic" context (Kameda 1989).

The study of Nicole Le Douarin (1971) provided experimental

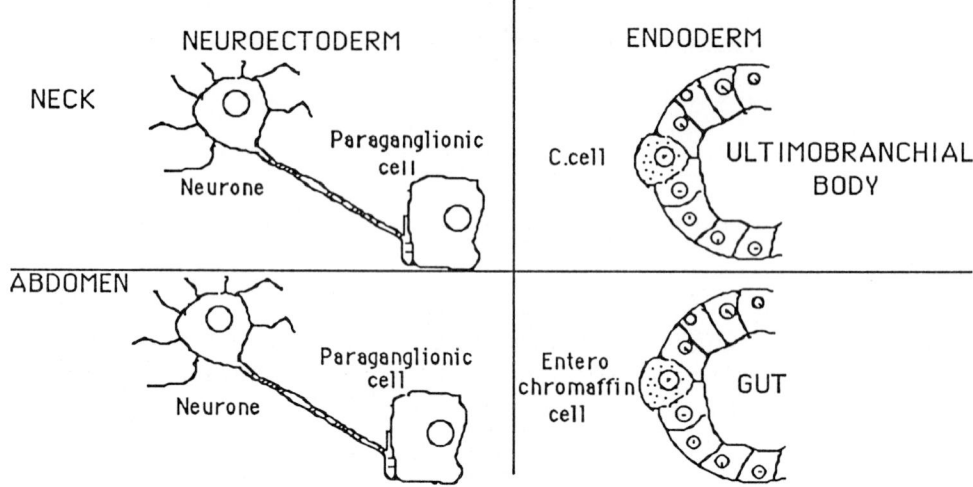

Fig.

evidence that there is a neuroectodermal cell which penetrates into the ultimobranchial body and which synthesizes calcitonin. However this study does not demonstrate that the parafollicular cell located inside the follicle is a derivative of the neural crest. We think that precise knowledge of the final topology of the cells is crucial to the elucidation of this question. In summary, we propose that there are two types of cells producing calcitonin in the neck: a paraganglionic cell of neuroectodermal origin and a parafollicular cell of endodermal origin.

Some authors have cast some doubts on the utility of these kinds of discussions. On the contrary, to accept that follicular cell and C cell have a common endodermal stem cell and as a consequence may share common genotypes and phenotypes appears to us of paramount importance both from the point of view of the clinician and the research scientist. For instance, the genetic programme of C cells is able to induce a truely follicular structure (Kameda,1981;Harach,1983). On the other hand, follicular cells which synthesize Tg can lose their usual spherical configuration and morphologically resemble medullary carcinoma.with a solid endocrinoid pattern (i.e. hyalinizing trabecular tumour). Holm et al.(1987) have in several cases of mixed follicular and medullary carcinoma indicated the presence of cells positive for both thyroglobulin and calcitonin. Today all these data have to be present in the mind of the pathologist who has the responsability of making an accurate diagnosis.

Conclusion

We suggest that the parafollicular C cell and the epithelial follicular thyroid cell could have a common endodermal stem cell. In our opinion, the whole spectrum of morphological features of medullary carcinoma makes more sense if it is considered as a tumour having the same origin as the other follicular tumours of the thyroid. We think that this approach is essential for the classification of different types of thyroid cancers and for accurate diagnoses. Moreover it seems that cytogenetists and molecular biologists should take these data into account to add arguments against or in favour of this concept.

References:

Böck, P.,(1982): The paraganglia. Handb. Mikr. Anat.VI/8 Sringer-Verlag Berlin
Caillou, B.,Calmettes, C., Talbot, M., Rougier, P., Lefevre, M.(1981) : Mise en evidence dans un cancer dela thyroide de formations vesiculaires comparables aux vesicules de type ultimobranchial decrites chez la souris. C.R. Acad.Sc.Paris. 292, 999-1004.
Caillou, B., Talbot, M., Schlumberger, M., Rougier, P., Bellet , D.Travagli, JP. (1983) :Usefulness of new methodological and conceptual approaches in thyroid carcinoma (especially in medullary carcinoma). Acta Endocrinol. Suppl. 252, 29-31.
Caillou, B., Talbot , M., Schlumberger, M., Rougier, P., Parmentier, C. (1984) : Etudes immunohistochimiques et ultrastructurales des cancers thyroidiens.Ann. Med. Int. 135, 365-368.
Caillou, B., Rougier, P., Schlumberger, M., Talbot, M., Parmentier, C. (1984) : Interet de l'immunohistochimie dans l'etude du cancer medullaire de la thyroide. Implication des resultats pour le concept de systeme "APUD" et d'"APUDOME". Bull. Cancer (Paris). 71, 2, 140-144.
Godwin, MC.(1937) : Complex IV in the dog with special emphasis on the relation of the ultimobranchial body to interfollicular cells in the post natal thyroid gland.Am. J. Anat. 60,299-339.
Hales, M., Roseneau, W., Okerlund, MD., Galante, M. (1982) : Carcinoma of the thyroid with a mixed medullary and follicular pattern. Cancer. 50,1352-1359.
Harach, HR., Williams, ED. : Glandular (tubular and follicular) variant of medullary carcinoma of the thyroid. Histopathology.7,83.
Hazard, JB., Hawk, WA. ,Crile, G.(1959) : Medullary (solid) carcinoma of the thyroid - A clinicopathologic entity.J. Clin. Endocr.Met. 19,152-161.
Holm, R., Sobrino-Simoes, M., Nesland, JM., Gould, VE., Johannessen, JV. (1987) : Medullary thyroid carcinoma with thyroglobulin immunoreactivity. A special entity ? Lab. Invest. 57, 258-268.
Horn, RC., (1951) : Carcinoma of the thyroid : description of a distinctive morphological variant and report of seven cases. Cancer 4, 697
Kameda, Y., (1982) : Immunohistochemical study of C cell follicles in dog thyroid glands.Anat. Rec. 204, 855-860.
Kameda, Y., (1989) : Occurrence of calcitonin-positive C cells within the distal vagal ganglion and the recurrent laryngeal nerve of the chicken. Anat. Rec. 224, 43-54.
Le Douarin, N., Le Lievre, C. (1970) : Demonstration de l'origine neurale des cellules a calcitonine du corps ultimobranchial chez l'embryon de poulet. C. R. Acad.Sci. (Paris).270, 2857-2860.
Ljungberg, O., Ericsson, UB.,Bondeson, L., Thorell, J.(1983) : A compound follicular parafollicular cell carcinoma of the thyroid, a new tumor entity ? Cancer 52, 1053-1061.
Pearse, AGE. (1966) : Common cytochemical properties of cells producing polypeptides hormones, with particular reference to calcitonin and thyroid C cells. Veterinary Res. 79, 587.
Pfaltz, M., Hedinger, CE., Muhtethaler, JP. (1983) : Mixed medullary and follicular carcinoma of the thyroid. Virchows arch. (Pathol.Anat.). 400, 43-59
Rode, J., Dhillon, AP., Papadaki, L., Griffiths, D.(1982) : Neurosecretory cells of the lamina propria of the appendix and their possible relationship to carcinoids. Histopathology.6, 69-79.
Schmidt, HG., Schmid, A., Lux, G.(1986): The neuro-endocrine complex NEC of the gastro intestinal tract.Gastroenterology 90, 1616A.
Tubiana, M., Milhaud, G., Coutris, G., Lacour, J , Parmentier, C., Bok, B.(1968) : Medullary carcinoma and thyrocalcitonin.Brit. Med. J. 4, 87-89.
Wetzel, BK., Wollman, SH. (1969) : Fine structure of a second kind of thyroid follicle in the C3H mouse. Endocrinology. 84, 563-570.
Williams, ED., (1966) : Histogenesis of medullary carcinoma of the thyroid. J. Clin. Path.19,114-118.
Wollman, SH., Neve, P., (1971) : Ultimobranchial follicles in the thyroid glands of rats and mice. Rec ProgHorm. Res. 27, 213-221.

Medullary carcinoma of the thyroid : a microfollicular carcinoma

Clara Sambade[1]*, Jahn M. Nesland[2], Ruth Holm[2] and Manuel Sobrinho-Simões[1]

[1] *Departments of Pathology, Medical Faculty, University of Porto, 4200 Porto, Portugal and* [2] *The Norwegian Radium Hospital and Institute for Cancer Research, 0310 Oslo, Norway*

* Author for correspondence

It has been repeatedly shown that medullary carcinomas of the thyroid (MCT) may secrete thyroglobulin together with calcitonin and other neuropeptides (cf.Holmes *et al*, 1986;1987). These findings suggest that some thyroid tumors originate from a common stem cell that could represent the precursor of both follicular and C cells (cf.Calmettes *et al*, 1982;Sobrinho-Simões *et al*, 1985).

Faced with complex cases that could not be easily categorized the pathologists have resorted to subclassifications and terms such as "trabecular thyroid carcinoma producing calcitonin" (Milhaud *et al*, 1970), "microfollicular thyroid carcinoma with amyloid rich stroma" (Valenta *et al*,1977), "glandular (tubular and follicular) variants of MCT"(Harach & Williams, 1983), "differentiated thyroid carcinoma, intermediate type" (Ljungberg *et al*, 1984) , and "mixed medullary and follicular carcinoma of the thyroid"(Hales *et al*, 1982; Pfaltz *et al*, 1983) . There is, however, no general agreement whether the descriptive terminology is actually relevant for the clinical workup of patients.

In view of the fact that follicles may indeed occur not only in follicular and papillary carcinomas but also in MCT we extended our previous electron microscopy study of MCT (Sobrinho-Simões *et al*, 1990) in order to determine the prevalence of lumina in ordinary MCT as well as the morphological features of such structures in several light microscopic variants of MCT.

MATERIAL AND METHODS

Light microscopy: Sections from formalin-fixed , paraffin-embedded specimens of 27 MCT were stained with haematoxylin and eosin, Congo and periodic acid-Schiff with and without prior diastase digestion (D-PAS and PAS, respectively). *Lectin histochemistry* was performed in 12 MCT as described previously (Sobrinho-Simões & Damjanov, 1986). Results were expressed as strongly positive (+++), positive (++), weakly positive (+), or negative (-). The data from 13 follicular and papillary carcinomas previously studied were available for comparison with the present findings. *Electron microscopy*: Fresh tumour tissue from the 27 tumours was immediately fixed in a cacodylate-buffered mixture of 4% paraformaldehyde and 1% glutaraldeyde or in a cacodylate-buffered solution of 3% glutaraldyde, or in a phosphate-buffered solution of 4% formaldehyde, post-fixed in buffered 1% osmium tetroxide, dehydrated in graded ethanols and embedded in Epon or in an Epon/Araldite mixture. From each case ultrathin sections from two to four blocks were examined under the transmission electron microscope. *Immunoelectron microscopy:* The indirect single immunogold staining method according to Varndell *et al* (1982) was employed to identify calcitonin and calcitonin-gene-related-peptide as previously described (Holm *et al*, 1989).

RESULTS

All the cases were scrutinized by *light microscopy* to determine whether they contain any follicular structures. Follicles, if found, were denoted either as empty or filled with eosinophilic diastase resistant colloid-like material. According to this approach the 27 cases were classified into three categories: a) Follicular MCT (n=4), here defined as tumors displaying abundant follicles by light microscopy. These corresponded to the so-called Tubular variant of Harach and Williams (1983). One of these MCT had areas of mucinous differentiation; b) MCT with minute rosettes and abortive follicles within a predominantly solid growth pattern (n=9); c) Solid MCT without any obvious follicular structure by light microscopy (n=14). Two of these MCT displayed signet ring cells.

Electron microscopy study disclosed microfollicles in all four follicular MCT, in all rosette-like MCT and in 12 of the 14 tumours without discernible follicular structures by light microscopy. The lumina in the latter group did not differ from those in the other two groups except in frequency and size. The three types of lumina previously described were observed: well defined glandular lumina (Figs.1,2), moderately defined glandular lumina (Fig. 3) and, finally, poorly defined lumina (Figs.1,3).

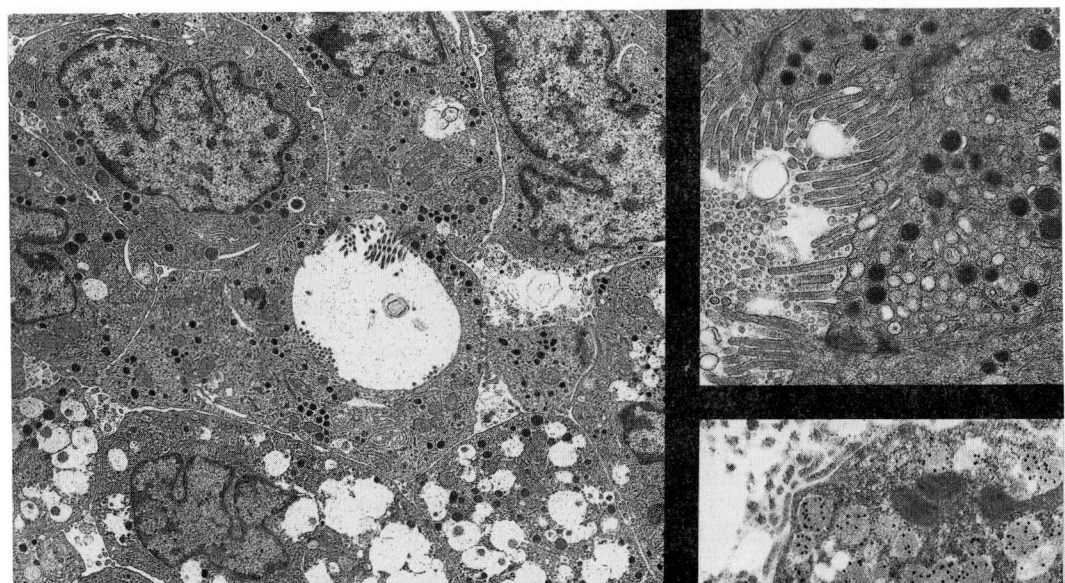

Fig.1. The cluster of neoplastic cells is centered by a well formed and two poorly formed lumina (x6160) *Upper inset.* Detail of a well formed lumen with tight junctions and numerous slender microvilli containing vesicles and granules (x13,800). *Lower inset.* Calcitonin immunoreactivity in apical, medium electron dense granules (Immunoelectron microscopy, x17,600).

Table 1 - Lectin binding to luminal content of MCT and colloid of follicular and papillary carcinomas*.

Lectin	Luminal content (n=12)	Colloid (n=13)	Lectin	Luminal content (n=12)	Colloid (n=13)
DBA	-	2/+**	RCA-II	11/+	13/+++
LAA	-	1/+	PHA-E	12/++	13/+++
LTA	-	-	PHA-L	12/++	13/+++
GSA-I	-	-	PNA	7/++	2/+++
GSA-II	-	-	SBA	6/++	7/++
HAA	4/+++	4/+++	STA***	3/+	11/++
HPA	4/+++	4/+++	SucConA	12/++	13/+++
LCA***	3/+++	13/+++	UEA-I***	3/++	9/++
MPA	5/++	13/+++	VVA	4/++	1/+++
RCA-I	10/+	13/++			

* Data on colloid of follicular and papillary carcinomas from Sobrinho-Simões & Damjanov (1986)
** Results are expressed in nº of positive cases/staining intensity
*** $p<0.05$

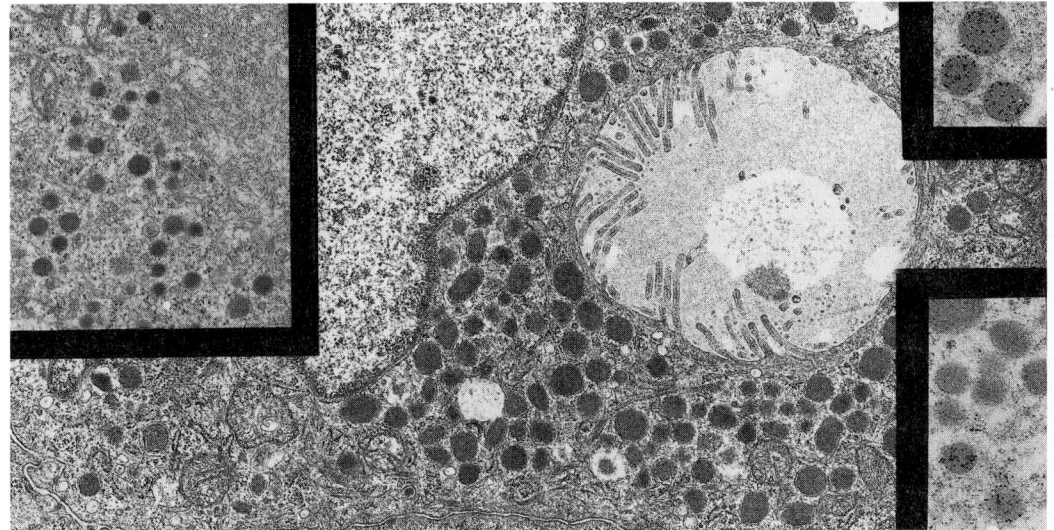

Fig. 2. Well formed glandular lumen (intercellular? intracellular?) (x13,200). *Upper right inset.* Calcitonin immunoreactivity in the three granules (Immunoelectron microscopy, x32,000). *Lower right inset.* Calcitonin-gene-related-peptide in two of several granules (Immunoelectron microscopy, x32,000). *Left inset.* No cell membrane separates the cytoplasm of the neoplastic cell and the amyloid fibrils (x17,600).

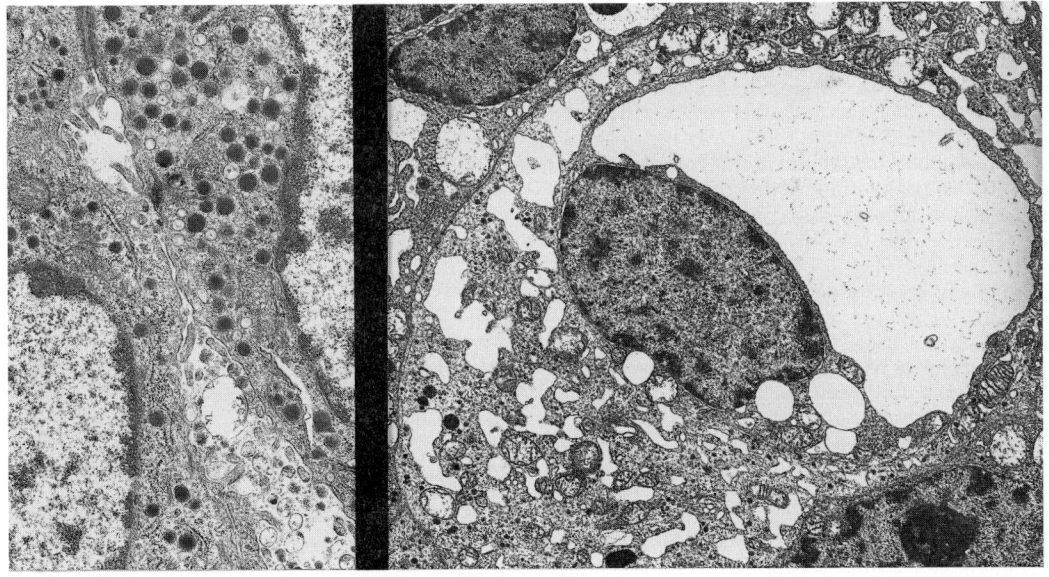

Fig. 3. *Left.* A moderately well formed lumen and a poorly formed lumen in seen between these two neoplastic cells (x13,200). *Right.* The signet ring cell appearance of this MCT cell is due to a large cytoplasmic vacuole (x6160).

61

Neurosecretory granules were accumulated in the apical parts of cytoplasm of the cells lining all three types of lumina although less conspicuously in the latter than in the two other types of lumina (Figs.1-3).The signet ring cell appearance was due to the presence of intracytoplasmic lumina or large cytoplasmic vacuoles (Fig. 3).Amyloid deposits were found in the stroma of most cases. In a few cases, however, amyloid deposits were intimately apposed to the apical pole of neoplastic cells and occasionally even without the presence of a cell membrane (Fig. 3).
Immunoelectron microscopy revealed that the apical neurosecretory granules contained calcitonin and/or calcitonin-gene-related-peptide (Figs.1,2).
The results of the *lectin histochemistry study* are summarized in Table 1 and show that the luminal content of MCT reacts with most lectins like the colloid of follicular and papillary carcinomas.

DISCUSSION
This electron microscopy study has shown follicular structures in most of MCT including the 12 out of 14 MCT (86%) displaying an exclusively solid growth pattern by light microscopy . It is therefore tempting to reinforce our previous conclusion (Sobrinho-Simões *et al*, 1990) that most if not all MCT display small lumina by electron microscopy and thus represent microfollicular carcinomas with a predominantly solid or trabecular growth pattern.
This finding shows that in thyroid tumours, as in tumours of other organs (i.e. "exocrine" and "neuroendocrine" tumors of the gut) there is no clear cut distinction between glandular and trabecular/solid growth patterns. Our data also clarify some of the controversy pertaining to some features considered "unusual" or atypical for MCT. Thus, the "trabecular thyroid carcinoma producing calcitonin" reported by Milhaud *et al* (1970) and the "MCT with atypical pattern" described by Bussolati & Monga (1979) that had ultrastructural features suggesting follicular carcinoma despite being calcitonin positive and amyloid rich, should not be regarded in this context as atypical MCT, but simply as tumors falling within the spectrum of usual MCT. Accordingly, the so-called Follicular variant of MCT should be considered as a "macrofollicular MCT".
We have shown once more the accumulation of neurosecretory granules in the apical parts of MCT cells lining follicles and demonstrated, furthermore, that these apical granules contain, regardless of their size and electron density, calcitonin and calcitonin-gene-related-peptide. The meaning of these findings has been discussed in detail elsewhere (Holm *et al*, 1989).
We have previously stressed that the high prevalence of well-developed lumina in MCT supports the assumption that an active process of secretion and/or storage of proteins, putatively linked to the biosynthesis or secretion of calcitonin and other polypeptide secretory products of C-cells, occurs in these tumours (Sobrinho-Simões *et al*, 1990)
This assumption fits with the finding of small follicles composed of C-cells in normal dog thyroids (Kameda *et al*, 1980). The cells lining these lumina are linked by tight junctions and equipped with microvilli and a colloid-like material is stored within the lumina. Kameda *et al* (1979; 1980) stressed, moreover, that C-cells, like follicular cells, not only have the ability to form follicles, but can also accumulate the secretory material into the lumina.
Alternatively, the luminal extracellular spaces of MCT just serve as sites for deposition of waste products of the synthesis and/or secretion of calcitonin. The D-PAS positive material that frequently fills the follicles and small acini of MCT has been found to be consistently and strongly positive for a large protein (MW of approximately 260×10^4 daltons - 32S), designated as C-thyroglobulin (C-Tg) by Kameda *et al* (1979). According to these authors MCT cells, as well as normal C-cells, in addition to calcitonin show distinct immunoreactivity for C-Tg. Kameda *et al* (1979) also showed that intense immunoreaction of MCT cells for C-Tg increases markedly after induced hypercalcemia, and that the appearance of C-Tg in fetal dog C-cells precedes that of calcitonin. Taking all these findings together, Kameda & Ikeda (1979) suggested that C-Tg might be a biosynthetic precursor form of calcitonin.
We have also found a striking similarity between the lectin binding to the luminal content of MCT and to the colloid of follicular and papillary carcinomas even in what concerns the absence or extreme rarity of binding sites to the lectins from *L.alpinum, G. simplicifolia (I,II), D.biflorus* and *L.tetragonolobus* (Table 1). Whether or not this resemblance points to the involvement of similar glycoproteins in the "synthesis" "storage" and/or "secretion" of both thyroglobulin and calcitonin, as previously suggested (Sobrinho-Simões *et al*, 1990)), remains to be seen.

REFERENCES

Bussolati, G. and Monga, G. (1979): Medullary carcinoma of the thyroid with atypical pattern .*Cancer* 44:1769-1777.

Calmettes, C., Caillou, B. Moukhtar,M.S., Milhaud,G., Gerard-Marchant,R. (1982): Calcitonin and carcinoembryonic antigen in poorly differentiated follicular carcinoma. *Cancer* 49:2342-2348.

Hales, M., Rosenau, W., Okerlund,M.D. and Galante,M (1982): Carcinoma of the thyroid with a mixed medullary and follicular pattern. *Cancer* 50:1352-1359.

Harach,H.R. and Williams,E.D. (1983): Glandular (tubular and follicular) variants of medullary carcinoma of the thyroid. *Histopathology* 7:83-89.

Holm,R., Ferrants,G.W., Nesland,J.M., Sobrinho-Simões, M., Jorgensen,O.G. and Johannessen,J.V. (1989): Ultrastructural and electron immunohistochemical features of medullary thyroid carcinoma. *Virchows Arch. A Pathol. Anat.414:* 375-384.

Holm, R. , Sobrinho-Simões,M. ,Nesland,J.M. and Johannessen, J.V.(1986): Concurrent production of calcitonin and thyroglobulin by the same neoplastic cells. *Ultrastruct. Pathol. 10:* 241-248.

Holm,R. , Sobrinho-Simões, M., Sambade,C., Nesland,J.M. and Johannessen, J.V. (1987): Medullary thyroid carcinoma with thyroglobulin immunoreactivity: a special entity? *Lab. Invest.* 57:258-268.

Kameda,Y., Harade,T. , Iko,K. and Ikeda,A. (1979): A immunohistochemical study of the medullary thyroid carcinoma with reference to C-thyroglobulin reaction of the tumor cells. *Cancer* 44:2071-2082.

Kameda,Y. and Ikeda,A.(1979): C cell (parafollicular cell) immunoreactive thyroglobulin: purification, identification and immunological characterization. *Histochemistry* 66:155-168.

Kameda, Y., Shigemoto,H. and Ikeda,A. (1980): Development and cytodifferentiation of C-cell complexes in the dog fetal thyroids. *Cell. Tissue Res.*206:403-415.

Ljungberg, O., Bondeson, L. and Bondeson,A.G.(1984): Differentiated thyroid carcinoma, intermediate type: a new tumor entity with features of follicular and parafollicular cell carcinoma. *Hum. Pathol.* 15:218-228.

Milhaud,G., Calmettes,C., Dreyfus,G. and Moukhtar,M.S. (1970): An unusual trabecular thyroid carcinoma producing calcitonin. *Experientia* 26:1381-1383.

Pfaltz,M. , Hedinger, C., Muhlethaler,J.P. (1983): Mixed medullary and follicular carcinoma of the thyroid . *Virchows Arch. A Pathol.Anat. 400:* 53-57.

Sobrinho-Simões,M.and Damjanov,I.(1986): Lectin histochemistry of papillary and follicular carcinoma of the thyroid gland. *Arch.Pathol. Lab. Med.* 110:722-729.

Sobrinho-Simões,M. , M., Nesland,J.M. and Johannessen, J.V.(1985): Farewell to the dual histogenesis of thyroid tumors. *Ultrastruct. Pathol.* 8(2-3):iii-v.

Sobrinho-Simões,M., Sambade, C.,Nesland,J.M., Holm,R. and Damjanov,I. (1990): Lectin histochemistry and ultrastructure of medullary carcinoma of the thyroid gland. *Arch.Pathol.Lab.Med. 114:* 369-375.

Valenta,L.J., Michel-Bechet,M., Mattson,J.C. and Singer,F.R.,(1977): Microfollicular thyroid carcinoma with amyloid rich stroma, resembling medullary carcinoma of the thyroid (MCT). *Cancer* 39:1573-1586.

Varndell,I.M., Tapia,F.J., De Rey,J., Rush,R.A., Bloom, S.R., Polak,J.M. (1982): Electron immunocytochemical localization of enkephalin-like material in catecholamine-containing cells of the carotid body, the adrenal medulla, and pheochromocytomas of man and other mammals. *J. Histochem. Cytochem.* 30:682-690.

De la cellule C au CMT. Les cancers thyroïdiens à sécrétions peptidiques

André Pages* and Brigitte Franc

* Service Central d'Anatomie Pathologique, CHR Saint-Eloi-Gui de Chauliac, 34059 Montpellier Cedex, France

SUMMARY
Results of systematic immunostaining in thyroid tumors pointed out several questions and disturbed some assessments.
Are we allowed to call MTC tumors morphologically identical but without calcitonin ? Follicular carcinomas with secreting peptides are they similar to the mixt form of MTC. Several hypothesis are discussed without any determinant argument against a neuroectodermic origin for C cells.

L'utilisation des techniques immuno-cytochimiques dans l'étude des cancers de la thyroïde a suscité de nouvelles interrogations et remis en question certaines notions qui semblaient définitivement acquises. Nous allons tenter d'en rapporter brièvement l'analyse.

. **Les cancers médullaires de la thyroïde (C.M.T.) sans calcitonine :**
Lors de la réunion de San-Miniato (1984), le problème de l'absence de calcitonine dans une tumeur de morphologie médullaire a été abordé (Albores-Saavedra et al). Même dans une tumeur peu différenciée, un tel diagnostic peut être accepté, s'il existe un contexte de maladie familiale ou une hyperplasie à cellules C. Dans les autres cas, il convient d'être plus prudent, même si la quantité de calcitonine intra tumorale peut être trop faible pour être détectée, ou trop rapidement dégradée ou excrétée. Plusieurs séries de la littérature ont rapporté des cas sans calcitonine, mais renfermant d'autres peptides comme le C.G.R.P., l'A.C.T.H, la neurotensine, la somatostatine, la sérotonine, la chromogranine etc... Il s'agissait de tumeurs à type de C.M.T. classique ou au contraire plus indifférenciées (Eusébi et al 1990, Garcia et al 1990, Nakamura et al 1987, Uribe et al 1985). La mise en culture de l'une d'entre elles n'a pas montré de sécrétion de calcitonine (Nakamura et al 1987). Les substances produites étaient analogues à celles retrouvées en dehors de la calcitonine dans de nombreux C.M.T et certaines cellules C à l'état normal. Ces substances sont aussi produites par d'autres éléments du Systéme Endocrinien Diffus. On peut voir coexister au sein d'une même lésion des sécrétions peptidiques variées. Ces tumeurs sont-elles développées à partir des cellules C usuelles ou d'un autre contingent plus minoritaire, qui à l'état normal élabore d'autres hormones ? Faut-il classer ces carcinomes sans sécrétion de calcitonine parmi les C.M.T.? Dans l'affirmative, doit-on faire une enquête familiale et une recherche de polyoncose endocrinienne ? de quel type ?
A la première question, on peut répondre que le terme de C.M.T. ne possédait pas la signification sécrétoire qu'il a acquise par la suite. Il constitue au niveau de la thyroïde le groupe des tumeurs développées aux dépens du contingent cellulaire para-folliculaire. Il suffirait d'en distinguer les différentes variétés par leur sécrétion, comme cela a été fait dans la nomenclature des tumeurs du pancréas endocrine ou du S.E.D par l'O.M.S. Quant à la suite à donner à la découverte de telles tumeurs sans calcitonine, il est malaisé de l'envisager. Cependant, de même qu'au niveau des tumeurs du reste du S.E.D, le champ des pathologies associées à explorer est peut-être plus large que celui des N.E.M de type II, et englobe les N.E.M de type I et les neurofibromatoses (Duhq et al 1987).

. Comment nommer les tumeurs de souche vésiculaire (quelles que soient leurs morphologies) qui comportent des sécrétions peptidiques analogues à celles rencontrées dans les CMT ou équivalents ?
Deux situations doivent être envisagées. Dans la première, il ne s'agit pas d'une sécrétion des cellules tumorales mais de l'incorporation au sein de la tumeur de cellules C résiduelles, parfois hyperplasiques, que la tumeur n'a pas encore détruites. Les cellules C apparaissent en effet assez résistantes, puisque l'on peut les retrouver sur du matériel autopsique dans des thyroïdes entièrement détruites par de la fibrose. Dans la seconde, il existe d'indéniables sécrétions peptidiques dans les différentes formes de tumeurs de souche vésiculaire. La présence de cellules endocrines a été rapportée dans plusieurs types de tumeurs épithéliales non endocrines. Comme la thyroïde, elles sont de souche endodermique (poumon, estomac, pancréas, prostate), ou mésodermique (endomètre, ovaire...). Différentes hypothèses ont tenté de l'expliquer. Nous en discuterons deux.
La première vient d'être magistralement résumée par Wright (1990). Il semble que dans les tumeurs endodermiques une même cellule souche puisse se différencier dans plusieurs directions et produire des cellules endocrines, qui peuvent être prédominantes. Elles donnent alors naissance à des tumeurs de type carcinoïde. Dans les tumeurs digestives, certains auteurs ont tenté de démontrer (Auböck et al 1983) qu'elles pouvaient provenir d'autres systèmes cellulaires. Ont ainsi été décrites dans l'appendice (Auböck et al 1983) des cellules endocrines extra-épitheliales intra-neurales. De telles distinctions sont-elles possibles dans les tumeurs thyroïdiennes de souche vésiculaire ? Existe-t-il dans le tissu thyroïdien des dispositifs analogues à ceux décrits dans l'appendice ? Les tumeurs dont nous venons de parler constituent un groupe morphologique très hétérogène, que Ljungberg (1984) a proposé de classer en carcinomes intermédiaires. Cette solution d'attente est probablement un peu simplificatrice, et mélange certains carcinomes insulaires (Carcangiu et al 1984), très carcinoïdes d'aspect, à des tumeurs sans rapport manifeste (Lebodic et al 1989, Ljungberg et al 1984). Quant aux dispositifs endocrines intra-neuraux, ils n'ont jamais été formellement démontrés. Nous avons cependant observé très récemment dans la thyroïde d'un embryon de 3,5 mois des terminaisons nerveuses en contact étroit avec une cellule à calcitonine et, au contact d'un micro-cancer médullaire, des cellules à calcitonine dans des filets nerveux juxta-tumoraux. Comment expliquer de surcroît la production de thyroglobuline par ces tumeurs ? Ce sont, avec les goîtres ovariens, les seules tumeurs ayant cette double aptitude.

. Faut-il assimiler ces tumeurs à double composante à la variante dite mixte des C.M.T. ?
Lors de l'embryogenèse de la thyroïde, on assiste à la fusion entre une ébauche médiane impaire, venant du canal thyréoglosse, et une ébauche paire latérale, venant des corps ultimo-branchiaux (C.U.B.). Ces premiers constituants sont identiques et se présentent comme des canaux à épithélium cylindrique cilié et mucipare émanant de l'entoderme pharyngien. Depuis 1970, Mesdames Le Douarin et Lelièvre ont démontré l'origine neurale des cellules à calcitonine du C.U.B de l'embryon de poulet. Aucun autre travail n'a réfuté cette hypothèse. Il faut donc admettre que les C.U.B colonisés par ces cellules les transporteront dans la thyroïde lors de leur fusion. L'étude de 41 dysgénèses thyroïdiennes, par Williams et al. en 1989, a permis de constater que lorsqu'il existe un trouble de migration de l'ébauche médiane, les C.U.B. ne peuvent fusionner et donnent naissance à des éléments vestigiaux et à des formations cellulaires marquées par la calcitonine et le C.G.R.P., et dans un cas à des follicules thyroïdiens marqués par la thyroglobuline. Ainsi est démontré que le C.U.B participe pour une petite partie à la formation de la thyroïde. Nous avons pu examiner au sein de la thyroïde d'un embryon de 3,5 mois un C.U.B comportant un revêtement de type cilié en métaplasie pavimenteuse partielle. L'immunomarquage par l'A.C.E. et la calcitonine a permis de constater que certaines formations pleines, situées un peu à distance, étaient marquées très positivement par l'A.C.E., de même que cette formation ciliée et pavimenteuse. A l'inverse, les cellules à calcitonine étaient peu nombreuses, dispersées dans les mêmes territoires autour de quelques vésicules thyroïdiennes. Une seule cellule à calcitonine était présente en périphérie de la formation en métaplasie pavimenteuse. Le contingent A.C.E. positif était beaucoup plus important que les cellules à calcitonine. Représente-t-il des cellules interfolliculaires précurseurs ? Elles seraient véhiculées par le C.U.B dans l'ébauche thyroïdienne d'où elles se répandraient en exprimant ensuite de la calcitonine. D'où viennent les cellules qui ont colonisé les C.U.B.? Mérida-Velasco et al. (1989), étudiant des embryons humains aux stades 14 et 15 d'O'Rahilly, montrent que les C.U.B dérivent de la 5ème poche entodermique. Ils sont colonisés au stade 14 par des cellules qui viennent de la partie la plus caudale de la placode épibranchiale. Dans le même temps, Kaméda (1990) démontre chez le poulet la présence de cellules C dans les fibres du nerf laryngé récurrent et dans le ganglion vagal distal. Elles ne sont retrouvées que si ces 2 structures sont en relation étroite avec le

C.U.B. Ces cellules, intitulées par l'auteur "vagal paraganglionic cell", synthétisent et sécrètent de la calcitonine ; elles ne sont pas chémoréceptrices. Ces travaux ne permettent ni d'exclure ni d'affirmer l'origine neuroectodermique des cellules C. Les rapports entre crête neurale et placode sont très étroits, tant par leur topographie que du point de vue induction et fonction (Weston 1970). Dans l'observation de Mme Patey, présentée ce matin, le C.U.B. en position extra-thyroïdienne, sans migration homolatérale de cellules C intra-thyroïdienne, est accompagné de cartilage. La participation à ces ébauches du mésenchyme céphalique doit être envisagée, en particulier celui du "squelette" des arcs branchiaux. Il s'agit du mésectoderme. Fontaine (1979), chez la souris, avait signalé des pré-cellules C dans la composante mésenchymateuse du 4ème arc branchial jusqu'au stade à 28 somites.

- La colonisation du C.U.B. par des cellules venant de la crête neurale ou de placodes constitue un faisceau d'arguments en faveur du caractère mixte des C.U.B. S'il en est ainsi, les néoformations comportant des cellules C et des cellules folliculaires sont authentiquement mixtes ou, comme le suggérait Wright (1990), des hybridomes. Suivant les situations, la cellule hybridante serait, soit une cellule C soit une cellule vésiculaire.

BIBLIOGRAPHIE

ALBORES-SAAVEDRA J, LIVOLSI V.A, WILLIAMS E.D. Medullary carcinoma.
Sem in Diagn Path, 1985, 2, 2, 137-146
AUBOCK L, HOFLER H. Extra epithelial intraneural endocrine cells as standing-points for gastro-intestinal carcinoids.
Virch Arch (Pathol Anat), 1983, 401, 17-33
CARCANGIU M.L, ZAMPI G, ROSAI J. Poorly differentiated ("insular") thyroid carcinoma.
Am J Surg Pathol, 1984, 8, 655-668
DUHQ Y, HYBARGER C.P, GEIST R, GAMSU G, GOODMAN Ph.C, GOODING G.A.W, CLARK O. Carcinoids associated with multiple endocrine neoplasia syndromes.
Am J Surg, 1987, 154, 142-148
EUSEBI V, DAMIANI S, RIVA C, LLOYD R.V, CAPELLA C. Calcitonin free oat-cell carcinoma of the thyroid gland.
Virch Arch A (Pathol Anat) 1990, 417, 267-271
FONTAINE J. Multistep migration of calcitonin cell precursors during ontogeny of the mouse pharynx.
Gen Compar Endocr, 1979, 37, 81-92
GARCIA A, MARTIN F, GARCIA C.F, CAVANZO F.J. Medullary carcinoma of the thyroid in Colombia : an immunohistochemical and clinicopathological study of 26 cases.
Surg Pathol, 1990, 3, 19-29
KAMEDA Y. Occurence of calcitonin. Positive C cells within the distal vagal ganglion and the recurrent laryngeal nerve of the chicken.
The Anat Rec, 1989, 224, 43-54
LEBODIC M.F, AILLET G, FICHE M, CHOMARAT H, CHARBONNEL B, VISSET J. Les carcinomes "mixtes" (vésiculaires et paravésiculaires) de la thyroïde. Etude histologique et immunocytochimique de 5 cas.
Ann Pathol 1989, 9, 1, 38-43
LE DOUARIN N, LE LIEVRE Ch. Démonstration de l'origine neurale des cellules à calcitonine du corps ultimo-branchial chez l'embryon de poulet.
C.H.Hebd. Scanc. Acad. Sci. Paris, 1970, 270, 2857-2860
LJUNGBERG O, BONDESON L, BONDESON A.G. Differentiated thyroid carcinoma, intermediate type : a new tumor entity with features of follicular and parafollicular cell carcinoma.
Hum Pathol, 1984, 15, 218-228
MERIDA-VELASCO J.A, GARCIA-GARCIA J.D, ESPIN-FERRA J, LINARES J. Origin of the ultimobranchial body and its colonizing cells in human embryos.
Acta Anat, 1989, 136, 325-330
NAKAMURA A, KAKUDO K, WATANABE K. Establishment of a new human thyroid medullary carcinoma cell line. Morphological studies.
Virchows Arch B, 1987, 53, 332-335

URIBE M, BRIMES M, FENOGLIO-PREISER C.M, FEIND C. Medullary carcinoma of the thyroid gland.
Am J Surg Pathol, 1985, 9, 8, 577-594
WESTON J.E. The migration and differenciation of neural crest cells.
Advances in Morphogenesis, VIII, 1970
WILLIAMS E.D, BROWN C.L, DONIACH I. Pathological and clinical findings in a serie of 67 cases of medullary carcinoma of the thyroid.
J Clin Pathol, 1966, 19, 103-113
WILLIAMS E.D, TOYN C.E, HARACH H.R. The ultimobranchial gland and congenital thyroid abnormalities in man.
J of Path, 1989, 159, 135-141
WRIGHT N.A. Endocrine cells in non endocrine tumours.
J of Pathol, 1990, 161, 85-87.

RESUME

Les résultats de l'immunomarquage systématique des tumeurs thyroïdiennes posent plus de questions qu'ils ne peuvent en résoudre.
Comment classer les carcinomes de morphologie médullaire de la thyroïde sans calcitonine ? Doit-on considérer les carcinomes vésiculaires à sécrétions péptidiques comme analogues aux variantes mixtes des CMT ? Plusieurs hypothèses sont discutées. Il n'existe pas d'argument décisif contre une origine neuroectodermique des cellules C.

III. Diagnostic means of the disease
III. Les méthodes de diagnostic de la maladie

Biochemical factors

Facteurs biochimiques

Calcitonine et ACE pour le dépistage et le suivi des CMT

Denis Guilloteau[1] and D. Bellet[2]

[1] INSERM U 316 et Laboratoire de Biophysique Médicale et Pharmaceutique, UFR Tours, 3702 Tours Cedex, France.
[2] Laboratoire d'Immunologie, Institut Gustave-Roussy, 94805 Villejuif Cedex, France

ABSTRACT

C cells secrete physiological calcitonin and CEA. CEA is a non specific marker of MTC, but is informative on the pronostic. Calcitonin is the specific marker of MTC. Assays of calcitonin may be performed by RIA or IRMA. Large difference exists between calcitonin level measured by RIA and IRMA. Both of these methods are efficiency for MTC (original or recurrent tumor) diagnoses. But IRMA provides a greater sensitivity to pentagastrine test and a better indentification of microcarcinoma in hereditary cases of MTC.

Les rôles d'un marqueur tumoral sont de signer la présence d'une tumeur, de permettre le dépistage des sujets atteints dans une population à risque, de permettre de faire le bilan et le suivi thérapeutique d'un cancer diagnostiqué. Dans le cas du cancer médullaire de la thyroïde (CMT) deux marqueurs sont classiquement utilisés : la calcitonine et l'ACE. Quelles sont les informations apportées par chacun de ces traceurs ? Comment et quand doit-on réaliser ces examens biologiques ? Que peuvent-ils apporter, en particulier au niveau du dépistage des formes familiales ? Nous allons tenter d'apporter des éléments de réponse en tenant compte de l'évolution technologique des méthodes de dosage.

I- LES MARQUEURS

La calcitonine

La calcitonine est un peptide de 32 acides aminés, dont la biosynthèse s'effectue essentiellement au niveau des cellules C de la thyroïde. Elle est sécrétée physiologiquement en dehors de toute pathologie tumorale, elle joue un rôle au niveau de l'équilibre phosphocalcique (Austin *et al.*, 1981) et probablement au niveau du système nerveux central, en effet des récepteurs spécifiques ont pu être mis en évidence au niveau cérébral. Il existe aussi une sécrétion de calcitonine extrathyroïdienne : des taux de calcitonine non négligeables ont été retrouvés chez des patients thyroïdectomisés (Silva *et al.*, 1973, Body *et al.*, 1983) et une immunoréactivité a pu être détectée au niveau de certains tissus et organes (hypophyse, poumons, thymus) (Austin *et al.*, 1981). Au niveau des cellules, la calcitonine est stockée dans des granules et libérée par des phénomènes d'exocytose. Les mécanismes de cette exocytose ne sont pas complètement élucidés : rôle du calcium ? rôle des agents sécrétagogues comme la pentagastrine ? existe-t-il des agents capable de freiner cette libération ?

La mise en évidence d'une importante sécrétion de calcitonine associée au CMT date de 1968 (Milhaud *et al.*, 1968, Cunliffe *et al*.,1968). La calcitonine, sécrétée normalement par des cellules C, va pouvoir être utilisée comme marqueur des tumeurs dérivées de ces cellules C et en particulier du cancer médullaire de la thyroïde.

Sur le plan structural la calcitonine n'est pas homogène, en effet, les dosages radioimmunologiques ont mis en évidence une grande hétérogénité des formes circulantes. Après étude chromatographique, il a été retrouvé des formes de poids moléculaires très supérieurs à celui des monomères, de l'ordre de 60 KD. Ces formes correspondent vraisemblablement à des précurseurs de la calcitonine (Dermody *et al.*, 1981). Au niveau des dosages ces différentes formes vont poser problème car elles seront reconnues de manière différente en fonction de la spécificité des anticorps utilisés.

L'ACE

L'antigène carcinoembryonnaire (ACE) décrit par Gold *et al.*, 1965), est une glycoprotéine associée aux membranes. Cet antigène est présent dans les cellules C normales (Kodama *et al.*,1983). L'ACE n'est pas spécifique du CMT, on le retrouve sécrété par d'autres tumeurs au niveau du colon en particulier. De plus les taux d'ACE peuvent être aussi légèrement élevés en dehors de toute pathologie comme chez le fumeur par exemple (Mériadec *et al.*, 1976).

En conclusion, la calcitonine est le marqueur spécifique du CMT, l'ACE est un marqueur aspécifique, cependant chacun aura son propre intérêt, nous allons tenter de déterminer la valeur qu'il faut accorder à ces deux marqueurs d'une part au niveau du diagnostic et du suivi et d'autre part du pronostic.

II- DOSAGES DES MARQUEURS DU CMT

La calcitonine

1) Dosage biologique

Le premier dosage décrit fut un dosage biologique basé sur l'effet hypocalcémiant de la calcitonine. Il est possible de mettre en évidence une relation entre la baisse de la calcémie chez le jeune rat et la quantité de calcitonine injectée (Kumar *et al.*, 1965). Ce dosage qui a le mérite d'avoir permis la mise en évidence de la sécrétion de calcitonine par le CMT (Milhaud, *et al.*,1968) est difficile à mettre en oeuvre et manque de sensibilité. Il n'est donc pas utilisable pour le suivi et le dépistage des CMT.

2) Le dosage radioimmunologique

Ce dosage est basé sur le principe de la compétition entre la calcitonine à doser et la calcitonine radiomarquée vis-à-vis d'un anticorps spécifique. De nombreux systèmes ont été décrits depuis 1969 (Clark *et al.*, 1969). Malgré les progrès apportés à cette technologie un certain nombre de problèmes persistent avec l'utilisation de ces différents immunodosages.

Le problème de sensibilité : les taux de calcitonine de quelques dizaines de picogrammes sont difficiles à détecter, ce qui pose un problème au niveau du dépistage des formes familiales. Différentes procédures ont été proposées pour améliorer cette sensibilité : - Une monoextraction de la calcitonine avant dosage, mais c'est une technique lourde et dont la reproductibilité est difficile à contrôler (Body *et al.*, 1983). - Une incubation séquentielle des différents réactifs. C'est une technique longue, pouvant prendre quelques jours mais utilisable en biologie clinique, les quantités minimum détectables sont de l'ordre de 100 pg/ml (Calmette *et al.*, 1986).

<u>Problème de spécificité des anticorps</u> : la variabilité de spécificité des anticorps polyclonaux utilisés dans les différents systèmes d'une part et l'hétérogénéité des formes circulantes de calcitonine d'autre part rendent très complexes l'interprétation et la comparaison des résultats d'un laboratoire à un autre. Avant toute interprétation il faudra donc parfaitement connaître la spécificité des anticorps utilisés et les valeurs de la population de référence.

3) <u>Dosage immunoradiométrique</u>

Ce dosage est basé sur l'utilisation de deux anticorps monoclonaux, l'un fixé sur une phase solide servant à l'immunoextraction, l'autre radiomarqué permettant la révélation et la quantification de l'antigène (calcitonine). Le premier dosage de ce type a été décrit par Motte *et al.*, 1988.

Les avantages d'un tel système sur un système RIA classique sont :
- la parfaite connaissance de l'analyte, le monomère de calcitonine dans le cas présent.
- la meilleure sensibilité (limite de détection de l'ordre de 5 pg/ml).

Il est fondamental de comparer et de discuter les résultats obtenus avec cette nouvelle technologie avec ceux obtenus avec les RIA classiques et de définir les nouvelles règles d'interprétation.

L'ACE

Il est dosé par méthode immunoradiométrique classique utilisant deux anticorps monoclonaux.

III- TEST DE STIMULATION

L'ACE est une substance dont la sécrétion ne semble pas sous l'influence d'agent sécrétagogue, donc seul son taux de base sera déterminé.

En revanche la calcitonine qui est stockée au niveau de granules peut être libérée sous l'action d'agents sécrétagogues, il va donc être possible de déterminer soit son taux de base, soit son taux après stimulation. Différents agents sécrétagogues ont été proposés et utilisés : le calcium, l'alcool et la pentagastrine. L'alcool induit des réponses faibles et inconstantes. L'injection de calcium et de pentagastrine sont deux épreuves de stimulation efficaces. Le test à la pentagastrine (*) donne les réponses des plus importantes. Il a l'avantage d'être rapide, mais peut engendrer des sécrétions désagréables transitoires. Il est le test conseillé pour le suivi et le dépistage (Milhaud *et al.*,1975).

IV- RESULTATS

1) <u>Population de référence</u> : Les taux de base de calcitonine et d'ACE ainsi que les taux de calcitonine après stimulation ont été déterminés chez une population de référence.

Taux de base de l'ACE :
Dans une population de référence, les taux de base d'ACE sont inférieurs à 6 ng/ml.

---

*) Protocole test à la pentagastrine :
  Petavlon, 5 µg/kg de poids, injecter en 3 minutes, prélèvement au temps -10, -0, 3, 5, 10, 11.

Taux de base de la calcitonine :
Les résultats sont fonction de la méthodologie utilisée RIA ou IRMA (ELSA-hCT Cis Bioindustries) et de la spécificité des anticorps. Les valeurs obtenues avec trois méthodes RIA différentes sont les suivantes: 95 pour cent des sujets ont un taux inférieur à 250 pg/ml avec deux des méthodes et inférieur à 160 pg/ml avec la troisième. Avec la méthode IRMA, utilisant deux anticorps monoclonaux l'un dirigé contre la séquence 11-17 et l'autre contre la séquence 24-32, les valeurs de référence sont inférieures à 10 pg/ml (tableau 1). Les taux de base plus bas chez les sujets normaux avec la méthode IRMA s'expliquent par le fait que ce dosage ne reconnaît qu'une seule forme de calcitonine : le monomère, contrairement aux méthodes RIA utilisant des anticorps polyclonaux.

Stimulation par la pentagastrine :
Un test de stimulation a été réalisé chez des volontaires sains âgés de 20 et 35 ans. Les résultats rapportés dans le tableau 2 ont été obtenus par méthodes IRMA et RIA. Ils sont exprimés soit par la valeur de la différence entre le taux de base et le pic à 3 mn (Δ) soit par le rapport de la valeur de ce pic au taux de base (S). Avec les méthodes RIA, les tests sont considérés comme positifs quand S est supérieur à 2,5. Avec la méthode IRMA, il est difficile d'utiliser S car les taux de base sont en général non détectables. Il faudra donc dans ce cas utiliser l'expression Δ. Avec la méthode RIA une augmentation du taux de calcitonine après stimulation n'a été détectée que chez un seul sujet (S = 3,2). En revanche avec la méthode IRMA, chez 9 des 18 sujets nous avons pu mettre en évidence une élévation de la calcitonine plasmatique après stimulation, dont 7 avec une valeur de Δ comprise entre 10 et 28 pg/ml.

2) CMT : tumeur primitive ou récidive

Taux de calcitonine
Dans cette population les taux de calcitonine sont toujours élevés quelque soit le dosage utilisé, RIA ou IRMA. Cependant il existe de grandes variations des valeurs absolues de calcitoninémie entre les méthodes RIA et IRMA. Ces variations sont liées à la spécificité des anticorps et à la ou les formes de calcitonine reconnues (Guilloteau *et al.*, 1990).

Taux d'ACE
En présence de tumeur ou de métastase il y a en général production d'ACE, accompagnant la production de calcitonine (Calmettes *et al.*, 1977). Alors qu'un taux élevé de calcitonine est pathognomonique du CMT, l'ACE n'est pas spécifique de cette affection. Il peut éventuellement apporter un élément de pronostic, une élévation du taux d'ACE en présence d'une relative stabilité de la calcitonine serait un témoin de la dédifférenciation donc d'un mauvais pronostic (Calmettes *et al.*, 1979).

Dépistage des forme familiales
Dans ce cas, seul le dosage de la calcitonine après stimulation n'a d'intérêt. Une récente étude multicentrique (Guilloteau *et al.*, 1990) a montré que des taux de calcitonine plasmatique de 38 pg/ml détectés par méthode IRMA après stimulations pouvaient être le reflet de microcarcinome. Certaines formes familiales dans cette étude n'avaient pas été détectées par la méthode RIA (4 cas sur 8) (Guilloteau *et al.*, 1990).
Le problème actuellement est de fixer la limite entre sujets normaux et sujets sains. Avec les techniques classiques on ne mettait en évidence que des élévations relativement importantes qui étaient toujours le reflet de microcarcinome ou de carcinome (Calmettes *et al.*, 1984). La meilleure sensibilité des méthodes IRMA permet de détecter les sécrétions des cellules normales. L'interprétation avec la méthode IRMA est plus délicate puisque des sujets sains peuvent présenter une valeur de S égale à 28 pg/ml et un microcarcinome peut être associé à une valeur de 30 pg/ml.

Fréquence des tests
Il semble raisonnable de répéter les tests dont la réponse est limite dans un délai maximal de 6 mois et les tests négatifs dans un délai de 3 ans.

DISCUSSION

Les cellules C sécrètent en quantité importante de la calcitonine et en quantité plus faible de l'ACE. L'ACE, dont le dosage ne pose pas de problème particulier, est un marqueur aspécifique du CMT, mais peut apporter des informations au niveau du pronostic.

La calcitonine est le marqueur spécifique du CMT. Son dosage qui a subi de grandes évolutions peut poser des problèmes d'interprétation, en fonction de la méthodologie et des anticorps utilisés. Les valeurs trouvées par les méthodes RIA et IRMA sont très différentes du fait des différentes formes immunoréactives reconnues. Ceci ne pose pas de problème pour le diagnostic et le suivi des tumeurs, les taux étant, quelque soit la méthode de dosage, très élevés. En revanche pour le diagnostic des formes familiales, où seule la détermination des taux de calcitonine après stimulation est informative, les interprétations seront différentes selon la méthode utilisée (RIA ou IRMA).

Avec les méthodes RIA, il est souhaitable d'exprimer les résultats en rapport (S) et de considérer une réponse comme pathologique au delà de 2,5. Avec la méthode IRMA, du fait de la non détection des taux de base, il est souhaitable d'exprimer les résultats en valeur absolue (Δ).

A ce jour nous pouvons retenir les critères d'interprétation suivants :

$S < 30$ pg/ml   Sujets sains
$30 < S < 100$ pg/ml Très forte suspicion d'hyperplasie ou de microcarcinome
                     à interpréter avec d'autres critères familiaux, génétiques...
$S > 100$ pg/ml   Hyperplasie ou microcarcinome

$S = $ (Taux à 3 mn) - (Taux de base)
Méthode IRMA ELSA hCT Cis Bioindustrie

Il est important de s'interroger sur la possibilité d'interférence de certaines substances sur la réponse à un test à la pentagastrine - blocage des phénomènes d'exocytose par exemple. A ce jour seule l'action inhibitrice de la cimétidine a été rapportée. (Ericsson *et al.*, 1981).

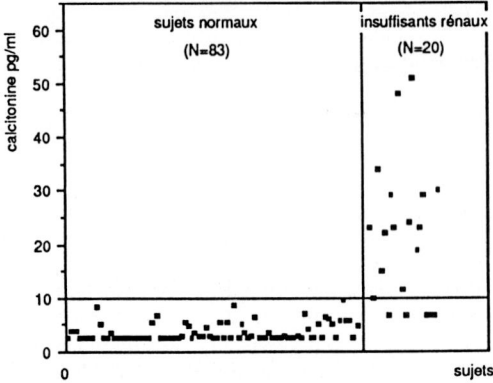

Tableau 1 : Calcitonine plasmatique déterminée par méthode IRMA chez 83 sujets sains et 20 insuffisants rénaux. Notons l'élévation rencontrée dans cette dernière pathologie.

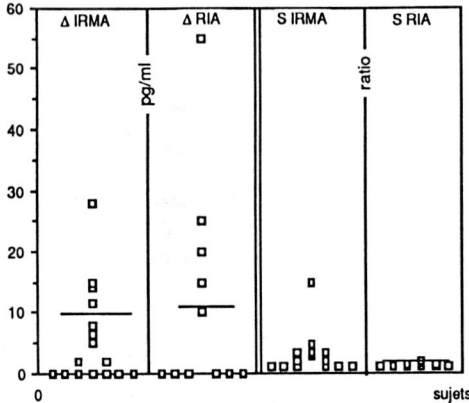

Tableau 2 : Résultats des tests à la pentagastrine réalisés chez 18 sujets sains avec deux méthodes RIA et IRMA. Les résultats sont exprimés sur le rapport de la valeur du pic antérieur de base (Δ) ou par la différence entre ces deux valeurs (S).

REFERENCES

Austin, LA, Heath, H. (1981) : Calcitonin : physiology and pathology. N Engl J Med., **304**, 269-278.
Body, JJ and Heath, III H. (1983) : Estimates of circulating monomeric calcitonin : physiological studies in normal and thyroidectomized man. J Clin.Endocrinol Metab, **57**, 5, 897-903.
Calmettes C, Guilloteau D, Baulieu JL, Besnard JC, Milhaud G. (1984) : Cancer médullaire de la thyroïde : nécessité du dépistage de la forme familiale par dosage de la calcitonine après stimulation. J Biophys Med Nucl., **8**, 123-125.
Calmettes C, Guilloteau D, Bouyge N, Philippe M. (1986) : Dosage de la calcitonine plasmatique. Applications en physiologie et dans la détection précoce des cancers médullaires familiaux de la thyroïde. Colloque sur les actualités en immunoanalyse. 159-160.
Calmettes C, Cressent M, Mouktar MS, Milhaud G. (1977) : Carcinoembryonic antigen and calcitonin in medullary carcinoma of the thyroïd. Acta Endocrinol, suppl. **212**, 198.
Calmettes C, Mouktar MS, Milhaud G. (1979) : Calcitonine et antigène carcionembryonnaires : marqueurs tumoraux au cours du cancer médullaire de la thyroïde. La Nouvelle Presse Médicale., **8**, 48, 3947-3950.
Catherwood BD, Deftos LJ. (1979) : Reactivity of ACTH and synthetic ACTH peptides with antisera to human calcitonin. J Immunol Methods., **31**, 315-319.
Clark MB, Boyd GW, Byfield PGH, Foster GV. (1969) : A radioimmunoassay for human calcitonin M. Lancet., **2**, 74-77.
Cunliffe MB, Black MM, Hall R, Johnson IDA, Hudgson P, Shuster S, Gudmundsson TV, Joplin GF, Williams ED, Woodhouse NJY, Galante L, MacIntyre I. (1968) : A calcitonin-secreting thyroid carcinoma. Lancet., 63-66.
Dermody WC, Rosen MA, Ananthaswamy R, Mc Cormick WM, Levy AG. (1981) : Characterization of the major forms of human calcitonin in tissue and serum. J clin endocrinol Metab., **52**, 1090-1098.
Ericsson M, Ingemansson S and Järhult J. (1981) : Regulatory Peptides, **2**, 175-180.
Ericsson M, Ingemansson S and Järhult J. (1981) : Cimetidine inhibits the pentagastrin-induced release of calcitonin in normocalcaemic man. Regulatory Peptides, **2**, 175-180.
Gold P, and Freedman SO. (1965) : Specific carcinoembryonic antigens of the human digestive system. J Exp Med.,122, 67-480.
Guilloteau D, Perdrisot R, Calmettes C, Baulieu JL, Lecomte P, Kaphan G, Milhaud G, Besnard JC, Pallet P and Bigorgne JC. (1990) : Diagnosis of medullary carcinoma of the thyroid (MCT) by calcitonin assay using monoclonal antibodies : criteria for the pentagastrin stimulation test in hereditary MCT. J Clin Endocrinol Metab., **71**, 4.
Kodama T, Fujino M, Endo Y, Obara T, Fujimoto Y, Oda T and Wada T. (1980) : Identification of carcinoembryonic antigen in the C-cell of the normal thyroid. Cancer., 45, 98-101.
Kumar MA, Slack E, Edwards A, Soliman H, Baghdiantz A, Foster GV, Mc Intyre I. (1965) : A biological assay for calcitonin. Science., **33**, 469-475.
Mériadec de Byans B, Ducimetière P, Richard JL, Salard JL and Henry R. (1976) : Variations in carcinoembryonic antigen levels correlated with t obacco consumption innormal subjects. Biomedicine, **25**, 197-198.
Milhaud G, Ribeiro FM, Calmettes C, Taboulet J, Coutris G, Moukhtar MS. (1975) : Epreuves de stimulation de la sécrétion de calcitonine. Intérêt dans les cancers médullaires de la thyroïde. La Nouvelle Presse Médicale., **4**, 24, 1793-1795.

Milhaud G, Tubiana M, Parmentier C, Coutris G. (1968) : Epithélioma de la thyroïde sécrétant de la thyrocalcitonine. C R Acad Sci (Paris) (D), **266**, 608-610.

Motté P, Vauzelle P, Gardet P, Ghillani P, Caillou B, Parmentier C, Bohuon C, Bellet D. (1988) : Construction and clinical validation of a sensitive and specific assay for serum mature calcitonin using monoclonal anti-peptide antibodies. Clin Chim Acta.,**174**, 35-54.

Rougier P, Calmettes C, Laplanche A, Travagli JP, Lefevre M, Parmentier C, Milhaud G, Tubiana M. (1983) : The values of calcitonin and carcinoembryonic antigen in the treatment and management of non familial medullary thyroid carcinoma. Cancer., **51**, 855-862.

Silva OL, Becker KL, Primack A, Doppman J and Snider RH. (1973) : Ectopic production of calcitonin. Lancet, 2, 317.

Stevenson JC. (1980) : The structure and function of calcitonin. Invest Cell Pathol., **3**, 187-193.

RESUME :

Les cellules C sécrètent physiologiquement de la calcitonine et de l'ACE. Ces deux substances peuvent être utilisées comme marqueur tumoral du CMT. L'ACE est un marqueur non spécifique, apportant une information sur le pronostic. La calcitonine est le marqueur spécifique du CMT. La mesure peut se faire soit par la méthode utilisant des anticorps polyclonaux (RIA) ou des anticorps monoclonaux (IRMA). Les taux de base déterminés par méthode RIA ou IRMA sont élevés en cas de tumeur avec récidive. En revanche pour le diagnostic des formes familiales seul un dosage après un test à la pentagastrine est informatif. Avec la méthode RIA un rapport de la valeur du pic au taux de base de 2,5 est considéré comme pathologique. Avec la méthode IRMA, des valeurs de la différence entre taux de base et pic inférieurs à 30 pg/ml sont trouvés chez des sujets normaux, des valeurs supérieures à 100 pg/ml évoquent la présence d'une hyperplasie ou d'un microcarcinome. Des valeurs entre 30 et 100 pg/ml sont très en faveur de la présence d'hyperplasie ou de microcarcinome, mais doivent actuellement être interprétées avec d'autres éléments familiaux, génétiques par exemple.

Somatostatin and other peptides in medullary thyroid cancer

Furio Pacini, Fulvio Basolo*, Laura Fugazzola, Arianna Cola* and Aldo Pinchera

Istituto di Endocrinologia and *Istituto di Anatomia Patologica, University of Pisa, Pisa, Italy

Medullary thyroid cancer (MTC) has the peculiar property to synthesize and to release into the circulation calcitonin (CT), the hormonal product of the normal parafollicular C cells of the thyroid from which it arises (De Lellis et al, 1978; Hazard, 1977; Tashjian et al, 1970; Williams, 1966). Furthermore, neoplastic C cells are also able to produce several other hormonal and non-hormonal substances (Uribe et al, 1985) which sometimes can be detected in elevated concentrations in the blood by immunological methods, or at the cellular level by immunohistochemistry or tissue extraction. The mechanism(s) and the biological relevance of such an heterogenous peptides production are not known, but for some peptide a paracrine role as modulator of the cell growth has been advocated.

In this study we have chosen to investigate the production of six separate antigens associated with MTC in order to clarify the relationship between their cellular expression and their presence in the circulation and the relationship with the tumor outcome.

Patients and methods

Eighteen patients (8 males and 10 females) were studied. They have been followed-up for a mean of 70.7 months and 50% of them died of their disease. The antigens studied were: calcitonin (CT), CEA, neuron specific enolase (NSE), calcitonin gene related peptide (CGRP), somatostatin (SMS) and thyroglobulin (Tg). They were measured in the blood using specific radioimmunoassays or immunoradiometric assays and in the primary and metastatic tumoral tissues by immunohistochemistry with specific antisera (Hsu et al, 1981). In these experiments both the number of positive cells (from 0 to 100%) and the degree of tissue staining (from - to +++) were recorded and correlated with the tumor outcome and other paramethers

Results

By immunoistochemistry both primary tumors and the metastases expressed CT and CEA in all cases with percent positivity usually higher than 40% of the neoplastic cells and with a strong degree of staining. The other peptides were expressed in varying percentages and degree of staining. In summary CGRP and NSE had an intermediate positivity while SMS and Tg had the lowest positivity both in terms of positive cells and degree of staining. As shown in the following table, except for CT and CEA, for the other peptides the positivity was higher in the primary tumors than in the metastases.

Table : Expression of the 6 antigen studied in the primary tumor or in the metastases.

Antigen	Primary tumor(%)	Metastases(%)
CT	100	100
CEA	100	92.8
NSE	90	71.4
CGRP	66	73.3
SMS	63	38.5
Tg	58	13.3

Measurements of the peptides in the circulation showed that CT and CEA were always increased in patients with metastases and normal in patients in remission after initial treatment. CGRP was increased in 73% of patients, NSE in 47% and SMS in 50%. Serum Tg levels were always undetectable. Increased levels of NSE and SMS were usually observed in patients with advanced metastatic involvement. The expression of an antigen in the metastatic tissue was associated with increased levels of the same antigen in the blood only in the case of CT and CEA. For the other peptides the expression in the tissue was not necessarely associated with hypersecretion in the circulation.

When looking at the tumor outcome, no correlation was found between the expression of CT, CEA, CGRP, NSE or Tg and the survival. On the contrary, SMS positive patients had better survival rates, 100% and 50% at 5 and 7 years respectively, while SMA negative patients had survival rates of 25% both at 5 and 7 years. This finding prompted us to investigate whether SMS could have inhibitory effect on the cell growth and CT production. Five patients were treated with a long-acting SMS analogue (SMS-201-995, Sandoz) at doses ranging between 100 µg and 1000 µg /day , for 3 months. Unespectedly no patient had a reduction in plasma CT concentrations nor a decrease in tumor border.

Discussion

Of the several substances expressed by MTC we decided to study CT and CEA because they are the best characterized and well defined markers for this disease (De Lellis et al, 1978), and could be used as comparison for the less define new markers. CGRP has been recently associated with MTC (Girgis et al, 1985; Morris et al, 1984); CGRP is also present in the normal C cells and is coded for by the same gene coding for CT by alternative splicing. NSE is potentially interesting since is an energy-providing enzyme actively expressed in neuroendocrine cells of the APUD system to which MTC belongs (Kameda, 1985; Pacini et al,1986). SMS was selected because our previous study indicating that it is present in MTC and that short term infusion of SMS can lower the increased levels of CT of MTC patients with metastatic involvement (Buffa et al, 1979; Pacini et al, 1989). Finally, Tg was considered in view of several recent reports (Holm et al, 1986) indicating the unexpected coexpression in few cases of MTC of CT (specif marker for parafollicular cells) and Tg (specific marker for follicular cells of the thyroid).

Our results indicate that while CT and CEA are almost equally expressed in the primary and metastatic tumor, the other antigens are often unexpressed in the metastases. This finding may signify that during the process of metastasizing the cells loose the property to expres a given antigen or that only cell clones not expressing that antigen are able to metastasize. Furthermore not in all cases the expression of an antigen was associated with the hypersecretion into the circulation, indicating that probably the mechanism(s) leading to the secretion of the antigen are impaired in the neoplastic cell. This was particularly true in the case of Tg which was expressed in more than 50% of the tumor but was never detected in the blood.

Regarding the clinical application of antigens meaurement in the serum, no one of the novel antigen we studied resulted superior to CT and CEA for monitoring the evolution of the disease. On the other hand, the immunostaining of the primary tumors indicated that SMS, but not CT and CEA, had a prognostic meaning, since SMS positive patients had significantly better survival rates than SMS negative patients. The importance of this finding dictates the need for further studies in larger series of patients, also in view of possible therapeutic implications.

References

Buffa, R., Chayvialle, J.A., Fontana, P., Ubellini, L., Capella, C., Solcia, E. (1979):
    Parafollicular cells of rabbit thyroid store both calcitonin and somatostatin and resemble gut D cells ultrastructurally. Histochem. 62, 281-285.

De Lellis, R.A., Rule, A.H., Spiler, I., Nathanson, L., Tashjian, A.H., Wolfe, H.J. (1978): Calcitonin and carcinoembryonic antigen as tumor markers in medull ary thyroid carcinoma. Am. J. Clin. Pathol. 70, 587-594.

Girgis, S.I., Mac Donald, D.W.R., Stevenson, J.C., et al. (1985): Calcitonin gene related peptide: potent vasodilator and major product of calcitonin gene. Lancet ii, 14-16.

Hazard, J. B. (1977): The C-cells (parafollicular cells) of the thyroid gland and medullary thyroid carcinoma. Am. J. Pathol. 88, 214-250.

Holm, R., Sobrinho-Simoes, M., Nesland, J.M., Johannessen, J.V. (1986): Concurrent production of calcitonin and thyroglobulin by the same neoplastic cells. Ultrastruct. Pathol. 10, 241-248.

Hsu, S.M., Raine, L., Fanger, H. (1981): A comparative study of the peroxidase antiperoxidase method and an avidin-biotin complex method for studying polypeptide hormones with radioimmunoassay antibodies. Am. J. Clin. Pathol. 75, 734-738.

Kameda, Y. (1985): Increased level of immunoreactive neuron-specific enolase in thyroid C cells from dogs and guinea pigs after chronic hypercalcemia. Endocrinol. 117, 1239-1245.

Morris, H.R., Panico, M., Etienne, T., Tippins, J. R., Girgis, S. I., MacIntyre I. (1984): Isolation and characterization of human calcitonin gene-related peptide. Nature 308, 746-748.

Pacini, F., Elisei, R., Anelli, S., Gasperini, L., Schipani, E., Pinchera, A. (1986): Circulating neuron-specific enolase in medullary thyroid cancer. Int. J. Biol. Markers 2, 85-88.

Pacini, F., Elisei, R., Anelli, S., Basolo, F., Cola, A., Pinchera, A. (1989): Somatostatin in medullary thyroid cancer: in vivo and in vitro studies. Cancer 63, 1189-1195.

Tashjian, A.H., Howland, B.G., Melvin, K.E.V., Hill, C.S. (1970): Immunoassay of human calcitonin: clinical measurement, relation to serum calcium and studies in patients with medullary carcinoma. New Engl. J. Med. 283, 890-895.

Uribe, M., Grimes, M., Fenoglio-Preiser, C.M., Feind, C. (1985): Medullary carcinoma of the thyroid gland: clinical, pathological and immunohistochemical features with review of the literature. Am. J. Surg. Pathol. 9, 577-594.

Williams, E.D. (1966): Histogenesis of medullary carcinoma of the thyroid. Clin Pathol. 19, 114-118.

In vitro and in vivo identification of somatostatin receptors in medullary thyroid carcinomas, pheochromocytomas and paragangliomas

J.C. Reubi[1] [*], E. Modigliani[2], C. Calmettes[3], L. Kvols[4], E.P. Krenning[5] [6] and S.W.J. Lamberts[5]

[1] Sandoz Research Institute Bern Ltd., BO Box, 3001 Bern, Switzerland
[2] Département d'Endocrinologie, Hôpital Avicenne, Bobigny, France
[3] INSERM U113, Hôpital Saint-Antoine, Paris, France
[4] Mayo Clinic, Rochester, MN, USA
Depts. of Internal Medicine[5] and Nuclear Medicine[6], Erasmus University, Rotterdam, The Netherlands

* Author for correspondence

It has recently been shown that somatostatin (SRiF) receptors are markers for various types of neuroendocrine tumors: most GH and TSH producing pituitary adenomas contain SRiF receptors as well as a significant proportion of endocrine inactive pituitary adenomas (1); most endocrine hormone-producing gastroenteropancreatic (GEP) tumors (1); numerous differentiated brain tumors of neuronal, glial or meningial origin (1); some small cell lung cancers (1); a limited number of breast tumors which have been shown to be positive for neuroendocrine markers and of favourable prognosis (1). Interestingly, many of the above-mentioned tumors belong to the group of apudomas, i.e. tumors having the APUD cell as common origin (2). Since medullary thyroid carcinomas (MTC), but also pheochromocytomas and paragangliomas, are also suspected to have APUD features, it was our goal to test whether SRiF receptors, which may be a general marker for neuroendocrine tumors, are present in these types of cancer.

Surgically removed samples of MTC, pheochromocytomas or paragangliomas were obtained from the French Group of Medullary Thyroid Tumor, Paris, the Mayo Clinic, Rochester (USA), and the Erasmus University Hospital, Rotterdam. All tumors were analysed for their content in SRiF receptors using receptor autoradiography with a SRiF-28 analogue and/or the SRiF octapeptide [Tyr^3]-SMS 201-995 as iodinated radioligands, as described previously (3).

In MTC, 6 out of 26 cases were SRiF receptor positive with the SRiF octapeptide radioligand. These cases as well as 4 additional tumors (10/26) were also positive with the SRiF-28 radioligand ^{125}I-[Leu^8, D-Trp^{22}, Tyr^{25}]-SRiF-28. High affinity binding sites pharmacologically specific for bioactive SRiF analogues were identified, specifically located on tumor tissue (Fig. 1). In some cases the SRiF receptors were distributed in a non-homogenous pattern, labelling occurring preferentially in highly differentiated tumor regions. Numerous cases were shown to have a high tumoral SRiF content measured by radioimmunoassay or immunohistochemical technique (4). However, there was no correlation between SRiF receptor status and tumor levels of endogenous SRiF (4). No correlation was seen between the clinical outcome or the survival of the patients and their tumoral SRiF receptor content. Whereas some medullary thyroid carcinomas seem to be a target for SRiF, the SRiF function in these tumors remains unclear.

Among 52 pheochromocytomas, 38 cases (73%) were shown to contain SRiF receptors, measured with the $[Tyr^3]$-SMS 201-995 radioligand. The receptors, often present in high density, were located on tumor cells exclusively.

The highest incidence of SRiF receptors was found in paragangliomas, since 11 out of 12 of these tumors tested in vitro (92%) were shown to have a high density of specific, high affinity SRiF receptors.

These data indicate that SRiF receptors may represent a useful morphological and pathobiochemical marker in these 3 groups of neuroendocrine tumors. Therefore, all tumor types belonging to the so-called apudomas, namely pituitary adenomas, carcinoids, islet cell carcinomas, small cell lung tumors, MTC, pheochromocytomas and paragangliomas possess, although not always in a 100% incidence, SRiF receptors. Whereas we know that SRiF analogues such as octreotide (SMS 201-995) are particularly beneficial in patients with SRiF receptor positive carcinoids, islet cell carcinomas or pituitary adenomas (5,6), it is at present unknown whether such drugs will also positively affect the symptoms of MTC, pheochromocytoma or paraganglioma patients having SRiF receptor positive tumors.

An exciting new diagnostic opportunity for SRiF receptor containing tumors is the possibility to visualize such tumors and their metastases in vivo. Krenning et al. have recently shown that after intravenous injection of ^{123}I-$[Tyr^3]$-SMS 201-995 SRiF receptor positive tumors and metastases can be localized by scanning the patient with a -camera (7). This method has been shown to be extremely successful for the visualization of carcinoids, islet cell tumors or meningiomas (7). Also SRiF receptor positive pituitary adenomas were identified. We have recently extended this technique to paragangliomas which were shown to be strongly visualized in all cases (8); the method is particularly valuable for paragangliomas since their multiple sites of location are all identified. Preliminary data suggest that also SRiF receptor positive MTC and their metastases can be visualized in the patient; the same is true for pheochromocytomas. Therefore, SRiF receptor imaging may be an attractive diagnostic tool in these tumor types.

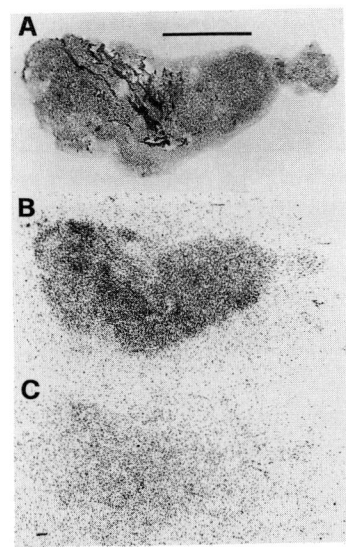

Figure legend

Fig. 1: Somatostatin receptors in one case of medullary thyroid carcinoma.
A: Hematoxylin-eosin stained section
B: Autoradiogram showing total binding of ^{125}-[Tyr^3]-SMS 201-995.
C: Non-specific binding (in presence of 10^{-5} M [Tyr^3]-SMS-201-905.
Bar = 1 mm.

References

1. Reubi, J.C., Kvols, L., Krenning, E. and Lamberts, S.W.J.
   Distribution of somatostatin receptors in normal and tumor tissue
   Metabolism 39 (Suppl.):78-81 (1990).
2. Pearse AGE, The APUD concept and hormone production. In: Clinics in Endocrinology, Abe, K. (ed)., Saunders, Philadelphia, 211-222 (1980).
3. Reubi, J.C., Haecki, W.H. and Lamberts, S.W.J.
   Hormone-producing gastrointestinal tumor contain high density of somatostatin receptors
   J Clin Endocrinol Metab 65:1127-1134 (1987).
4. Reubi, J.C., Chayvialle, J.A., Franc, B., Cohen, R., Calmettes, C. and Modigliani, E.
   Somatostatin receptors and somatostatin content in medullary thyroid carcinomas
   Lab. Invest. (1991) (in press)
5. Reubi, J.C. and Landolt, A.M.
   The growth hormone responses to octreotide in acromegaly correlate with adenoma somatostatin receptor status
   J Clin Endocrinol Metab 68:844-850 (1989).
6. Reubi, J.C., Kvols, L.K., Waser, B., Nagorney, D.M., Heitz, P.U., Charboneau, J.W., Reading, C.C. and Moertel, C.
   Detection of somatostatin receptors in surgical and percutaneous needle biopsy samples of carcinoids and islet cell carcinomas
   Cancer Res 50:5969-5977 (1990).
7. Krenning, E.P., Bakker, W.H., Breeman, W.A.P., Koper, J.W., Kooij, P.P.M., Ausema, L., Lameris, J.S., Reubi, J.C. and Lamberts, S.W.J.
   Localization of endocrine-related tumours with radioiodinated analogue of somatostatin
   Lancet I:242-244 (1989).
8. Lamberts, S.W.J., Bakker, W.H., Reubi, J.C. and Krenning, E.P.
   The value of somatostatin receptor imaging in the localization of endocrine and brain tumors
   New England J Medicine 323:1246-1249 (1990).

Bombesin/gastrin-releasing peptide in medullary thyroid carcinoma

Jean-Alain Chayvialle

INSERM U 45, Hôpital Edouard-Herriot, Lyon, France

Summary Gastrin-releasing peptide (GRP) - like components are synthetized by most medullary thyroid carcinomas, as a result of inappropriate GRP gene expression. Their potential roles, as regards autocrine stimulation of cell proliferation and/or synthesis of other secretory products by C cells, remains to be delineated.

Beside calcitonin, various peptides are occasionally synthetized by neoplastic C cells (Deftos et al., 1980 ; Uribe et al., 1985). Gastrin-releasing peptide (GRP), the mammalian counterpart of amphibian bombesin, is detected in a large majority of medullary thyroid carcinomas (MTC) both at immunocytochemistry and by radioimmunoassay of tumor extracts (Kameda et al., 1983 ; Yamaguchi et al., 1984 ; Ghatei et al., 1985). In contrast to unmeasurably low GRP concentrations in normal thyroid tissue, Yamaguchi et al. (1985) found significant amounts of immunoreactive GRP in every of 10 primary MTCs and in 92 % of 12 metastatic tumors. Modigliani et al. (1990 a) recorded abnormally high values (i.e. greater than 62 pmol/g wet weight, up to 7800 pmol/g) in 32 of 34 MTCs.

The GRP gene is expressed in neoplastic C cells (Suzuki et al.,1987 ; Sunday et al.,1988). Interestingly GRP mRNAs are detected in up to 80 % of C cells in fetuses and neonates, but in only 5 % of C cells in adults, GRP gene expression and thyroid GRP concentrations being positively correlated among the various age groups (Sunday et al.,1988). This pattern closely resembles GRP gene expression in lung, with abnormal expression in small cell carcinomas (Yamaguchi et al.,1983).

The high incidence of GRP synthesis in MTCs raises several issues, among which i) the potential use of plasma GRP concentration as a marker of dedifferentiation and/or tumor mass, ii) the possibility that C cells retaining GRP gene expression during adult life are those prone to neoplastic growth , and iii) the presumptive paracrine or autocrine role of GRP within the tumor. Bombesin stimulates the growth of several cell types, including endocrine cells (Rozengurt and Sinnett-Smith, 1983 ; Weber et al., 1985 ; Lhoste el al., 1986 ; Lehy and Puccio, 1990). Moreover, evidence was provided for an autocrine, growth-stimulating, role of bombesin in small-cell lung carcinoma cell lines (Cuttitta et al., 1985). It is thus tempting to speculate that similar effects are exerted by GRP in MTCs.

Beside its potential role on tumor growth, GRP could modulate the secretory activity of neoplastic C cells, because the peptide, like bombesin, stimulates several endocrine cell types (Ghatei et al.,1982 ; Vagne et al., 1987 ; Vaysse,1988). In this respect, the significant positive correlation between log concentrations of immunoreactive GRP and somatostatin in tissue extracts from 34 MTC cases recently reported (Modigliani et al.,1990 a) suggests that GRP may stimulate somatostatin synthesis within the tumor. Indeed, tissue somatostatin concentrations significantly greater than the values in normal thyroid tissue are observed in a majority of MTCs (Modigliani et al., 1990 b). Whether C cell-borne GRP stimulates as well somatostatin release within MTCs, as bombesin does in digestive tract, remains to be established. The possible local interaction between a stimulatory, growth-promoting peptide such as GRP, and an inhibitory mediator such as somatostatin obviously is of utmost importance for the understanding of MTC pathophysiology. Significant advances in the delineation of GRP contribution are awaited from the use of potent bombesin antagonists (Coy et al., 1989 ; Wang et al., 1990) since they already have proved useful for a reappraisal of bombesin physiology (Cuber et al., 1990).

Résumé . Des peptides apparentés au gastrin-releasing peptide (GRP) sont synthétisés par la plupart des cancers medullaires de la thyroide, du fait d'une expression inappropriée du gène du GRP. Leurs rôles potentiels en tant que facteurs de croissance autocrines et/ou de régulateurs d'autres produits de sécrétion des cellules C restent à élucider.

REFERENCES

Coy, D.H., Taylor, J.E., Jiang, N.Y., Kim, S.H., Wang, L.H., Huang, S.C., Moreau, J.P., Gardner, J.D., and Jensen, R.T. (1989) : Short-chain pseudopeptide bombesin receptor antagonists with enhanced binding affinities for pancreatic acinar and swiss 3T3 cells display strong antimitotic activity. *J. Biol. Chem.* 264 : 14691-14697.

Cuber, J.C., Bernard, G., Coy, D.H., Bernard, C., and Chayvialle, J.A. (1990) : Blockade of bombesin receptors with [Leu14-psi (CH2NH)-Leu13] bombesin fails to suppress nutrient-induced CCK release from rat duodenojejunum. *Peptides* . 11 : 255-258.

Cuttitta, F., Carney, D.N., Mulshine, J., Moody, T.W., Fedorko, J., Fischler, A., and Minna, J.D. (1985) : Bombesin-like peptides can function as autocrine growth factors in human small-cell lung cancer. *Nature* . 316 : 823-826.

Deftos, L.J., Bone, H.G. III, and Parthemore, J.G. (1980) : Immunohistological studies of medullary thyroid carcinoma and C-cell hyperplasia. *J. Clin. Endocrinol. Metab.* 51 : 857-862.

Ghatei, M.A., Jung, R.T., Stevenson, J.C., Hillyard, J., Adrian, T.E., Lee, C., Chrisotfides, N.D., Sarson, D.L., Mashiter, K., McIntyre, I., and Bloom, S.R. (1982) : Bombesin action on gut hormones and calcium in man. *J. Clin. Endocrinol. Metab.* 54 : 980-985.

Ghatei, M.A., Springall, D.R., Micholl, C.G., Polak, J.M., and Bloom, S.R. (1985) : Gastrin releasing peptide like immunoreactivity in medullary thyroid carcinoma. *Am. J. Clin. Pathol.* 84 : 851-856.

Kameda, Y., Besshot, T., Tsumuraya, M., Yamaguchi, K., Abe, K., Schimosato, Y., Yanaihara, N. (1983) : Production of gastrin releasing peptide by medullary carcinoma of the thyroid, an immunohistochemical study. *Virchows Arch. (Pathol.Anat.).* 401 : 99-108.

Lehy, T., and Puccio, F. (1990) : Promoting effect of bombesin on the cell proliferation in the rat endocrine pancreas during the early postnatal period. *Regul. Peptides* . 27 : 87-96.

Lhoste, E., Aprahamian, M., Pousse, A., Hoeltzel, A., and Stock-Damge, C. (1986) : Combined effect of chronic bombesin, secretin and cholecystokinin on the rat pancreas. *Peptides* . 6 : 83-87.

Modigliani, E., Casanova, S., Chayvialle, J.A., Bernard, C., Franc, B., Cohen, R., and Calmettes, C. (1990 a) : Immunoreactive gastrin-releasing peptide in medullary thyroid carcinoma. *J. Clin. Endocrinol. Metab.* 71 : 831-835.

Modigliani, E., Alamowitch, C., Cohen, R., Calmettes, C., Guliana, J.M., Franc, B., Bernard, C., and Chayvialle, J.A. (1990 b) : The intratumoral immunoassayable somatostatin concentration is frequently elevated in medullary thyroid carcinoma. *Cancer* . 65 : 224-228.

Rozengurt, E., and Sinnett-Smith, J. (1983) : Bombesin stimulation of DNA synthesis and cell division of swiss 3T3 cells. *Proc. Natl.Acad. Sci. USA* . 80 : 2936-2940.

Sunday, M.E., Wolfe, H.J., Roos, B.A., Chin, W.W., and Spindel, E.R. (1988) : Gastrin-releasing peptide gene expression in developing, hyperplastic, and neoplastic human thyroid C-cells. *Endocrinology.* 122 : 1551-1558.

Suzuki, M., Yamaguchi, K, Abe, K., Adachi, N., Nagasaki, K., Asanuma, F., Adachi, I., Ki mura, S., Terada, M., Taya, Y., Matsuzaki, J., and Miki, K. (1987) : Detection of gastrin-releasing peptide mRNA in small cell lung carcinomas and medullary thyroid carcinomas using synthetic oligodeoxyribonucleotide probes. *Jpn. J. Clin. Oncol.* 17 : 157-163.

Uribe, M., Fenoglio Preiser, C.M., Orin, M., and Feind, C. (1985) : Medullary carcinoma of the thyroid gland : clinical, pathological and immunohisto-chemical features with review of the litterature. *Am. J. Surg. Pathol.* 9 : 577-594.

Vagne, M., Collinet, M., Cuber, J.C., Bernard, C., Chayvialle, J.A., McDonald, T.J., and Mutt, V. (1987) : Effect of porcine gastrin releasing peptide on gastric secretion and motility and the release of hormonal peptides in conscious cats. *Peptides* . 8 : 423-430.

Vaysse, N. (1988) : Les peptides de la famille bombesine : de la physiologie aux applications thérapeutiques potentielles. *Gastroenterol. Clin. Biol.* 12 : 447-453.

Wang, L.H., Coy, D.H., Taylor, J.E., Jiang, N.Y., Kim, S.H., Moreau, J.P., Huang, S.C., Mantey, S.A., Frucht, H., and Jensen, R.T. (1990) : Desmethionine alkylamide bombesin analogues : a new class of bombesin receptor antagonists with potent antisecretory activity in pancreatic acini and antimitotic activity in swiss 3T3 cells. *Biochemistry* . 29 : 616-622.

Weber, S., Zuckerman, J.E., Bostwick, D.G., Bensch, K.G., Sikic, B.I., Raffin, T.A. (1985) : Gastrin-releasing peptide is a selective mitogen for small cell lung carcinoma in vitro. *J.Clin. Invest.* 75 : 306-313.

Yamaguchi, K., Abe, K., Kameya, T., Adachi, I., Taguchi, S., Otsubo, K., and Yanaihara, N. (1983) : Production and molecular size heterogeneity of immunoreactive gastrin-releasing peptide in fetal and adult lungs and primary lung tumors. *Cancer Res.* 43 : 3932-3939.

Yamaguchi, K., Abe, K.,Adachi, I., Suzuki, M., Kimura, S.,Kameya, T., and Yanaihara, N. (1984) : Concomitant production of immunoreactive gastrin-releasing peptide and calcitonin in medullary carcinoma of the thyroid. *Metabolism* . 33 : 724-727.

Peptide regulatory factors in the thyroid C cell system : an updating

Lucio Scopsi

Division of Anatomical Pathology and Cytology, Istituto Nazionale per lo Studio e la Cura dei Tumori, Via G. Venezian, 1, 20133 Milano, Italy

While a number of non-calcitonin genes-derived neurohormonal peptides are produced by the C cells, the biological importance of this fact remains to be elucidated. However, there is a growing body of experimental evidence to suggest that at least some of these peptides could be important markers for 1) defining a subset of medullary carcinomas (MC's) with a less aggressive behaviour (Pacini et al., 1989; Scopsi et al., 1990a, Scopsi et al., 1990b), and 2) monitoring C cell activity (Sunday et al., 1988; Scopsi et al., submitted). Furthermore, since some of these peptides have direct effects on thyroid follicular cells (Ahren, 1989; Ahren and Hedner, 1989; Zerek-Melen et al., 1990), C cells could have a paracrine role in thyroid homeostasis by virtue of their neuropeptide gene products. Finally, these peptides could also be of value in the treatment of MC (Modigliani et al., 1989). Since an exhaustive review on C cell regulatory polypeptides has recently appeared (Scopsi, 1990), I will confine my discussion to the most recent acquisitions on pancreatic polypeptide (PP)-fold peptides, thyrotropin-releasing hormone (TRH), and cholecystokinin (CCK).

We have recently confirmed, by site-directed immunocytochemistry, the presence of PP and its C-flanking peptide in a few sparse cells of a minority of human MC's. On the same occasion, we provided evidence that a molecule closely related to pro-Neuropeptide Tyrosine (NPY) is present in both normal and pathologic human C cells. Interestingly, PP- and NPY-like immunoreactivities did not overlap, and no Peptide Tyrosine Tyrosine (PYY)-immunoreactivity was detected. Thus, at least two members of the PP-fold family seem to be present in separate cells of this neuroendocrine system, and for one of them the chemical identity with PP has been proved (O'Hare et al., 1986). However, since the archival source of our material (Scopsi et al., 1990b) precluded an adequate biochemical charaterization, it cannot be ruled out that part or even all of the NPY-like immunoreactivity found represents a yet unidentified member of this peptide family (Schwartz et al., 1989). However that may be, production of a NPY-like substance is a universal concomitant of MC and can be used as a marker of C cell activity, since -like that found for somatostatin (Pacini et al., 1989; Scopsi et al., 1990a)- high levels of expression of this peptide seem to define a subset of tumors with a less aggressive behaviour (Scopsi et al., 1990b).

Although the occurrence of TRH-like immunoreactivity in the thyroid was first described in the early 80's (Pekary et al., 1983; Iversen et al., 1984), it was not until the elucidation of the sequence of the TRH precursor that its chemical identity with TRH and its origin from the C cells were unequivocally demonstrated (Sevarino et al., 1988; Simard et al., 1989; Gkonos et al., 1989). Today we know that the TRH gene is expressed in the rat C cell system (Sevarino et al., 1988; Gkonos et al., 1989) and that the preproTRH is processed in a manner similar to what which occurs in the hypothalamus (Simard et al., 1989). However, TRH species other than the mature TRH-amide have been identified in both normal C cells (Gkonos et al., 1989) and MC (Sevarino et al., 1988), and the possibility also exists that a portion of the thyroidal TRH immunoreactivity represents a yet unidentified TRH-like peptide (Gkonos et al., 1989). It is also apparent that the thyroid TRH is mobilizable, since, e.g., dexamethasone stimulates TRH synthesis and secretion by the C cells (Tavianini et al., 1989). As to the role of TRH in the thyroid, TRH perfusion of dog thyroid tissue inhibits the normal TSH-induced cAMP response and secretion of thyroid hormones (Delbeke et al., 1983; Iversen & Laurberg, 1985), but does not affect the basal and Ca++ induced release of calcitonin and somatostatin (Iversen & Laurberg, 1985). Furthermore, chronic TRH or T4 treatment of euthyroid rats increases the thyroid content of TRH and of its precursor (Simard et al., 1989). In accordance with the findings on normal dog thyroid (Iversen & Laurberg, 1985), TRH administration does not affect plasma calcitonin (CT) levels in normal humans or in MC patients with low basal CT values (Haase et al., 1989; O'Connell et al., 1990). In MC patients with elevated basal CT values, TRH administration produces a rise in plasma CT levels, the magnitude of which is, however, far smaller than that observed with pentagastrin (Nakamura et al., 1987; O'Connell et al., 1990; Haase et al., 1989).

The homologous peptide hormones gastrin and CCK are associated with C cells in at least two ways: 1) because their common C-terminal pentapeptide amide stimulates the release of CT, and is, for this reason, a precious tool for the early diagnosis of MC, and 2) because gastrin/CCK immunoreactivity and a CCK mRNA have been detected in normal thyroid C cells and MC (see Scopsi, 1990 for review). The CCK precursor present in rat and human MC's is processed in a quite unusual way (Haun et al., 1989, Rehfeld et al., 1990), since only small molecular forms have been detected in both species. However, in the human tumors more than 90% of the amidated immunoreactivity eluted like non-sulphated CCK-8 or CCK-7 (Rehfeld et al., 1990), whereas the predominant form of immunoreactive CCK produced by a rat MC cell line is indistinguishable from synthetic CCK-8 sulphate (Haun et al., 1989). Although reliable immunocytochemical localization studies are still lacking, preliminary results in this direction would suggest that only very few sparse neoplastic cells react with CCK-specific antibodies in human MC's (Scopsi: unpublished), which is in keeping with the low amounts of radioimmunoassayable CCK found in the most tumors (Rehfeld et al., 1990). Taken together with the observation that CCK-5 is a potent CT secretagogue in several animal species, these findings raise the possibility that small non-sulphated CCK peptides are involved in the autocrine modulation of C cell activity.

It is unlikely that the control of any individual cellular event (e.g., development, proliferation, and differentiation) be dominated by a single agent. Thus, future studies should aim at disclosing the relationships among the diverse components of the C cell secretory cocktail. To understand the role of these C cell peptides, one must also know what are their stored and circulating forms, which means further physiological and biochemical characterization studies. Finally, it is reasonable to speculate that further analysis of C cell products could identify other peptide regulatory factors. One such peptide is neuromedin U, a novel neurotransmitter, distributed throughout the central and peripheral nervous systems and in the pituitary gland (Domin et al., 1990).

REFERENCES.

Ahren, B. (1989): Effects of gastrin-releasing peptide on basal and stimulated thyroid hormone secretion in the mouse. Acta Endocrinol. (Copenh.) 120,245-249.

Ahren, B., & Hedner, P. (1989): Effects of VIP and helodermin on thyroid hormone secretion in the mouse. Neuropeptides 13,59-64.

Delbeke, D., Van Sande, J., Cochaux, P., Decoster, C., and Dumont, J.E. (1983): Effect of thyrotropin-releasing hormone on dog thyroid in vitro. Biochem. Biophys. Acta 761,262-268.

Domin, J., Al-Madani, A.M., Desperbasques, M., Bishop, A.E., Polak, J.M., and Bloom, S.R. (1990): Neuromedin U-like immunoreactivity in the thyroid gland of the rat. Cell Tissue Res. 260,131-135.

Gkonos, P.J., Tavianini, M.A., Liu, C.-c., and Roos, B.A. (1989): Thyrotropin-releasing hormone gene expression in normal parafollicular cells. Mol. Endocrinol. 3,2101-2109.

Haase, R., Windeck, R., Benker, G., and Reinwein, D. (1989): Thyrotropin-releasing hormone enhances calcitonin secretion in medullary thyroid carcinoma. Abstract presented at the "Third International Workshop on Multiple Endocrine Neoplasia, type 2", September 28-30, 1989, Heidelberg, F.R.G.

Haun, R.S., Beinfeld, M.C., Roos, B.A., and Dixon, J.E. (1989): Establishment of a cholecystokinin-producing rat medullary thyroid carcinoma cell line. Endocrinology 125,850-856.

Iversen, E., & Laurberg, P. (1985): Thyrotrophin-releasing hormone (TRH) and hormone secretion from the folicular and C-cells of perfused dog thyroid lobes. Acta Endocrinol. (Copenh.) 109,499-504.

Iversen, E., Weeke, J., and Laurberg, P. (1984): TRH immunoreactivity in the thyroid gland. Scand. J. clin. Lab. Invest. 44,703-709.

Modigliani, E., Guliana, J.M., Maroni, M., Guillausseau, J.P., Chabrier, G., Dupont, J.L., Caron, J., Roger, P., Bentata Pessayre, M., Jacob, C., Baulieu, J.L., Guillausseau-Scholler, C., Delepine, N., Desbois, J.C., Siame Mourot, C., Charpentier, G., Sangalli, F., Tourniaire, J., Lalau, J.D., Deidier, A., et Calmettes, C. (1989): Effets de l'administration sous cutanee de la sandostatine (SMS 201.995) en sous cutane dans 18 cas de cancer medullaire du corps thyroïde. Ann. Endocrinol. (Paris) 50,483-488.

Nakamura, H., Someda, H., Mori, T., and Imura, H. (1987): Thyrotrophin releasing hormone induced calcitonin secretion in patients with medullary carcinoma of the thyroid. Clin. Endocrinol. (Oxford) 27,69-74.

O'Connell, J.E., Dominiczak, A.F., Isles, C.G., McLellan, A.R., Davidson, G., Gray, C.E., and Connell, J.M.C. (1990): A comparison of calcium pentagastrin and TRH tests in screening for medullary carcinoma of the thyroid in MEN IIA. Clin. Endocrinol. (Oxford) 32,417-421.

O'Hare, M.M.T., Shaw, C., Johnston, C.F., Russel, C.F.J., Sloan, J.M., and Buchanan, K.D. (1986): Pancreatic polypeptide immunoreactivity in medullary carcinoma of the thyroid: identification and characterisation by radioimmunoassay, immunocytochemistry and high performance liquid chromatography. Regul. Pept. 14,169-180.

Pacini, F., Elisei, R., Anelli, S., Basolo, F., Cola, A., and Pinchera, A. (1989): Somatostatin in medullary thyroid cancer. In vitro and in vivo studies. Cancer 63,1189-1195

Pekary, A.E., Richkind, M., and Hershman, J.M. (1983): Thyrotrophin releasing hormone and related peptides in canine tissues. J. Endocrinol. 98,299-306.

Rehfeld, J.F., Johnsen, A.H., Odum, L., Bardram, L., Schifter, S., and Scopsi, L. (1990): Non-sulphated cholecystokinin in human medullary thyroid carcinomas. J. Endocrinol. 124,501-506.

Schwartz, T.W., Fuhlendorff, J., Langeland, N., Thogersen, H., Jorgensen, J.Ch., and Sheikh, S.P. (1989): Y1 and Y2 receptors for NPY. The evolution of PP-fold peptides and their receptors. In Neuropeptide Y - 14th Nobel Symposium, eds. V. Mutt, T. Hökfelt, & K. Fuxe, pp.534-541. New York: Raven

Scopsi, L. (1990): Non-calcitonin genes-derived neurohormonal polypeptides in normal and pathologic thyroid C cells. Progr. Surg. Pathol. 11,185-229.

Scopsi, L., Ferrari, C., Pilotti, S., Holst, J.J., Rehfeld, J.F., Fossati G., and Rilke F. (1990a): Immunocytochemical localization and identification of prosomatostatin gene products in medullary carcinoma of human thyroid gland. Hum. Pathol. 21,820-830.

Scopsi, L., Pilotti, S., and Rilke, F. (1990b): Immunocytochemical localization and identification of members of the pancreatic polypeptide (PP)-fold family in human thyroid C cells and medullary carcinomas. Regul. Pept. 30,89-104

Scopsi, L., Di Palma, S., Ferrari, C., Holst, J.J., Rehfeld, J.F., and Rilke, F.: C cell hyperplasia accompanying thyroid diseases other than medullary carcinoma. An immunocytochemical study by means of antibodies to calcitonin and somatostatin. (submitted).

Sevarino, K.A., Wu, P., Jackson, I.M.D., Roos, B.A., Mandel, G., and Goodman, R.H. (1988): Biosynthesis of thyrotropin-releasing hormone by a rat medullary thyroid carcinoma cell line. J. Biol. Chem. 263,620-623.

Simard, M., Pekary, A.E., Smith, V.P., and Hershman, J.M. (1989): Thyroid hormone modulation of TRH precursor levels in rat hypothalamus, pituitary, thyroid and blood. Peptides 10,145-155.

Sunday, M.E., Wolfe, H.J., Roos, B.A., Chin, W.W., and Spindel, E.R. (1988): Gastrin-releasing peptide gene expression in developing, hyperplastic, and neoplastic human thyroid C cells. Endocrinology 122,1551-1558.

Tavianini, M.A., Gkonos, P.J., Lampe, T.H., and Roos, B.A. (1989): Dexamethasone stimulates thyrotropin-releasing hormone production in a C cell line. Mol. Endocrinol. 3,605-610.

Zerek-Melen, G., Lewinski, A., and Szkudlinski, M. (1990): Influence of somatostatin and epidermal growth factor (EGF) on the proliferation of thyroid follicular cells in culture. Regul. Pept. 28,293-300.

Cytology and imaging

Cytoponction et imagerie

Aspiration cytology of medullary thyroid carcinoma

Lennart Bondeson

Department of Cytology, General Hospital, S-214 01 Malmö, Sweden

Medullary thyroid carcinoma (MTC) shows a wide spectrum of growth patterns and cellular features giving rise to a most varied aspiration cytology. Nevertheless, the many variants do have certain features in common, which makes it possible to establish the diagnosis by fine needle aspiration in most cases according to the following guidelines.

Smear patterns

In general, smears of aspirates from MTC display a marked dissociation of the tumor cells, but more or less cohesive clusters are seen in most cases. These clusters are usually irregular in shape as well as cellular arrangement. It is noteworthy, however, that glandular variants of MTC do occur, and occasionally one sees pictures that are reminiscent of follicular neoplasia. When the dissociation is extreme, on the other hand, patterns looking similar to lymphoma may also be encountered. This likeness can be enhanced by plasmacytoid features of the tumor cells.

Cell types

A variety of rounded, polygonal, and spindle-shaped elements are seen in MTC. Sometimes the tumor cell population is uniform. More often, however, it is heterogenous with a characteristic mixture of polygonal and spindle-shaped elements. Irrespective of the predominating cell type, there is often a minor but distinctive component of triangular and bi-or multinucleated tumor cells.

Cellular details

In epitheloid cell variants from MTC, the nuclei are often situated eccentrically. The chromatin structure and the nucleoli are unpredictable, and the nuclear features may vary from quite bland to frankly malignant. A trait shared with the papillary type of thyroid carcinoma is the occurrence of intranuclear inclusions of cytoplasm in some of the tumor cells. Such "nuclear holes" can also be seen in rare benign thyroid tumors (the so called hyalinizing trabecular adenomas).

The appearance of the cytoplasm and its diagnostic significance depends on the method used. In this context, air-dried and Giemsa-stained smears give more information than ethanol-fixed material stained by hematoxylin-eosin or Papanicolaou. Giemsa (but not the other stains) demonstrates a distinctive metachromatic (azurophilic) pink to purple granulation of the cytoplasm in MTC. Such granulated cells are sometimes numerous, but usually they constitute a minority population and have to be searched for. The metachromatic granulation is highly characteristic but not pathognomonic of MTC. It occurs in other amine and/or peptide hormone producing tumors (such as paragangliomas and carcinoids), and granulation looking much the same can also be seen in metastases from melanoma and breast cancer.

Odd variants

Rare cases of MTC include features such as bizarre giant cells, clear cell changes, mucin production, oncocytic changes, squamous differentiation, and melanin production, which can be mistaken for evidence of metastases in the thyroid gland. Because of therapeutic consequences it is important that MTC is kept in mind as a differential diagnosis whenever unusual pictures of neoplasia are seen in thyroid aspirates.

Special diagnostic methods

If in doubt about the diagnosis on the basis of routine specimens, a suspected MTC can be verified by fine needle aspiration using the same special methods that are applied in histopathology. The simplest method is to demonstrate amyloid. In smears stained by hematoxylin-eosin, Papanicolaou or Giemsa, amyloid looks much the same as clumps of colloid. However, these two substances are readily distinguished from each other by alkaline Congo red. This stain can be applied to air-dried as well as ethanol-fixed smears, and even previously stained material can be used for this purpose after destaining.

Lack of amyloid does not exclude MTC, however, and the most specific way to establish the diagnosis preoperatively is to demonstrate production of calcitonin, either by measurement of serum levels, or by immunocytochemistry applied to fine needle aspirates.

Les différentes modalités de l'imagerie dans le diagnostic, le traitement et la surveillance du cancer médullaire de la thyroïde (CMT)

Marie-Joëlle Delisle

Service de Médecine Nucléaire, Institut Jean-Godinot, BP 171, 51056 Reims Cedex, France

SUMMARY

Serum CT dosages and histological examination provide the most reliable methods in the management of MCT but multimodality imaging remains essential at all stages. Evocative scintigraphic, ultrasonographic and cytological features allow for the isolation of a group of patients with a high probability of MCT. Such guidance makes possible preoperative diagnosis and intervention of a specialized multidisciplinary team for the search of an associated pheochromocytoma and optimal surgery. During the follow-up if the level of serum CT remains or becomes detectable, secreting tumor tissue must be detected by use of all available imaging methods conforming to a well-thought-out strategy : cervical and abdominal echography, CT scan, scintigraphies with different radiotracers in order to detect recurrence or distant metastases as early as possible and propose an adequate treatment.

INTRODUCTION

En présence d'une anomalie cervicale clinique, le dosage de la calcitonine plasmatique suffit dans la plupart des cas à assurer le diagnostic de cancer médullaire de la thyroïde (CMT) pour peu qu'il ait été évoqué. Il est peu d'autres exemples d'un marqueur tumoral aussi sensible et spécifique et dont on puisse disposer aussi aisément. Il en est de même pour les cas familiaux dépistés à l'occasion d'une enquête. Pourtant, l'imagerie, à l'échelon microscopique et au niveau macroscopique dans ses différentes modalités ultrasonique, radiologique, scintigraphique et par résonance magnétique nucléaire, est un élément indispensable à toutes les étapes du diagnostic, du traitement et de la surveillance des cancers à calcitonine (CT), isolés ou intégrés dans un tableau de néoplasie endocrinienne multiple.

IMAGERIE ET DIAGNOSTIC DU CMT

Etant donné l'extrême fréquence des anomalies morphologiques thyroïdiennes, le dosage de la CT plasmatique n'est pas réalisé de façon systématique, en dehors de très rares centres, pour des raisons économiques, bien qu'il eut pu remplacer avec profit les dosages de T3, T4 et TSH dans un grand nombre de nodules hypofixants chez des patients euthyroïdiens. Dans la masse des bilans thyroïdiens, **l'imagerie permet de définir une population à risque avec une forte probabilité de CMT** chez laquelle le diagnostic sera assuré par le dosage de la CT.

Sur la **scintigraphie thyroïdienne** au Tc 99m et à l'I123, le CMT apparait comme un nodule hypofixant à la partie moyenne et externe (Baulieu, 1984) (Fig. 1).Le risque est encore plus grand si le nodule est bilatéral (Fig. 2) et/ou s'accompagne d'adénopathies cervicales.

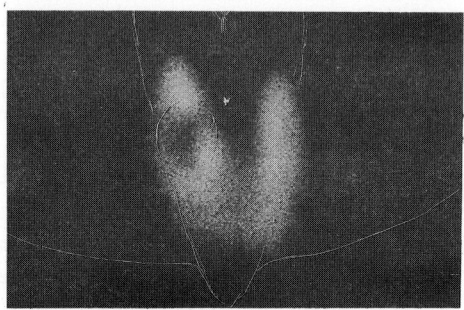

Figure 1 : Scintigraphie au Tc 99m. Nodule froid à la jonction des 1/3 supérieur et moyen du lobe droit.

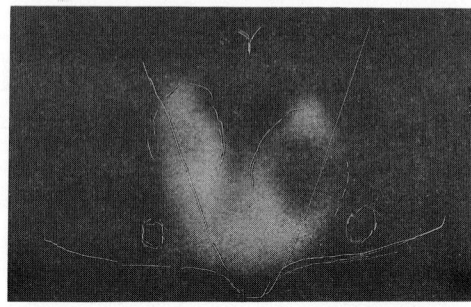

Figure 2 : Scintigraphie au Tc 99m. Nodule froid bilatéral et ganglions sus claviculaires droit et gauche.

En **échographie**, le CMT apparait volontiers comme un nodule médiolobaire, hypoéchogène avec des mouchetures hyperéchogènes disséminées, souvent accompagné d'images ganglionnaires qui ont les mêmes caractères d'échostructure (Delisle, 1988) (Fig. 3 et 4), ces multiples foyers hyperéchogènes brillants, générateurs de cônes d'ombre correspondraient à des petites calcifications entourées de substance amyloïde. Ces aspects évocateurs ne sont cependant pas spécifiques.

Dans le cadre d'une enquête familiale l'échographie permet de visualiser des lésions de quelques millimètres, non palpables et n'apparaissant pas sur la scintigraphie (Fig. 5).

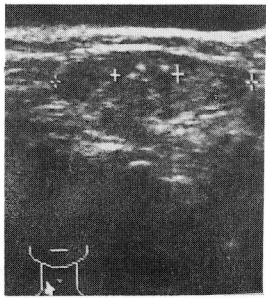

Figure 3 : Echographie latérocervicale droite. Coupe sagittale. Mouchetures hyperéchogènes.

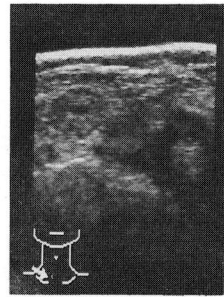

Figure 4 : Echographie sus-claviculaire droite. Envahissement ganglionnaire confirmé histologiquement.

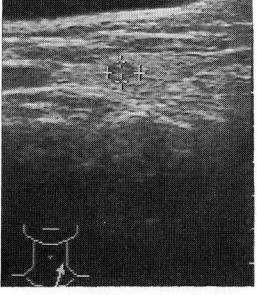

Figure 5 : Echographie cervicale gauche : coupe sagittale. Nodule hypoéchogène de 9 mm.

L'examen cytologique par ponction à l'aiguille fine orientée par l'échographie amène des indices importants en faveur du diagnostic en découvrant des cellules polygonales ou en fuseau avec un cytoplasme granuleux, qui expriment une réactivité aux études immunocytochimiques avec des anticorps anti-CT et anti-ACE (Geddie, 1984 ; Rastad, 1987) (Fig. 6).

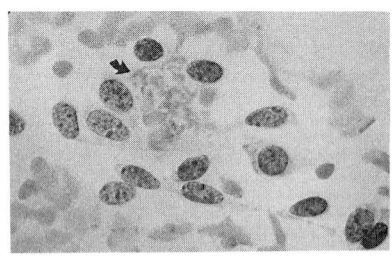

Figure 6 : Examen cytologique par ponction à l'aiguille fine sans aspiration.

L'un ou l'autre de ces éléments, à plus forte raison quand ils sont associés, justifie les dosages conjoints de la CT et de l'ACE qui conjuguent spécificité et sensibilité pour infirmer ou confirmer le diagnostic de CMT.

Il existe bien évidemment des aspects qui s'écartent de cette description : un petit CMT peut être, sur une scintigraphie, masqué par un nodule chaud (Fig. 7) ou associé à un autre nodule froid de localisation banale. Un CMT très évolué s'étend à tout le lobe et peut même en dépasser les limites (Fig. 8). En échographie, on peut observer des aspects kystisés (Mey, 1988) (Fig. 9). Enfin, le CMT n'échappe pas aux difficultés de prélèvements adéquats pour l'examen cytologique qui nécessite un nombre de cellules suffisant.

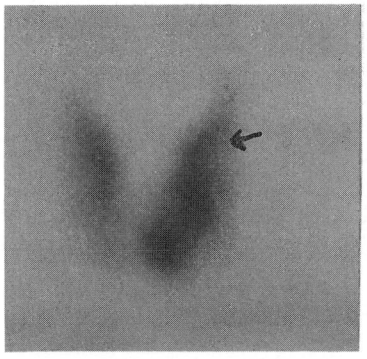

Figure 7 : Scintigraphie thyroïdienne à l'123I. Petit CMT de 15 mm dans un goitre multinodulaire, associé à 2 adénomes bénins du lobe gauche.

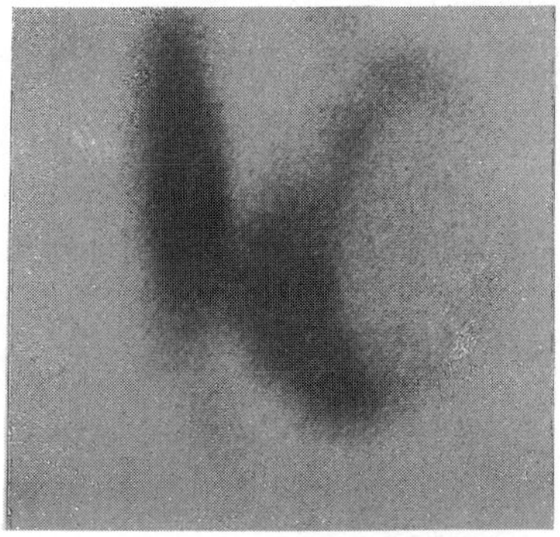

Figure 8 : Scintigraphie au 99m Tc. Volumineux CMT à extension extracapsulaire.

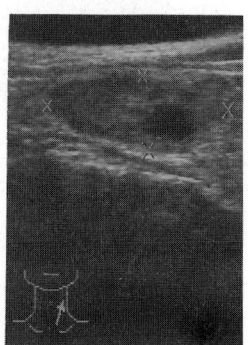

Figure 9 : Echographie cervicale. Coupe sagittale gauche. Volumineux CMT de 55 mm avec plage kystique.

IMAGERIE ET TRAITEMENT DU CMT

L'orientation par l'imagerie permet dans la presque totalité des cas de faire un diagnostic pré-opératoire avec des conséquences très appréciables à l'étape thérapeutique en autorisant la prise en charge du patient, puis éventuellement de sa famille, par une équipe spécialisée multidisciplinaire. Deux raisons majeures justifient cette attitude : le risque de phéochromocytome associé et la nécessité d'une chirurgie initiale thyroïdienne et ganglionnaire parfaite :

1. L'appartenance à une **néoplasie endocrinienne multiple de type II** doit être systématiquement envisagée avant tout acte chirurgical, la cure de l'anomalie surrénalienne étant recommandée avant l'exérèse du CMT. Outre l'étude des catécholamines plasmatiques et urinaires, le bilan comportera un bilan morphologique surrénalien, échographie, scanner et au moindre doute, scintigraphie à la MIBG qui permet une étude du corps entier (Fig. 10).

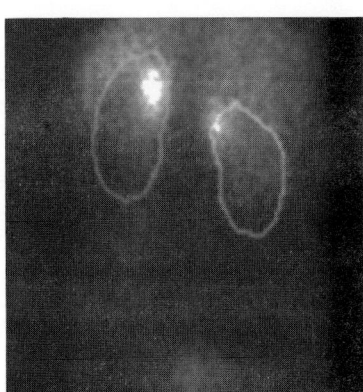

Figure 10 : Phéochromocytome bilatéral asymptomatique découvert par le bilan endocrinien préopératoire d'un CMT, dépisté par une enquête familiale.

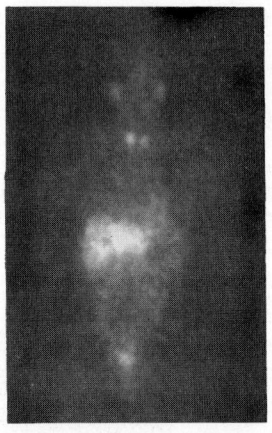

On peut profiter de l'injection de ce traceur très spécifique pour étudier sa fixation sur le CMT bien qu'elle soit inconstante et souvent peu intense (Fig. 11). L'imagerie, orientée par le bilan phosphocalcique peut objectiver un adénome parathyroïdien dont l'exérèse supposera une attention particulière du chirurgien et de l'anatomo-pathologiste.

Figure 11 : Fixation de la MIBG-131I sur un CMT bilatéral dans le cadre d'un NEM II a (même patient que figure 10).

2. Au stade thérapeutique, l'imagerie est indispensable pour préciser l'extension locale et planifier une chirurgie réglée et rigoureuse qui constitue la meilleure chance de guérison, évitant les chirurgies dites de rattrapage, plus dangereuses et moins efficaces. Le choix de la thyroïdectomie totale dans tous les cas de CMT (Marmousez, 1990) s'est imposé mais l'importance de l'extension ganglionnaire est telle (Delisle, 1984) et donc la nécessité d'une chirurgie ganglionnaire minutieuse que le scanner cervico-médiastino-thoracique doit être réalisé systématiquement en pré-opératoire (Fig. 12). Il peut orienter le chirurgien vers une intervention cervicothoracique d'emblée avec, si nécessaire, une sternotomie (Sarrazin, 1990).

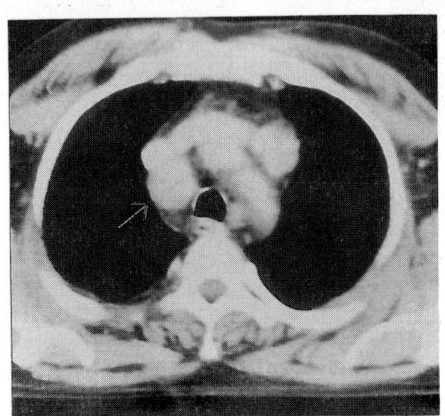

Figure 12 : Adénopathie hilaire droite métastatique ayant nécessité une cervicothoracotomie.

L'imagerie, en facilitant un diagnostic pré-opératoire, permet de mettre le malade dans les conditions optimales pour bénéficier d'un geste chirurgical curateur à l'abri du risque mortel que pourrait lui faire encourir un phéochromocytome méconnu.

IMAGERIE ET SURVEILLANCE DU CMT
Comme à l'étape diagnostique, le dosage de la calcitonine, couplé au dosage de l'antigène carcino-embryonnaire est l'élément fondamental de la surveillance post-opératoire. Son évolution dans le temps constitue le fil directeur de l'imagerie.

Si le **taux de CT reste indétectable à l'état basal et après stimulation par la pentagastrine** dans les jours puis les semaines qui suivent la thyroïdectomie totale, la guérison du malade est très probable. Il n'est besoin d'aucune exploration morphologique et on peut se contenter d'une surveillance clinique et surtout biologique.

Si le **taux de CT est détectable et évolutif**, la maladie n'est pas éradiquée même en l'absence de tout signe clinique. En effet, le marqueur tumoral étant très sensible, l'anomalie biologique peut précéder de plusieurs mois les anomalies de l'imagerie qui précèdent elles-mêmes le plus souvent les données cliniques pendant de longues périodes totalement asymptomatiques. Il est donc nécessaire de **traquer le tissu tumoral sécrétant** au niveau des récidives cervicales et des métastases à distance par toutes les modalités possibles de l'imagerie. Il est nécessaire de respecter une démarche logique mettant en oeuvre progressivement et selon une stratégie réfléchie des méthodes des plus simples et non invasives aux plus agressives et coûteuses. Le but est de découvrir récidives et métastases au stade le plus précoce possible pour envisager la thérapeutique la mieux adaptée à chaque localisation, chirurgie chaque fois que cela est possible, irradiation externe ou chimiothérapie.

L'échographie à fréquence élevée permet l'étude de la loge thyroïdienne et des aires ganglionnaires adjacentes à la recherche d'une récidive dans le lit de la thyroïdectomie ou au niveau d'un ganglion (Fig. 13, Fig. 14). Elle constitue la méthode la plus simple d'analyse du parenchyme hépatique (Fig. 15) (Gorman, 1987 ; Schverk, 1985). Comme au niveau de la tumeur primitive, les métastases cervicales ou hépatiques du CMT peuvent se présenter sous la forme de petits foyers hyperéchogènes. D'un coût modéré et non agressive, elle doit être la première investigation après l'examen clinique. Elle permet en outre la réalisation d'examens cytologiques par ponction guidée et donc la confirmation étiologique.

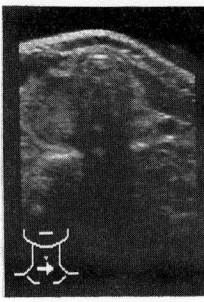
Figure 13 : Récidive latérocervicale droite.

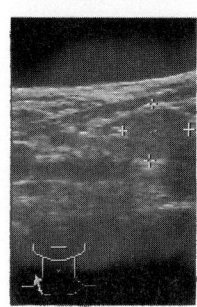
Figure 14 : Récidive ganglionnaire sus-claviculaire droite nécessitant une reprise chirurgicale.

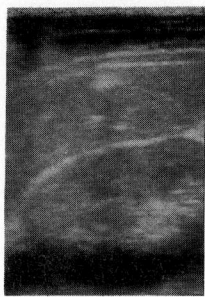
Figure 15 : Echographie hépatique avec foyers hyperéchogèniques durant la surveillance post-opératoire d'un patient à CT détectable.

L'étude tomodensitométrique est indispensable pour découvrir des lésions à un stade où elles ne sont pas encore visibles sur les clichés en radiologie conventionnelle. Le scanner cervico-médiastino-thoracique analyse le cou mais surtout le médiastin, le parenchyme pulmonaire, les plèvres et le squelette thoracique vertébrocostal. Le foie mérite un scanner en coupes fines à la recherche de petites calcifications multiples au sein des métastases (Bankoff, 1987 ; Mc Donnell III, 1986).

Les **techniques scintigraphiques** en acquisitions planes et si besoin tomographiques, centrées sur une région d'intérêt ou en balayage corps entier se prêtent particulièrement aux recherches de localisations cancéreuses à un stade infraclinique à condition de pouvoir disposer d'un traceur spécifique de la pathologie en cause. Depuis longtemps, les métastases osseuses et hépatiques du CMT ont pu être visualisées par les méthodes scintigraphiques classiques utilisant un traceur ostéotrope et les colloïdes radioactifs donc sans aucune spécificité (Johnson, 1984). La découverte d'une métastase osseuse à un stade précoce permet cependant, après éventuelle confirmation biopsique, l'application d'une irradiation externe à dose curative, si l'exérèse chirurgicale n'est pas réalisable. Les possibilités thérapeutiques sont moins évidentes quand il s'agit de métastases hépatiques que les tomoscintigraphies peuvent déceler en situation profonde et de petites tailles. Il a été rapporté l'accumulation d'un traceur technétié ostéotrope dans les métastases extraosseuses d'un CMT mais ces constatations restent anecdotiques (Shigeno, 1982).

Depuis quelques années, les travaux se sont concentrés sur quelques **molécules marquées susceptibles de se fixer de façon suffisante sur le tissu tumoral dérivant des cellules C** pour pouvoir passer d'un stade expérimental à une utilisation en routine.

- Le **Thallium 201**, peu utile au stade diagnostique, s'avère intéressant dans l'étude de la maladie résiduelle au niveau du cou, justifiant une ré-intervention (Fig. 16), ou à distance (Talpos, 1985 ; Arnstein, 1986 ; Hoefnagel, 1988).

- Le DMSA Tc 99m pentavalent proposé dès 1984 par le groupe de l'université de Kyoto a ses partisans (Clarke, 1987 et 1988 ; Guerra, 1989 ; Udelsman, 1989) et ses détracteurs (Hilditch, 1986). Le mécanisme de captation n'est pas parfaitement élucidé et l'utilisation est délicate car il est indispensable d'utiliser la forme pentavalente et non la forme trivalente des explorations isotopiques rénales. Les résultats publiés par les auteurs qui maîtrisent cette préparation sont intéressants mais rares sont les équipes en particulier françaises qui ont développé la méthode (Fig. 17, Fig. 18).

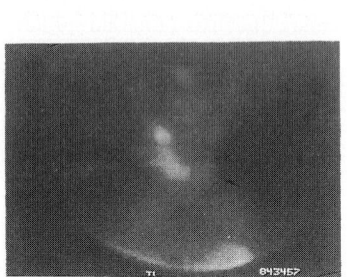 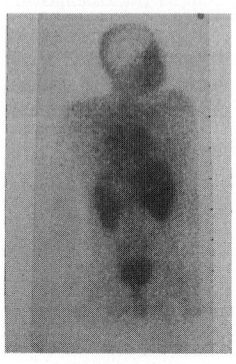 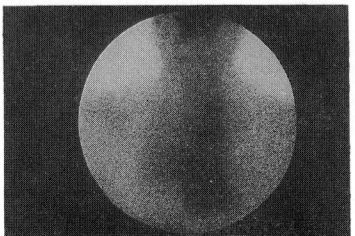

Figure 16 : Adénopathies cervicales au Tl 201. Dr J.L. BAULIEU, CHU TOURS.

Figure 17 : Adénopathies médiastinales DMSA 99mTc(V). Dr LUCOT, CAC TOULOUSE.

Figure 18 : Adénopathies cervico-médiastinales DMSA 99mTc(V). Dr J.L. BAULIEU, CHU TOURS.

- La méta-iodo-benzyl-guanidine marquée à l'iode 131 (131I MIBG) ou l'iode 123 (123I MIBG) accumulée dans les vésicules de stockage des cellules chromaffines est un marqueur potentiel de toutes les tumeurs qui dérivent du système APUD, sa captation par la tumeur thyroïdienne à calcitonine est inconstante et peu intense. Une étude française coopérative a démontré (Baulieu, 1987) qu'outre la visualisation du phéochromocytome avant la chirurgie, elle peut aider à localiser les récurrences et les métastases (Fig. 19, Fig. 20), tout particulièrement dans les formes familiales.

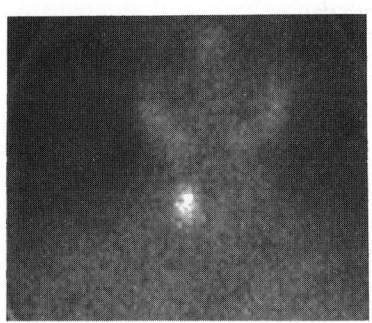 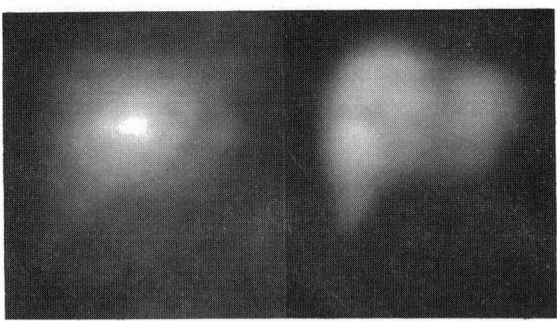

Figure 19 : Récidive cervicale droite avec fixation de la MIBG 131I.

Figure 20 : Fixation de la MIBG 131I au niveau d'une métastase hépatique.

L'évaluation de l'intensité de la captation peut être la première étape d'une utilisation thérapeutique encore limitée et à visée palliative. Les résultats des diverses séries affichent une très haute spécificité de la MIBG mais une sensibilité qui ne dépasse pas 30 à 40 % (Hoefnagel, 1988 ; Guerra, 1989 ; Troncone, 1988 et 1990). La scintigraphie à la MIBG devrait donc être réservée aux malades qui pourraient bénéficier d'une administration thérapeutique.

- **Les anticorps monoclonaux anti-ACE et anti-CT** ont un intérêt théorique incontestable. Les résultats sont encore préliminaires et de nombreux problèmes doivent être résolus (Lumbroso, 1983 ; Manil, 1989 ; Vuillez, 1990 ; Sandrock, 1990) (Fig. 21) avant d'envisager une large utilisation. Si les résultats sont probants, les anticorps monoclonaux pourraient devenir les vecteurs d'une immunoradiothérapie. Les possibilités de la détection scintigraphique en double spectrométrie permet de situer les foyers fixants la MIBG ou les anticorps marqués par rapport à des repères anatomiques osseux, hépatiques ou rénaux.

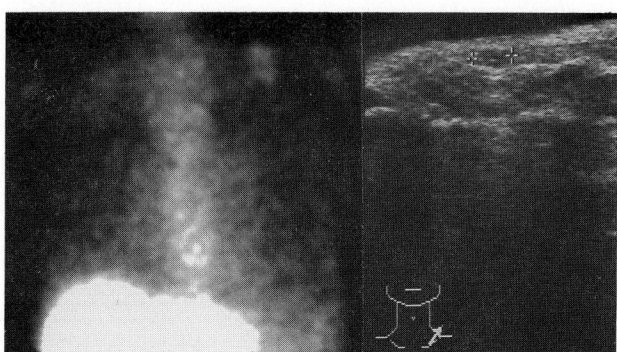

Figure 21 : Adénopathie cervicale découverte par l'immunoscintigraphie aux anticorps monoclonaux anti-ACE, confirmée secondairement par une échographie et un scanner, vérifiée par biopsie et examen histologique.

L'imagerie "multimodalités" trouve sa pleine expression dans les superpositions d'images, par exemple superposition d'une métastase signalée par une fixation sur la coupe tomodensitométrique correspondante (Fig. 22).

- **L'image par résonance magnétique nucléaire** est la méthode la plus fine pour l'étude des localisations nerveuses et vertébrales. Pour les autres sites, cette technique peut suppléer aux insuffisances des précédents explorations sur des dossiers sélectionnés. Enfin, la recherche des sites, sécrétant la calcitonine par la mise en évidence de gradients de concentration par le cathétérisme veineux étagé est la méthode la plus sophistiquée et la plus invasive. Elle sort du cadre de l'imagerie.

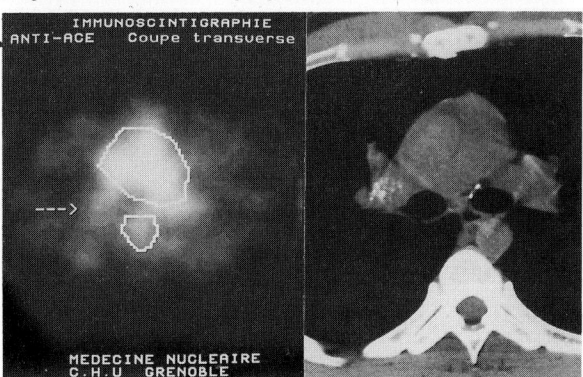

Figure 22 : Récidive médiastinale d'un CMT. Coupe immunoscintigraphique transversale (repérage activité vasculaire et osseuse) : foyer rétrocardiaque des anticorps anti-ACE F(ab')2 marqué à l'Indium 111. Coupe tomodensitométrique correspondante : opacité rétrocardiaque avec image de microcalcifications.

RESUME

Les dosages plasmatiques de CT et l'examen histologique sont les éléments clés du diagnostic et de la surveillance des CMT mais l'imagerie dans ses différentes modalités reste indispensable à tous les stades. La mise en évidence de signes évocateurs scintigraphiques, échographiques et cytologiques permettent de définir une population à risque. Cette orientation autorise un diagnostic préopératoire et donc la prise en charge par une équipe multidisciplinaire spécialisée pour la recherche et l'exérèse d'un phéochromocytome associé et la réalisation d'une chirurgie thyroïdienne et ganglionnaire d'emblée la plus complète possible. Si le taux de CT reste détectable durant la surveillance, il faut traquer le tissu secrétant par toutes les méthodes d'imagerie selon une stratégie raisonnée, la moins agressive et la moins coûteuse possible : échographie cervicale et abdominale, tomodensitométrie, scintigraphies avec différents traceurs, IRM, ceci dans le but de détecter les récidives et les métastases le plus tôt possible afin de leur opposer une thérapeutique adaptée.

REFERENCES

Arnstein, N.B., Juni, J.E. et al (1986): Recurrent MCT Demonstrated by Thallium-201 Scintigraphy. J Nucl Med 27,1564-1568.

Bankoff, M.S., Tuckman, G.A. et al (1987): CT Appearance of Liver Metastases from MCT. J Comput Assist Tomogr 11,1102-1103

Baulieu, J.L., Guilloteau, D. et al (1984): Imagerie du cancer médullaire de la thyroïde. Bull. Cancer 71,182-187

Baulieu, J.L., Guilloteau, D. et al (1987): Radioiodinated Meta-Iodobenzylguanidine Uptake in Medullary Thyroid Cancer. A French Cooperative Study. Cancer 60,2189-2194

Clarke, S., Lazarus, C. et al (1987): The role of technetium-99m pentavalent DMSA in the management of patients with medullary carcinoma of the thyroid. The British Journal of Radiology 60,1089-1092

Clarke, S., Lazarus, C. et al (1988): Pentavalent (99m Tc)DMSA, (131I)MIBG, and (99m Tc)MDP-An Evaluation of Three Imaging Techniques in Patients with Medullary Carcinoma of the Thyroid. J Nucl Med 29,33-38

Delisle, M.J. (1988): Circonstances diagnostiques, moyens thérapeutiques et surveillance au long cours des CMT. Ann Endocrinol 49,51-60

Delisle, M.J., Gardet, P. et al (1984): Les signes cliniques des CMT. Bull Cancer 71,165-171

Duh, Q.Y., Sancho, J.J. et al (1989): MCT. The Need for Early Diagnosis and Total Thyroidectomy. Arch Surg 124,1206-1210.

Edington, H.D., Watson, C.G. et al (1988): Radioimmunoimaging of metastatic MCT using an indium-111-labeled monoclonal antibody to CEA. Surgery 104,1004-1010

Geddie, W.R., Bedard, Y.C. et al (1984): MCT in Fine-needle Aspiration Biopsies. Am J Clin Pathol 82,552-558

Gorman, B., Charboneau, J.W. et al (1987): MCT : Role of High-Resolution US[1]. Radiology 162,147-150

Guerra, U., Pizzocaro, C. et al (1988): The use of 99mTc(V)DMSA as imaging for MTC. J Nucl Med Allied Sci 32,242-247

Guerra, U.P., Pizzocaro, C. et al (1989): New tracers for the imaging of the MCT. Nucl Med Comm 10,285-295

Hilditch, T.E., Connell, J.M.C. et al (1986): Poor Results with Technetium-99m (V) DMS and Iodine-131 MIBG in the Imaging of MCT. J Nucl Med 27,1150-1153

Hoefnagel, C.A., Delprat, C.C. et al (1988): New Radionuclide Tracers for the Diagnosis and Therapy of MCT. Clin Nucl Med 13,159-165

Johnson, D.G., Coleman, R.E. et al (1984): Bone and liver images in MCT : concise communication. J Nucl Med 25,419

Lumbroso, J., Berche, C. et al (1983): Utilisation en tomoscintigraphie d'anticorps monoclonaux radio-marqués pour la détection chez l'homme des cancers digestifs et des CMT. Bull Cancer 70,96

Manil, L., Boudet, F. et al (1989): Positive Anticalcitonin Immunoscintigraphy in Patients with MCT. Cancer Research 49,5480-5485

Marmousez, T., Mellière, D. et al (1990): Actualisation de la prise en charge chirurgicale des CMT. Lyon Chir.86/2

McDonnell III, C.H., Fishman, E.K. et al (1986): CT Demonstration of Calcified Liver Metastases in Medullary Carcinoma. J Comput Assist Tomogr 10,976-978

Mey, P., Minier, J.F. et al (1988): Aspect inhabituel du CMT : deux observations. La Presse Médicale 17,1364

Mojiminiyi, O.A., Udelsman, R. et al (1990): Clinical application fo 99mTc(V)DMSA scintigraphy in patients with MCT. Eur J Nucl Med 16, 406

Ohta, H., Endo, K. et al (1984): A new imaging agent for MCT. J Nucl Med 25,323

Rastad, J., Wilander, E. et al (1987): Cytologic Diagnosis of a MCT by Sevier-Munger Silver Staining and Calcitonin Immunocytochemistry. Acta Cytologica 31,45-47

Sandler, M.P., Patton, J.A. et al (1989): Multimodality imaging of the thyroid gland. Baillière's Clinical Endocrinology and Metabolism 3,89-119

Sandrock, D., Steinröder, M. et al (1990): Scintigraphy with different methods in patients with MCT. Eur J Nucl Med 16,406

Sarrazin, R., Roux, J.F. et al (1990): Curage cervico-médiastinal dans les CMT. Lyon Chir. 86/2

Schwerk, W.B., Grün, R. et al (1985): Ultrasound Diagnosis of C-Cell Carcinoma of the Thyroid. Cancer 55,624-630

Shigeno, C., Fukunaga, M.et al (1982): Accumulation of Tc-99m phosphorus compounds in MCT : report of 2 cases. Clin Nucl Med 7,297

Talpos, G.B., Jackson, C.E. et al (1985): Localization of residual MCT by thallium/technetium scintigraphy. Surgery 98,1189-1196

Troncone, L., Rufini, V. et al (1988): The possible use of radioiodinated metaiodobenzylguanidine (MIBG) in MCT. Thyroidology 1,45-53

Trocone, L., Rufini, V. et al (1990): The diagnostic and therapeutic utility of radioiodinated metaiodobenzylguanidine (MIBG) ; 5 years of experience. Eur J Nucl Med 16, 325-335

Udelsman, R., Mojiminiyi, O.A. et al (1989): MCT : management of persistent hypercalcitonaemia utilizing 99mTc (V) dimercaptosuccinic acid scintigraphy. Br J Surg 76,1278-1281

Vuillez, J.Ph., Peltier, P. et al (1990): Immunoscintigraphy (IS) uding In 111-labeled anti CEA monoclonal antibody (MAb) F(AB')2 fragments for detection of medullary thyroid carcinoma (MTC). Eur J Nucl Med 16,406

Nuclear medicine techniques for imaging medullary thyroid carcinoma (MTC)

Susan E.M. Clarke

Department of nuclear medicine, Guy's Hospital, London, United Kingdom

SUMMARY

Various radionuclide techniques have been developed over the past few years that are contributing to the management of patients with MTC. The recent developments include the use of 201Thallium, 123I and 131I Metaiodo benzylguanidine (MIBG) and 99mTechnetium v Dimercaptosuccinic Acid (DMSA). The use of these techniques in primary diagnosis and follow up is becoming established as well as the already established non-specific nuclear techniques for imaging bone, brain and liver metastases.

201 Thallium has been extensively investigated and sensitivities of detection of recurrent disease upto 90% have been reported. Unfortunately, poor imaging characteristics, high whole body radiation doses (24 mSv) and relative expense make this radiopharmaceutical less than ideal.

123I and 131I MIBG have also been used to detect both primary and recurrent disease but the sensitivity of detection of tumour even when tomographic imaging is used with 123I MIBG is only 40%. In those patients whose tumours take up MIBG, however, therapy becomes an option.

99mTechnetium v DMSA has also been used to image both primary and recurrent disease. Sensitivities of tumour detection of 80% are being achieved but it is evident that the method of preparation of this radiopharmaceutical is critical and some poor results have been reported and may well be due to low levels of Pentavalent DMSA in the final preparation. Work is at present being undertaken to determine the sensitivities of the various 99mTechnetium v DMSA preparations that are now commercially available. With high levels of 99mTechnetium v DMSA in the prepared radiopharmaceutical, excellent quality images can be obtained with a radiation dose of 8 mSv.

It is surprising, given the rarity of MTC, that so much radiopharmaceutical research is at present being undertaken. Radionuclide techniques at present provide a cost effective method of investigating patients with MTC particularly those in whom calcitonin levels start to rise following removal of the primary tumour.

Pheochromocytoma detection

Dépistage du phéochromocytome

Biochemical tests for phaeochromocytoma : diagnostic yield of the determination of urinary metanephrines, plasma cathecholamines and plasma neuropeptide Y

Pierre-François Plouin[1], Gilles Chatellier[1], Eliane Billaud[2], Eric Grouzmann[3], Etienne Comoy[4] and Pierre Corvol[1]

Département d'Hypertension et INSERM U 36[1], département de Pharmacologie et INSERM U194[2], Hôpital Broussais, Paris, France. Division d'Hypertension[3], CHUV, Lausanne, Switzerland. Laboratoire de Biologie Clinique[4], Institut Gustave-Roussy, Villejuif, France

Phaeochromocytoma (PH) is a rare and potentially lethal disease. Although its most frequent expression is hypertension, either paroxysmal or sustained, PH is present in less than one per 1.000 hypertensive patients. However, since hypertension is a common condition, biochemical screening for PH using specific costly biochemical tests is not practicable in unselected hypertensive patients. Our strategy for diagnosing PH is therefore a stepwise approach that includes 1) Clinical screening of a subgroup of patients considered to be at high risk of PH, 2) biochemical tests for these patients, and 3) localization procedures for those with positive biochemical tests only. This paper will focus on the management of the screening and biochemical tests.

PATIENTS AND METHODS

PH was diagnosed and surgically confirmed in 109 of the 26.262 consecutive patients referred to the Broussais-Saint Joseph Hypertension Clinic from 1976 to 1989. This prevalence of 0.42% probably overestimates the true prevalence of PH, as the disease is conceivably more frequent in patients referred to a specialized clinic than among the general hypertensive population. Among these 109 cases, PH was malignant in 15 (14%), ectopic in 17 (16%), combined with phakomatosis in 9 (8%), or with multiple endocrine neoplasia type 2 (MEN 2) in 7 (6%).

The methods of detection and diagnosis used in our Clinic have been described elsewhere (Grouzmann et al., 1989, Plouin et al., 1981a, 1981b, Trouvin & Billaud-Mesguich, 1987). Briefly, for each hypertensive patient, the circumstances of the diagnosis of hypertension, and its symptoms and signs, including recumbent and orthostatic pulse rate and blood pressure (BP), were noted in a computerized record. Total urinary metanephrines (MN) were determined for each patient suspected to have PH. In addition, the levels of plasma cathecholamines (CA) and neuropeptide Y (NPY) were measured in the routine work-up of PH suspects or carriers in 1980 and 1985 respectively. To assess the value of each of these techniques of detection or diagnosis, we compared the results obtained in suitably matched groups of PH carriers and subjects with essential hypertension.

SCREENING CRITERIA

An effective screening test should be sensitive (especially when the disease is severe) and specific (especially when it is rare), involve no risk for the patient, and be easily available and inexpensive. With these objectives in mind, we tested the diagnostic usefulness of detecting symptoms and signs frequently associated with PH. Among a population of 2.585 hypertensive subjects, the presence of the symptomatic triad comprising sweating, headaches and palpitations enabled a group of 170 hypertensive PH suspects to be singled out; we found that the sensitivity and specificity of this triad for detection of PH were respectively 91 and 92%, whereas the permanent or paroxysmal character of hypertension (i.e. whether or not BP was always over 160/95 mmHg) had no diagnostic value (Plouin et al., 1981a). We also assessed this value for orthostatic hypotension (difference of more than 10 mmHg between systolic BP in the recumbent and standing positions) by comparing 39 PH carriers to 21 patients with essential hypertension (Plouin et al., 1988). Orthostatic hypotension measurement lacked sensitivity, although its specificity was excellent (95%) when the symptomatic triad was present.

These results indicate that biochemical tests for PH are especially useful in hypertensive subjects who complain of sweating, headaches and palpitations, particularly when combined with orthostatic hypotension. Other signs and symptoms might be useful for PH detection, although their diagnostic value has not been quantitatively assessed. This applies, for instance, to refractory hypertension or to rare conditions associated with a high prevalence of PH, such as Von Recklinhausen and Von Hippel-Lindau phakomatoses and MEN 2.

BIOCHEMICAL DIAGNOSIS

Urinary determinations

High CA levels in the urine of patients with PH were reported in 1950 by Engel & von Euler. However, measurement of CA was soon supplanted by that of their chief metabolites - vanillymandelate acid (VMA) and MN - which are more abundant and easier to measure. VMA measurement has become the routine test for PH detection because of its relative simplicity, but it lacks specificity, as the presence of an aromatic nucleus in various foods or drugs entails the risk of false positives. Hamilton et al. (1978) claimed that an increase in the urinary adrenaline fraction was a characteristic feature of the PH associated with MEN 2, and that measurement of this fraction was a reliable and sensitive screening test in afflicted families. Their result was obtained from 7 members of the same family but the values for MN excretion were not reported. In 9 patients with PH combined with MEN 2, whose urinary CA and MN had been measured, Carney et al. (1976) found 6 false negatives for CA and 1 for MN. Measurement of MN excretion is generally acknowledged to be a better test than urinary CA measurement (Manu & Runge, 1984), one possible reason being that in PH, metanephrines are directly secreted by the tumour (Crout & Sjoerdsma, 1964). As many PH tumours exhibit methylating activity, MN constitute both a tumour marker and a marker of plasma conversion of CA to MN. The Table shows the mean values for urinary VMA, CA and MN determined during the same 24-hour period in 39 patients with PH and in 21 essential hypertensive patients, and demonstrates that MN determination is the most sensitive.

Interpretation of urinary determinations must allow for BP; if the latter is high and the results, normal, the possibility that PH is responsible for the high BP may be ruled out. On the other hand, if BP and MN levels are normal, it is impossible to say definitely whether or not PH is present, since it might be in a quiescent phase. In such cases, urinary CA must be measured within three hours of a surge of high BP. For this purpose, the patient should be supplied with a jar containing one ml of hydrochloric acid, and with instructions to empty the bladder and discard the urine at the very beginning of the paroxysmal episode and to collect the urine three hours later. According to

Engelman (1977), normal CA excretion during a period of high BP means that PH cannot be present, and conversely, CA levels are enormously high when PH is present. Note that measurement of MN or VMA would not be suitable for this type of test because of the latency connected with their metabolic conversion from CA.

Measurement of plasma CA

The major limitation for the measurement of plasma CA arises from the intermittent secretion exhibited by certain PH tumours. This variable secretion, combined with the brief half-life of CA, explains why a single measurement of the latter may be negative if blood is sampled during the intervals between surges of high BP (Jones et al., 1980, Plouin et al., 1981). Conversely, stress raises plasma CA in a non-specific fashion (Bravo & Gifford, 1984). These elements explain why the sensitivity and specificity of plasma CA measurement are limited for purposes of diagnosis, despite the high specificity of such measurement on the biochemical level. The Table shows the mean values for urinary MN and plasma CA in 30 patients with PH and 35 with essential hypertension. Mean levels of MN, noradrenaline and adrenaline were more than ten times higher in the patients with PH than in those with essential hypertension, but individual plasma CA levels were extremely scattered, and included normal levels in several patients. Determination of urinary MN was therefore more sensitive than that of plasma CA.

Plasma CA determination should be confined firstly, to patients who are hypertensive at the time of sampling, which avoids the risk of false negative results in cases of intermittently secreting PH (Plouin et al, 1981), and secondly, to the interpretation of the clonidine suppression test, since the latter enables false positive results due to stress to be disregarded (Bravo & Gifford, 1984).

Table. Means ± 1 standard deviation and sensitivity for diagnosis of phaeochromocytoma of the measurement of catecholamines (CA) and their metabolites, vanillyl-mandelic acid (VMA) and metanephrines (MN).

		patients with phaeochromocytoma	essential hypertensives	sensitivity %
Urinary determinations				
n=		39	21	
VMA	μmol/24h	110.5±71.7	19.7±6.10	76
CA	μmol/24h	13.4±24.5	0.43±0.13	89
MN	μmol/24h	33.8±29.4	1.66±0.71	98
Plasma CA vs urinary MN				
n=		30	35	
Adrenaline	nmol/l	6.8±16.6	0.58±0.43	40
Noradrenaline	nmol/l	27.4±45.9	1.29±0.67	80
MN	μmol/24h	36.0±35.6	2.05±0.87	100

Pharmacological tests

Pharmacological provocative tests are designed to improve the sensitivity of basal determinations of CA or CA metabolites, and suppression tests, to improve their specificity. Provocative tests are useless when PH is combined with permanent hypertension, because in such cases basal urine tests are always positive (Engelman, 1977). They might be useful to identify small PH or adrenal medullary hyperplasia in normotensive patients with MEN 2 whose basal plasma CA levels and urine MN excretion are normal. Unfortunately, however, provocative tests have proved disappointing for this indication. Thus, among 6 patients with MEN 2 and PH who had had MN determinations and various provocative tests, Carney et al. (1976) reported one false negative result for MN determination, 2/4 for the histamine provocative test and 4/4 for the glucagon provocative test. Hamilton et al. (1978) reported a false negative glucagon test in 7 patients of the same kindred with MEN 2 and PH.

Suppressor tests are designed to improve the specificity of basal determinations, and especially to avoid false positive tests due to stress. The best standardized test is the clonidine test, which is indicated in hypertension with high CA levels when there is doubt as to whether the abnormality is of adrenal or sympathetic origin (Bravo & Gifford, 1984). However, false positive or false negative results have been reported (Taylor et al, 1986), and the specificity of the clonidine suppression test is in fact limited when patients have intermittently secreting PH (Plouin et al., 1985, Elliot & Murphy, 1988).

Other markers for PH

Storage vesicles in the adrenal medulla contain a number of enzymes and proteins in addition to CA, including chromogranins A and B, and NPY. As the mechanism of CA release from PH is partly exocytotic, measurement of these proteins in circulating blood may provide a useful PH marker. Preliminary studies (Corder et al., 1986) have shown that, in half the PH tumours investigated, plasma NPY was abnormally high, as was circulating chromogranin A in 12 out of 15 patients with PH studied in another investigation (O'Connor & Deftos, 1986). The clinical usefulness of these PH markers should be determined by comparing it with that of CA and CA metabolites. Here, we measured the concentrations of plasma NPY, adrenaline and noradrenaline as well as urinary MN excretion in 34 patients with PH, and found that the sensitivities of NPY, adrenaline, noradrenaline, and MN determination were 41, 41, 76 et 100 % respectively (Plouin & Grouzmann, unpublished data) (Figure).

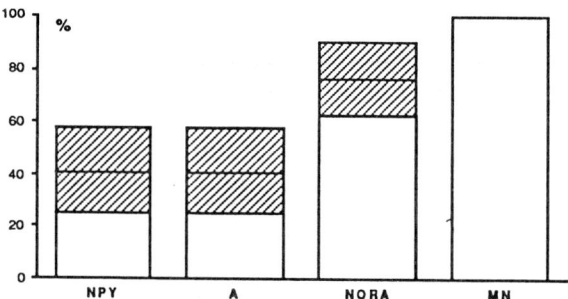

Figure. Sensitivities of neuropeptide Y (NPY), Adrenaline (A), Noradrenaline (NorA), and metanephrines (MN) determination in 34 patients with pheochromocytoma. Hatched bars are 95% confidence intervals

SUMMARY AND CONCLUSION

Isolation of suspected cases of phaeochromocytoma (PH) from a population of hypertensive subjects is based on the presence of the symptomatic triad combining sweating, headaches and palpitations, particularly in patients with systolic orthostatic hypotension. Biochemical investigations for PH should be confined to patients meeting these criteria, to those with severe hypertension resistant to treatment, and those with multiple endocrine neoplasia type 2, phakomatosis or familial PH. Positive diagnosis of PH is chiefly based on the measurement of urinary metanephrines (MN), as this test is more sensitive than measurement of urinary catecholamines (CA) or vanillymandelate acid or the determination of plasma CA or neuropeptide Y. If the patient is hypertensive at the time of urinary MN measurement, pathological or normal excretion will confirm or refute the diagnosis of PH. If hypertension is paroxysmal and MN are measured during a period of normotension, pathological excretion will confirm the diagnosis, but normal excretion will not enable it to be refuted. In such cases, urinary CA should be measured during the hours following paroxysmal manifestations. In view of the availability of accurate urinary assays, there is little need to subject patients to the hazard of provocative pharmacological tests.

REFERENCES

Bravo, E.L. & Gifford, R.W. (1984): Pheochromocytoma: diagnosis, localization and management. *N. Engl. J. Med.* 311, 1298-1303.
Carney, J.A., Sizemore, G.W. & Sheps, S.G. (1976): Adrenal medullary disease in multiple endocrine neoplasia, type II: pheochromocytoma and its precursors. Am. J. Clin. Path. 66, 279-90.
Corder, R., Shapiro, H., Lowry, P.J. et al. (1986): Relationship between tumour and plasma concentrations of neuropeptide Y in patients with adrenal medullary phaeochromocytoma. *J. Hypertension* 4 (suppl 6), 193-5.
Crout, R. & Sjoerdsma, A. (1964): Turnover and metabolism of catecholamines in patients with pheochromocytoma. *J. Clin. Invest.* 43, 853-4.
Elliot, W.J. & Murphy, M.B. (1988): Reduced specificity of the clonidine suppression test in patients with normal catecholamine levels. *Am. J. Med.* 84, 419-24.
Engel, A. & von Euler, U.S. (1950): Diagnostic value of increased urinary output of adrenaline and noradrenaline in phaeochromocytoma. *Lancet* 2, 387.
Engelman, K. (1977): Pheochromocytoma. *Clin. Endocr. Metab.* 6, 769-97.
Grouzmann, E., Comoy, E. & Bohuon, C. (1989): Plasma neuropeptide Y concentrations in patients with neuroendocrine tumors. *J. Clin. Endocrinol. Metab.* 68, 808-13.
Hamilton, B.P., Landsberg, L. & Levine, R.J. (1978): Measurement of urinary epinephrine in screening for pheochromocytoma in multiple endocrine neoplasia type II. *Am. J. Med.* 65, 1027-32.
Jones, D.H., Reid, J.L., Hamilton, C.A. et al. (1980): The biochemical diagnosis, localization and follow up of phaeochromocytoma: the role of plasma and urinary catecholamine measurements. *Quarterly J. Med.* 195, 341-61.
Manu, P. & Runge, L.A. (1984): Biochemical screening for pheochromocytoma: superiority of urinary metanephrine measurements. *Am. J. Epidemiol.* 120, 788-90.
Plouin, P.F., Degoulet, P., Tugayé, A., Ducrocq, M.B. & Ménard, J. (1981): Dépistage du phéochromocytome: Chez quels hypertendus ? Etude sémiologique chez 2585 hypertendus dont 11 ayant un phéochromocytome. *Nouv. Presse Med.* 10, 869-872.
Plouin, P.F., Duclos, J.M., Ménard, J. et al. (1981): Biochemical tests for diagnosis of phaeochromocytoma: urinary versus plasma determinations. *Br. Med. J.* 282, 853-854.
Plouin, P.F., Chatellier, G., Ménard, J. & Comoy, E. (1985): Diagnosis of pheochromocytoma. *N. Engl. J. Med.* 312, 721-2 (letter).
Plouin, P.F., Chatellier, G., Rougeot, M.A. et al. (1988): Recent developments in pheochromocytoma diagnosis and imaging. *Adv. Nephrol.* 17, 275-86.
Taylor, H.C., Mayes, D. & Anton, A.H. (1986): Clonidine suppression test for pheochromocytoma: examples of misleading results. *J. Clin. Endocrinol. Metab.* 63:238-42.
Trouvin, J.H. & Billaud-Mesguich E. (1987): Determination of urinary metanephrines in man using liquid chromatography with electro- chemical detection. *J. Liquid Chromatogr.* 10, 731-47.

Chromogranin A in pheochromocytoma[1]

H.P.H. Neumann[*], R.J. Hsiao[**], R.J. Parmer[**], J.A. Barbosa[**] and D.T. O'Connor[**]

[*] Department of Medicine, Albert-Ludwigs-University of Freiburg, Freiburg im Breisgau, Germany
[**] Department of Medicine, Veterans Administration Medical Center, San Diego, California, USA
[1] published in full length : Am. J. Med. (1990) 88, 607-613.

Summary

Chromogranin A, co-released with catecholamines from the adrenal medullary and sympathetic neuronal vesicles, is elevated in plasma from patients with pheochromocytoma. We assessed its diagnostic screening value in familial pheochromocytoma and sporadic pheochromocytoma. The sensitivity and specificity of Chromogranin A's diagnostic value for pheochromocytoma were established through one kindred with familial pheochromocytoma associated with von Hippel-Lindau syndrome (13 available members) and in seven subjects with sporadic pheochromocytoma. Chromogranin A was measured by radioimmunoassay based in purified pheochromocytoma Chromogranin A. In this kindred with six pheochromocytoma and ten non-pheochromocytoma patients and in seven sporadic pheochromocytomas and 45 controls, elevations of Chromogranin A (greater than 52 ng/mL) were sensitive (84 %) and specific (100 %) in detecting pheochromocytoma. These diagnostic values comparable to those achieved by conventional evaluations for pheochromocytoma, such as urinary catecholamines, urinary catecholamine metabolites or imaging methods. Elevated levels of plasma Chromogranin A specifically indicated pheochromocytoma, rather than von Hippel-Lindau syndrome gene carrier status. We conclude that plasma Chromogranin A is a valuable (sensitive and specific) diagnostic tool in detecting both familial and sporadic pheochromocytoma.

Introduction

Chromogranin A was originally described as the major soluble protein in the core of catecholamine storage vesicles of the adrenal medulla (SMITH & WINKLER 1967, SMITH & KIRSHNER 1967). Chromogranin A is now known to have a wide-spread neuroendocrine distribution, wherein it may be stored and released with various polypeptide hormones (O'CONNOR et al. 1983, COHN et. al. 1984). In 1984 O'CONNOR and BERNSTEIN described a radioimmunoassay for Chromogranin A. Subsequently Chromogranin A was found to be elevated in patients with pheochromocytoma and other peptide producing endocrine neoplasms (O'CONNOR & DEFTOS 1986). In this study we evaluated plasma or serum Chromogranin A concentration as a diagnostic tool for pheochromocytoma.

Subjects and Methods

Von Hippel-Lindau syndrome was diagnozed in descendants of one family in Freiburg. Members of the kindred manifest angiomatosis of the retina and pheochromocytoma but no other cysts or tumors. The screening program included assessment of blood pressure, heart rate, and neurologic status, ophthalmoscopic

examination, and performance of abdominal ultrasound and urinary catecholamine assay. Suggestive history, examination, laboratory values, or the finding of pheochromocytoma prompted special investigations, such as computed tomographic scanning of the abdomen, or MIBG scintigraphy of the adrenal glands.
To assess the sensitivity and specificity of Chromogranin A as a diagnostic tool in evaluating familial and sporadic pheochromocytoma, we obtained samples from the following groups: healthy adult control subjects (n=40; 10 men, 21 women); patients with essential hypertension (not members of families at risk for pheochromocytoma) in whom pheochromocytoma had been ruled out by negative findings on MIBG scintigraphy (n=22; 9 men, 13 women); preoperative subjects from the Freiburg area with sporadic pheochromocytoma (n=7); and the von Hippel-Lindau kindred. This kindred consists of 23 members in four genetations. Fourteen of these were evaluated for pheochromocytoma, and the concentration of Chromogranin A was measured in 13 of these: six preoperative subjects with pheochromocytoma, three of whom had both preoperative and postoperative plasma samples; two other subjects with a past history of pheochromocytoma resection and no recurrence; and five subjects without evidence of pheochromocytoma on history or examination.
Human Chromogranin A was isolated and charaterized from chromaffin granules of human pheochromocytomas, as previously described (O'CONNOR et al. 1984, O'CONNOR & DEFTOS 1986). Human Chromogranin A was measured by a rapid modification (O'CONNOR et al. 1989).
Concentrations of 24-hour urinary catecholamines (epinephrine and norepinephrine) were measured by spectrofluorometry while vanillylmandelic acid (VMA) was measured spectrophotometrically.

Results
Subjects with familial or sporadic pheochromocytoma did not differ in mean plasma Chromogranin A levels (affected familial n=6, 118 $\pm$ 26 ng/mL, sporadic affected n=7, 184 $\pm$ 46 ng/mL plasma Chromogranin A; p>0.1). Table I displays the sensitivity and specificity of these parameters as well as those of imaging methods in detecting familial and sporadic pheochromocytoma. In familial pheochromocytoma, Chromogranin A had a sensitivity of 83 % with a specificity of 100 % for the detection of pheochromocytoma, whereas in sporadic pheochromocytoma, the sensitivity was 86 % with a specificity of 100 %. Compared with other tests, Chromogranin A emerged as a useful diagnostic tool for evaluating pheochromocytoma.

Table I: Sensitivity and Specificity of Diagnostic Tests for Familial and Sporadic Pheochromocytoma

Test	Familial Pheochromocytoma Sensitivity	Specificity	Sporadic Pheochromocytoma Sensitivity	Specificity
Chromogranin A (normal 15-52 ng/ml)	83 % (5/6)	100 % (10/10)	86 % (6/7)	100 % (45/45)
Urinary norepinephrine (normal <124 µg/day)	80 % (4/5)	100 % (9/9)	100 % (7/7)	96 % (27/28)
Urinary epinephrine (normal <18.5 µg/day)	20 % (1/5)	100 % (9/9)	71 % (5/7)	93 % (26/28)
Urinary vanillylmandelic acid (normal <9.4 mg/day)	40 % (2/5)	100 % (7/7)	100 % (5/5)	100 % (20/20)
Ultrasound	100 % (5/5)	82 % (9/11)	86 % (6/7)	100 % (6/6)
Computerized tomography	100 % (5/5)		86 % (6/7)	100 % (2/2)
Magnetic resonance imaging	100 % (5/5)	0 % (0/1)	100 % (6/6)	50 % (1/2)
MIBG scintigraphy	100 % (5/5)	100 % (3/3)	86 % (6/7)	100 % (22/22)

In one known gene carrier who had only angiomatosis of the retina but not pheochromocytoma, the concentration of plasma Chromogranin A was within normal limits. In three other patients who had both pheochromocytoma and angiomatosis of the retina, the initial plasma Chromogranin A concentration was elevated, but then declined into the normal range after pheochromocytoma resection (mean, 25 ± 5 ng/mL). Thus, an elevation in the Chromogranin A concentration in a kindred member seems to specifically indicate pheochromocytoma, rather than positive gene carrier status.

Comments

Approximately 14 % of the gene carriers for von Hippel-Lindau syndrome develop pheochromocytoma (NEUMANN 1987). Since the appearance of pheochromocytoma at a young age in von Hippel-Lindau syndrome is associated with an increased incidence of multiple tumors and guarantees the gene-carrier status of such patients (SHARP & PLATT 1971), early and effective family screening for pheochromocytoma becomes all the more urgent to facilitate effective treatment and follow-up. We compared traditional measures such as urinary catecholamines and catecholamine metabolites with plasma Chromogranin A in evaluating pheochromocytoma in several subjects from one von Hippel-Lindau kindred, and we found that Chromogranin A had a sensitivity and specificity comparable to those of other diagnostic methods (Table I). Thus, Chromogranin A may be a useful diagnostic tool in the evaluation of suspected pheochromocytoma in the familial as well as the sporadic context. Because the concentration of plasma Chromogranin A declines into the normal range after pheochromocytoma resection in subjects with von Hippel-Lindau, and because subjects with angiomatosis of the retina without pheochromocytoma have normal plasma Chromogranin A concentrations, we further conclude that an elevation in the Chromogranin A concentration specifically indicates the presence of pheochromocytoma.

References

Cohn, D.V. et al. (1984): Selective localization of the parathyroid secretory protein - J adrenal medulla chromogranin A protein family in a wide variety of endocrine cells of the rat. Endocrinology 114, 1963-1974.

Neumann, H.P.H. (1987): Basic criteria for clinical diagnosis and genetic counselling in von Hippel-Lindau syndrome. Vasa 16, 220-226.

O'Connor, D.T., Bernstein K.N. (1984): Radioimmunoassay of chromogranin A in plasma as a measure of exocytotic sympathoadrenal activity in normal subjects and patients with pheochromocytoma. N. Engl. J. Med. 311, 764-770.

O'Connor, D.T. et al. (1983): Chromogranin A: Immunohistology reveals its universal occurrence in normal polypeptide hormone producing endocrine glands. Life Sci. 33, 1657-1663.

O'Connor, D.T., Deftos, L.J. (1986): Secretion of chromogranin A by peptide-producing endocrine neoplasms. N. Engl. J. Med. 314, 1145-1151.

O'Connor, D.T. et al. (1989): Rapid radioimmunoassay of circulating chromogranin A: in vitro stability, exploration of the neuroendocrine character of neoplasia, and assessment of the effects of organ failure. Clin. Chem. 35, 1631-1637.

Sharp, W.V., Platt, R.L. (1971): Familial pheochromocytoma, association with von Hippel-Lindau's disease. Angiology 22, 141-146.

Smith, W.J., Kirshner, N. (1967): A specific soluble protein from the catecholamine storage vesicles of bovine adrenal medulla. I. Purification and chemical characterization. Mol. Pharmacol. 3, 52-62.

Smith, A.D., Winkler, H. (1967): Purification and properties of an acidic protein from chromaffin granules of bovine adrenal medulla. Biochem. J. 103, 483-492.

Imagerie des phéochromocytomes

Jean-Louis Baulieu

Service de Médecine Nucléaire et Ultrasons, INSERM U 316, Hôpital Bretonneau, 37044 Tours, France

ABSTRACT :

Most of the pheochromocytomas associated with MTC (MEN II) develop from adrenomedullar hyperplasia. The current imaging procedures are non invasive and allow detection of tumors larger than 1 cm in diameter. Echotomography is easily performed in children. Scanner X and MRI provide regional anatomic studies. MRI provides tissue characterization by relaxation time T_2 measurement. MIBG scintiscan is a specific method for whole body imaging. MIBG uptake measuring in adrenal glands could indicate the presence of adrenomedullar hyperplasia. At the present time, pheochromocytoma imaging in MEN II takes advantage of complementarity and previous experience of scanner X and MIBG scintiscan.

Les techniques d'imagerie des phéochromocytomes ont considérablement évolué au cours des quinze dernières années, en se multipliant. Parallèlement s'est développée la notion d'hyperplasie des médullosurrénales, propre au syndrome de néoplasie endocrine multiple NEM (Delellis *et al.*, 1976). Ainsi se pose le problème du choix de la méthode ou de l'association de méthodes, la plus performante et la mieux adaptée.

MODALITES ET PERFORMANCES DES TECHNIQUES ACTUELLES

L'échotomographie des glandes surrénales est un examen simple facilement réalisable chez l'enfant. Les transducteurs habituellement utilisés ont une fréquence de 3,5 ou 5 MHz. L'exploration du côté gauche est parfois gênée par l'interposition de gaz intestinaux.

Les surrénales normales sont individualisables à droite dans près de 70% des cas et à gauche dans seulement 10% des cas (Päivänsalo *et al.*, 1988). Le phéochromocytome apparaît comme une échostructure bien circonscrite, d'échogénicité inférieure à celle du foie, souvent hétérogène en raison de remaniements nécrotiques.

La sensibilité de détection des tumeurs surrénaliennes en général d'un diamètre supérieur à 1cm, varie selon les auteurs de 82 à 97% (Chan & Wang, 1989). L'appartenance surrénalienne et la nature de la tumeur peuvent être difficiles à préciser.

L'atmosphère graisseuse péri-rénale est à l'origine d'un contraste spontané favorable à l'imagerie des glandes surrénales par la tomodensitométrie. Il n'est pas nécessaire d'injecter par voie veineuse de produit de contraste dont les risques sont connus en cas de phéochromocytome. L'exploration de l'abdomen à la recherche de localisations ectopiques peut être facilitée par

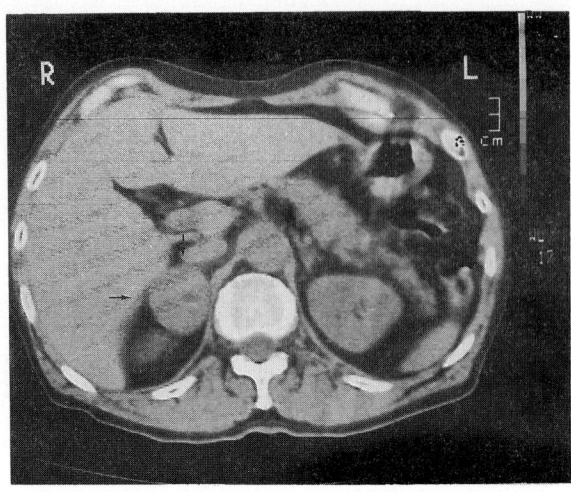

Fig. 1 : Phéochromocytome surrénalien droit (→) 3cm de diamètre. Tomodensitométrie. Présence de plages hypodenses témoignant de remaniements nécrotiques.

l'ingestion d'un produit de contraste digestif. Des coupes de 3 à 10 mm jointives sont pratiquées pour explorer les loges surrénaliennes.

Le phéochromocytome apparaît comme une masse arrondie ou ovalaire, parfois dépendante de la surrénale, de densité homogène, voisine de celle du foie et du pancréas. Une hypodensité centrale témoigne de remaniements nécrotiques (fig.1). Des calcifications peuvent être visibles (Chan & Wang, 1989). La sensibilité de détection des phéochromocytomes d'un diamètre de plus d'1cm est de 96%, ce qui correspond à la fréquence des localisations surrénales et péri-rénales (Bravo *et al.*, 1984). La mise en évidence des localisations ectopiques, des récidives et des formes métastatiques est plus difficile.

La méta-iodobenzylguanidine MIBG est un marqueur de la fonction de capture des monoamines dans le système nerveux sympathique et dans les tissus normaux et tumoraux, dérivés des crêtes neurales, appartenant au système APUD (Amine Precursor Uptake and Decarboxylation). A ce titre, il s'agit d'un marqueur spécifique des médullosurrénales et des phéochromocytomes. La fixation de la MIBG par ces tissus n'est pas directement reliée à la biosynthèse des catécholamines. Elle ne dépend pas non plus des capacités sécrétoires des tissus (Baulieu *et al.*, 1984).

La scintigraphie est effectuée 24 et 48 heures après injection de ^{131}I MIBG 37MBq ou 24 heures après injection de ^{123}I MIBG (37 à 130MBq). L'injection de la molécule radioiodée est précédée de la prise de solution de Lugol ou de perchlorate de potassium. L'iode 123 est trente fois moins irradiant que l'iode 131 (McEwan *et al.*, 1985) mais est d'un coût plus élevé. La ^{123}I MIBG est utilisée de préférence chez l'enfant. Pour faciliter la lecture des scintigraphies les reins sont repérés par un composé technetié approprié.

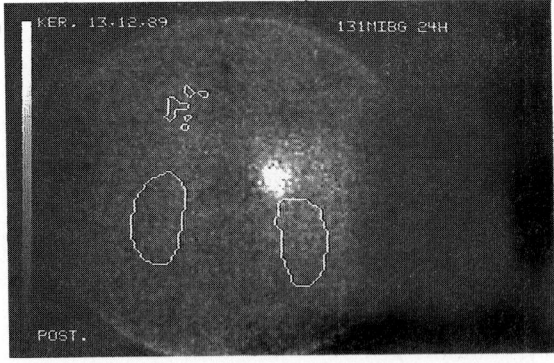

Fig. 2 : Même patient que fig. 1. Scintigraphie 24 heures après injection de ^{131}IMIBG 37 MBq. Incidence postérieure. Repérage du contour des reins par le ^{99m}Tc gluconate. Foyer de fixation exclusive au pôle supérieur du rein droit.

La visualisation des surrénales normales dépend de l'isotope utilisé, de l'activité administrée, des conditions de détection et du mode de traitement des images scintigraphiques.

Les images digitalisées obtenues 48 heures après injection de ^{131}I MIBG 37MBq, pendant 10 minutes permettent d'individualiser la surrénale gauche et la surrénale droite, respectivement chez 92% et 33% des sujets normaux (Baulieu *et al.*, 1984).

Le phéochromocytome est habituellement facilement identifié par un foyer intense au pôle supérieur du rein (fig.2).

Dans notre expérience, la sensibilité de détection est de 89% et la spécificité de 94% en accord avec les résultats des autres équipes (Shapiro et al., 1985). La possibilité d'interférence pharmacologique doit être envisagée devant un résultat négatif : en particulier, le labétalol agent $\propto_1$ et ß adrénergique est inhibiteur du captage des monoamines(Garnier et al.,1988).

Le repérage des localisations ectopiques en particulier médiastinales et vésicales est illustréepar de multiples observations (Shapiro *et al.*, 1984, Sakashita *et al.*, 1987). Dans les formes malignes la scintigraphie du corps entier permet de dénombrer et de localiser les métastases en particulier osseuses (Lynn *et al.*, 1986). Les performances sont excellentes : sensibilité 92%, spécifité 100% (Shapiro *et al* ., 1985).

L'imagerie par résonance magnétique (IRM) des glandes surrénales est réalisée à l'aide de champs de 0,26 T à 1 T. L'épaisseur des coupes est de 10mm. Le contraste de l'image dépend de la densité de protons des tissus et surtout des cinétiques de relaxation des moments magnétiques. Ces cinétiques de relaxation sont décrites par deux temps : le temps T_1 exploré par des séquences courtes d'une durée de l'ordre de 0,5 seconde qui montrent un signal élevé de la graisse, et le temps T_2 exploré par des séquences longues d'une durée de l'ordre de 2,5 secondes qui donnent un signal d'autant plus élevé que le tissu est riche en eau. L'examen dure de 35 à 50 minutes. La qualité des images peut être altérée par les mouvements respiratoires ou la présence de matériel ferro magnétique (Leroy-Willig & Luton, 1989).

La résolution anatomique est comparable à celle de la tomodensitométrie (Glazer *et al.*, 1986). L'intérêt de l'IRM est la possibilité d'une approche de la caractérisation tissulaire. Dès 1985, Fink et coll. observent chez 7 patients une forte intensité du signal sur les images de phéochromocytome pondérées en T_2. Ce signal est plus de deux fois plus intense dans le phéochromocytome que dans le foie. Il est ainsi possible de caractériser le phéochromocytome par rapport aux autres tumeurs surrénaliennes : métastases et adénomes (Glazer *et al.*,1986, Reinig *et al.*, 1986).

COMPARAISON DES TECHNIQUES

Echographie - Tomodensitométrie
Les tumeurs d'un diamètre supérieur à 2 cm sont visualisées en échographie et en tomodensitométrie. Les remaniements intra-tumoraux sont mieux analysés par l'échographie. Les tumeurs d'un diamètre inférieur à 1cm échappent à l'échographie (Yamakita *et al.*, 1985). La situation du phéochromocytome et ses rapports anatomiques sont mieux étudiés sur les coupes de tomodensitométrie.

Tomodensitométrie - Scintigraphie à la MIBG
Dans une étude multicentrique prospective portant sur 40 patients porteurs de phéochromocytome Chatal et Charbonnel (1985) ont comparé les résultats de la tomodensitométrie et de la scintigraphie : chez 32 patients les résultats étaient concordants, chez 4, la tomodensitométrie a montré des phéochromocytomes surrénaliens non révélés par la scintigraphie, chez 4 autres, la scintigraphie seule a montré un phéochromocytome surrénalien et 3 phéochromocytomes extra-surrénaliens.

En utilisant la MIBG marquée par l'iode 123 Bomanji et coll (1988) confirment la supériorité de la scintigraphie pour détecter les lésions extra-surrénaliennes.

Tomodensitométrie - Scintigraphie - IRM
Les 3 techniques ont été utilisées conjointement chez 19 patients en pré-opératoire (Quint *et al.*, 1987). Chez 15 patients les résultats étaient identiques, en accord avec les constatations opératoires. Dans 1 cas de localisations ectopiques et 1 cas de récidive post-opératoire, la tomodensitométrie était négative . Dans 1 cas d'hyperplasie signalée par la scintigraphie et vérifiée histologiquement , la tomoscintigraphie et l'IRM étaient toutes les deux négatives.

Dans une autre étude du même type portant sur 10 malades ayant un syndrome de NEM IIa (Mathieu *et al.*, 1987), l'IRM a permis d'établir un inventaire complet et correct des lésions, mais n'a pas apporté la confirmation d'une hyperplasie suspectée par la scintigraphie.

Au total, bien que les études restent limitées, l'IRM paraît équivalente à la scintigraphie pour reconnaître les localisations ectopiques et multiples, dans les limites des territoires qu'elle explore. La scintigraphie paraît plus sensible pour dépister l'hyperplasie des médullo-surrénales.

HYPERPLASIE DES MEDULLO-SURRENALES

Les méthodes d'imagerie morphologiques permettent une mesure des dimensions des surrénales. Cependant ces glandes se prêtent assez mal à une modélisation géométrique pour un calcul de volume. Il n'est pas possible de différencier cortex et médullaire. Le diagnostic d'hyperplasie par ces méthodes est donc aléatoire.

Bomanji et coll. (1988) ont montré que le taux de fixation de la MIBG est proportionnel à la concentration en granules de stockage de catécholamines, et reflète l'activité fonctionnelle des tissus chromaffines. Le calcul du taux de fixation de la MIBG dans les surrénales nécessite des corrections de bruit de fond et d'atténuation en profondeur. A partir de mesures effectuées sur 4 glandes normales et 2 glandes hyperplasiques, nous avons observé une relation linéaire ($r = 0,95$) entre le taux de fixation et le contraste scintigraphique. Le contraste scintigraphique est évalué par le rapport entre le nombre de coups dans le pixel d'activité maximum de l'image surrénalienne, et le comptage moyen d'une zone périphérique de bruit de fond. Dans les glandes normales, 24 heures après l'injection, il est inférieur à 1,4; dans les deux glandes hyperplasiques, il est supérieur à 1,5.

Chez 59 patients porteurs d'un carcinome médullaire de la thyroïde, nous avons observé une hyperplasie dans 2% (1/43) des formes apparemment sporadiques et 31% (5/16) des formes familiales.

CONCLUSION

L'imagerie des phéochromocytomes repose sur l'association tomodensitométrie - scintigraphie à la MIBG. Ces techniques complémentaires permettent respectivement une étude anatomique régionale et fonctionnelle globale. Leur utilisation à titre de dépistage dans les enquêtes familiales de NEM reste à discuter.

REFERENCES

Baulieu, JL., Guilloteau, D., Fetissof, F., Caron, J., Lecomte, P., Guilmot, JL., Lipinski, F., Baulieu, F., Itti, R., Pourcelot, L., Besnard, JC. (1984) : Paragangliomes sympathiques. Détection scintigraphique par une nouvelle molécule marquée, la méta-iodobenzylguanidine. Presse Méd., **13**, 1679-1682

Bomanji, J., Conry, BG., Britton, KE., Reznek, RH. (1988) : Imaging neural crest tumours with 123-I-meta-iodobenzylguanidine and X-ray computed tomography : a comparative study. Clinical Radiology, **39**, 502-506.

Bravo, EL., Gifford, RW, (1984) : Pheochromocytoma : diagnosis, localization and management. N. Eng. J. Med., **311**, 1298-1303.

Cho, KJ., Freier, DT., Mc Cormick, TL., Nishiyama, RH., Forrest, ME., Kaufman, A., Borlaza GS. (1980) : Adrenal medullary disease in multiple endocrine neoplasia type II, Am. J. Radiol., **134**, 23-29.

Chan, FL., Wang, C. (1989) : Imaging for adrenal tumours. Baillière's Clinical Endocrinology and Metabolism. **3**, 153-189.

Chatal, JF., Charbonnel, B. (1985) : Comparison of iodobenzylguanidine imaging with computed tomography in locating pheochromocytoma. J. Clin. Endocrinol. Metabol. **61**, 769-772.

Delellis, RA., Hubert, J., Wolfe, Robert, F., Gagel, Zoila, T., Feldman, BS, Miller, HH., David, L. (1976). Adrenal medullary hyperplasia. A morphometric analysis in patients with familial medullary thyroid carcinoma. Am. J. Pathol. **83**, 177-190.

Garnier, LF., Cosnay, P., Moquet, B., Doll, G., Robin, P., Baulieu, JL., Fauchier, JP., Raynaud, PA., Vandooren, M., Brochier, M.(1988) : Limites de la scintigraphie à la MIBG pour localiser les phéochromocytomes. Ann. Cardiol. Angéiol., **37**, 147-51.

Glazer, GM., Woolsey, EJ., Borello, J., Francis, IR., Aisen, AM., Bookstein, F., Amendola, MA., Gross, MD., Bree, RL., Martel, W. (1986) : Adrenal tissue characterization using MR imaging. Radiology, **158**, 73-79.

Guilloteau, D., Baulieu, JL., Vieil, JL., Valat, C., Baulieu, F., Chambon-Deschamps, C., Pourcelot, L., Itti, R., Besnard, JC., (1983) : Etude préliminaire d'un marqueur de la médullosurrénale et des terminaisons nerveuses sympathiques : la méta-iodobenzylguanidine. J. Biophys. Med. Nucl., **7**, 117-128.

Horne, T., Hawkins, LA., Britton, KE., Granowska, M., Bouloux, P., Besser, GM. (1984) : Imaging of pheochromocytoma and adrenal medulla with 123I- meta-iodobenzylguanidine. Nucl. Med. Communic., **5**, 763-8.

Leroy-Willig, A., Luton, JP. (1989) : L'imagerie par résonance magnétique des glandes surrénales. J. Urol., **95**, 305-308.

Lynn, MD., Braunstein, EM., Wahl, R., Shapiro, B., Gross, MD., Rabbani, R. (1986) : Bone metastases in pheochromocytoma : comparative studies of efficacy of imaging. Radiology, **160**, 701-706.

Mathieu, E., Despres, E., Delepine, N., Taieb, A. (1987) : MR imaging of the adrenal gland in Sipple disease. J. Comput. Assist. Tomogr., 11, **5**, 790-794.

Mc Ewan, AJ., Shapiro, B., Sisson, JC., Beierwaltes, WH, Ackery , DM. (1985) : Radio-iodobenzylguanidine for the scintigraphic location and therapy of adrenergic tumors. Sem. Nucl.Med., **15**, 132-53.

Päivänsalo, M., Merikanto, J., Kallioinen, M., Mc Ansh, G. (1988) : Ultrasound in the detection of adrenal tumours. Europ. J. Radiol. 8, 183-187.

Quint, LE., Glazer, GM., Francis, IR., Shapiro, B., Chenevert, TL. (1987) : Pheochromocytoma and paraganglioma : comparison of MR imaging with CT and I-131 MIBG scintigraphy. Radiology, **165**, 89-93.

Reinig, JW., Doppman, JL., Dwyer, AJ., Johnson, AR., Knop, RH.(1986) : Adrenal masses differentiated by MR. Radiology 158, 81-84.

Sakashita, S., Tanda, K., Togashi, M., Maru, A., Koyanagi, T., Tsukamoto, E., Itoh, K. (1987): Paraganglioma of urinary bladder, visualization with 131I-MIBG scintigraphy. Urol. Internat., **42**, 237-40.

Shapiro, B., Copp, JE., Sisson, JC., Eyre, PL., Wallis, J., Beierwaltes WH. (1985) : Iodine-131 metaiodobenzylguanidine for the locating of suspected pheochromocytoma : experience in 400 cases. J. Nucl. Med, **26**, 576-85.

Shapiro, B., Sisson, J., Kalff, V., Glowniak, J., Satterlee, W., Glazer, G., Francis, I., Bowers, R., Thompson, N., Orringer, M. (1984) : The location of middle mediastinal pheochromocytomas. J. Thor. Cardiovasc. Surg., **87**, 814-20.

Yamakita, N., Yasudo, K., Goshima, E., Murayama, M., Murase, H., Minamori, Y., Ishizuka, T., Miura, K. (1986) : Comparative assessment of ultrasonography and computed tomography in adrenal disorders. Ultrasound Med. Biol., **12**, 23-29.

RESUME :

La plupart des phéochromocytomes associés au CMT (NEM II) se développent à partir d'une hyperplasie des médullosurrénales. Les procédés d'imagerie sont devenus non invasifs et détectent les tumeurs surrénaliennes d'un diamètre de plus d'1 cm. L'échotomographie surrénalienne est bien adaptée à l'examen de l'enfant. La tomodensitométrie et l'IRM permettent une étude anatomique régionale. L'IRM apporte de plus une caractérisation tissulaire par la mesure du temps de relaxation T_2. La scintigraphie à la MIBG est une méthode spécifique et explore le corps entier. La mesure du pouvoir de concentration de la MIBG pourrait contribuer au diagnostic d'hyperplasie des médullosurrénales. En pratique, actuellement, l'imagerie des phéochromocytomes repose sur l'association scanner - scintigraphie à la MIBG, méthodes éprouvées et complémentaires.

Diagnostic means of the disease : discussion

Les méthodes de diagnostic de la maladie : discussion

DISCUSSION

BIOCHEMICAL FACTORS/*FACTEURS BIOCHIMIQUES*

L.Baldet (Montpellier) to **D.Guilloteau** (Tours): is there a good reproducibility of CIS IRMA calcitonin assay from one kit to another and is a CT value of 15-17 pg/ml always correctly interpreted ?
D.G.: I have sometimes to do again the assay because problems with some kits.
L.Baldet asks about the interpretation of CT peak when its occurs at 5 and not at 3 minutes after pentagastrin.
D.G. thinks that 5 minutes alevation may correspond to a slight delay in a blood puncture and that the peak in this case has to be interpreted as positive.
E.Modigliani (Paris): D.G. has shown us that a good correlation does exist between the results of CT with monoclonal and polyclonal assays. But, is it really true that MTC secrete mature CT rather than other CT forms ?
D.G.: it is in fact difficult to know exactly the predominant secretion in each cancer. In the litterature, the results show a great variability from a cancer to another. But, the fiability of the assay depends on the specificity of antibodies used therein.We have the feeling that monoclonal assays, even if they give CT lower levels, are not expressing a different type of secretion.
G.Andry (Bruxelles): why is CEA level of no interest in familial cases ?
D.G. familial cases are often detected at a precocious stage, that is why CEA, in my exprerience, is always normal. But, I agree that systematic CEA assay may be of interest from an evolutive point of view.
C.Mahler (Anvers): does a correlation beween CT and CEA levels exist ?
D.G.: they have usually the same evolution but it is not always the case.
C.Malher has observed a diminution of plasma CT without diminution of CEA level in patients treated with SMS 201-995. Physiologically, somatostatin inhibits only calcitonin. This point will be discussed in an other session.

M.Sobrinho-Simoes (Lisbonne) asks **F.Pacini**.(Pise) about the better outcome patients with positive somatostatin immuno-staining in their tumours : was this result controlled versus age and staging ?
F.P.: the results have been corrected for age and staging, but therapy may have been different. Anyway, on the beginning of their disease, the stage was the same. F.P. precises that he can't state positively that the prognosis is better. He only noticed that somatostatin-positive tumours had a better outcome.
E.Modigliani (Paris): did you find a difference in somatostatin staining between familial and sporadic forms ?
F.P.: I didn't find such difference but my cases were mostly sporadic, 2 familial cases of MTC excepted.

C.Jaffiol (Montpellier) to **J.C.Reubi** (Bern): it has been suggested that use of ^{131}I-somatostatin analog may be of potential use in therapy. What is the risk of irradiation of other organs with high levels of SMS receptors ?

J.C.R.: this is probably the weak point at the moment. However, the density of the receptors is much lower in normal tissue than that in tumoral tissue. It is not absolutely clear to which extend the role of somatostatin system is really crucial in the normal tissue compared to the cancer.
P.F.Plouin (Paris): you mentioned the SMS receptors were present in a lot of patients with pheochromocytomas. Do you mean that they were present in the tumors by autoradiography or in vivo by whole body imaging ?
J.C.R. it has been shown only in vitro, by autoradiography, in about 70% of the cases. To my knowledge, no pheochromocytoma has been visualized by ^{123}I-somatostatin analog.

CYTOLOGY AND IMMAGING/*CYTOPONCTION ET IMAGERIE*

E.D.Williams (Cardiff) asks **L.Bondeson** (Malmö). about his experience on fine needle aspiration (FNA) of mixed follicular tumours of the thyroid.
L. B. I have had so far too few of these tumours to be able to give a definitive description.
H.R.Harach (Cardiff) asks about the used of FNA in small, not palpable, lesions: at an asymptomatic stage, it may be found very small nodules on echography and FNA may be negative. If calcitonin is elevated after pentagastrin test, what is the message for indicating surgery ?
L.B.: If there is not any palpable nodule, negative FNA doesn't mean anything, especially in the case of familial detection. Surgery is indicated on the pathological CT results.

A.Garcia (Barcelona) to **S.E.M.Clarke** (London): How do you calculate the sensitivity of DMSA results?.Are all patients in whom DMSA imaging suspects some pathological results operated on ?
S.E.M.C. (London): many of them will be operated. Negative results correspond to very small tumours. Limit of sensitivity with DMSA is 0.5 cm diameter. Under this limit, the sensitivity goes right down.
D.Bergant (Ljubljana): how to obviate renal damage in the selenium DMSA treatment ?
S.E.M.C.: until now, 3 patients have been treated by this technique and we try to use preventive probenecid.
D.Sandrock (Gottingen) adds that we should not forget that immuno-scintigraphy gives also a good sensitivity and specificity. This may be followed in the future by a therapeutic approach.

PHEOCHROMOCYTOMA DETECTION/*DÉPISTAGE DU PHÉOCHROMOCYTOME*

E.Modigliani (Paris) asks **H.Neumann** (Fribourg) for the technical difficulties of chromogranin assay.
H.N.: it doesn't seem too difficult and there is now a commerciable available kit from Nichol's Institute in San Diego.

H.Neumann (Fribourg) asks **J.L.Baulieu** (Tours) about false positive results with MIBG scintigraphy in the french cooperative study group.
J.L.B. thinks that false positive results occur because of low uptake ground and the normal adrenal.

R. Mornex (Lyon) comments on the diagnosis of pheochromocytoma. He insists about doing morphologic investigations only after the establishment of hormonal hypersecretion of medullary adrenal. From his point of view, urinary methoxyamines have the best discriminative results for diagnosis of pheochromocytoma. Methoxyamines are calculated as the sum of normetanephrines and metanephrines, measured by HPLC. As 24-hours urinary collection is sometimes difficult to obtain, R.M. reports his results on blood methoxyamines in detection of pheochromocytoma. Normal range is below 1.4 ng/ml; hypertensive patients have somewhat higher levels. However, levels higher than 6 ng/ml are of value to detect more specifically pheochromocytomas, sporadic as well as MEN 2a forms.

IV. Epidemiology and genetics
IV. Epidémiologie et génétique

Clinical and molecular genetics of multiple endocrine neoplasia type 2A (MEN 2A)

L.M. Mulligan[1]*, E. Gardner[1], C. Jones[2], S.E. Mole[1], J. Moore[1], Y. Nakamura[3], I. Papi[1], H. Telenius[1] and B.A.J. Ponder[1]

[1] CRC Human Cancer Genetics Research Group, Department of Pathology, University of Cambridge, Cambridge CB2 1QP, UK.
[2] Eleanor Roosevelt Institute, Denver, Colorado 80262, USA.
[3] Division of Biochemistry, Cancer Institute, Tokyo 170, Japan
* Author for correspondence

MEN 2 is a clinically diverse syndrome comprising several distinct phenotypes including MEN 2A, MEN 2B and MTC-only MEN 2. The genetic relationship amongst these diseases is not clear. They may be the result of mutation of separate but closely linked genes or of different types of alteration within a single gene.

To distinguish these possibilities and to understand how these putative changes relate to the observed patient phenotypes we need to identify and characterize the MEN2 gene (or genes) and the type of mutations to which it is subject.

The locus for MEN 2A has been mapped to the centromeric region of chromosome 10 and recent evidence places the loci for MEN 2B and the MTC-only variety of MEN 2 in the same interval. While the region of interest is quite small with respect to the human genome it still represents a large genetic area within which to identify the gene of interest. It is therefore necessary to refine the genetic and physical map of the centromeric region of chromosome 10 to facilitate the search for the MEN 2 gene.

Our strategy has involved three complementary approaches:

1] Using genetic mapping techniques, to define the minimum interval in which the MEN 2 gene may lie.
2] To develop a series of mapped physical markers interspersed throughout this region.
3] To use these physical markers to examine DNA from germline and tumour samples from affected individuals for clues as to the localization and identity of the MEN 2 gene.

GENETIC LINKAGE MAPPING

The MEN 2 locus has been mapped to the centromeric region of chromosome 10 (10p11.2-q11.2) by genetic linkage analyses (Mathew et al, 1991). This region is defined by two loci, D10S34 (recognized by probe TB14.34) and RBP, which flank the MEN 2A locus at a sex averaged genetic distance of 3 centiMorgans (Fig. 1). Although the centromere lies within this region no recombination between it and the MEN 2 locus has been identified so we are presently unable to map the disease locus to the short or long arm of the chromosome.

POSITION OF MEN 2A

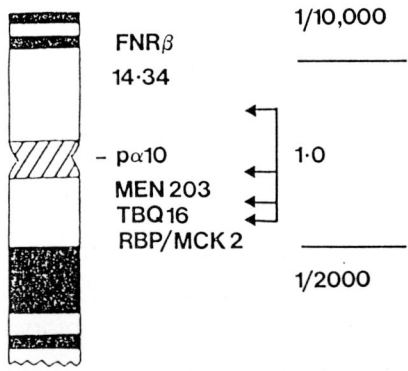

Fig.1. Map of the centromere region of chromosome 10 showing the approximate positions of markers determined by multipoint genetic linkage analysis in MEN 2 and reference families, and in situ hybridisation (FNRβ, RBP). The relative odds for the position of MEN 2A relative to these markers are derived from multipoint analysis in the family set.

In order to define the MEN 2 region more precisely we have identified new markers using probes isolated from a radiation hybrid which contains a part of chromosome 10 and the Y chromosome as its only human material. Probes which identified restriction fragment length polymorphisms (RFLPs) and which have been mapped to the appropriate region on a panel of somatic cell translocation hybrids, were used to test for recombinations in MEN 2 families which were already known to be recombinant with either D10S34 or RBP. To date, no further recombinants have been detected, and so we have been unable to narrow the MEN 2 region further.

PHYSICAL MAPPING

The resolution of genetic mapping techniques in the MEN 2 region is limited because of the proximity of the centromere. Therefore we are trying, in parallel, to develop a physical map based on chromosome breakpoints, either in radiation hybrids or in hybrids containing single copies of chromosome 10 which have undergone translocation with another chromosome.

Radiation hybrids have been prepared from hamster-human hybrids containing a] only human chromosome 10 + Y; b] 10q + Y; or c] human chromosome 10 only. Doses of radiation were varied (from 300 to 20,000 rads) in order to adjust the size of chromosome fragment generated. Clones were rescued by fusion with hamster cells and grown in the absence of selection. Probes for the pericentromeric region are currently being used to define the portion of chromosome 10 retained by 80 of these hybrids.

Another physical mapping resource is cell lines which have been prepared from EBV-transformed lymphocytes of individuals with a variety of naturally occurring translocations with a breakpoint in the pericentromeric region. Translocation chromosomes are being isolated in somatic cell hybrids using selectable markers for chromosome 10p (FNRβ) and 10q (proline auxotrophy). A summary of our current mapping of probes in respect of these translocation breakpoints is shown in Fig. 2.

PROBES MAPPED TO THE REGION OF CHROMOSOME 10q11

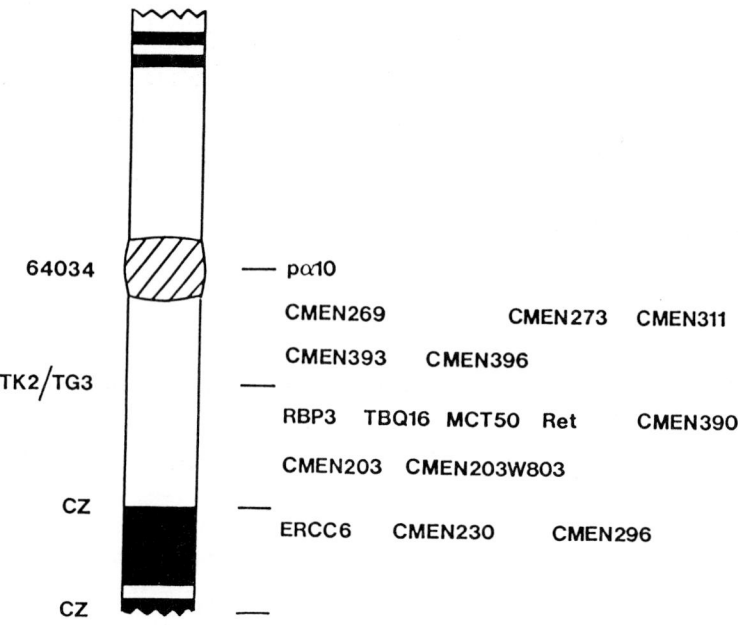

Fig. 2. The horizontal lines indicate breakpoints in the translocation or deletion hybrid cell lines 64034, TK2, TG3, and CZ : DNA probes have been mapped to the intervals defined by these breakpoints. The CMEN series are cosmid clones derived by Dr. Y. Nakamura : shown are those for which unique sequence fragments have been isolated and subcloned in our laboratory. p α10 is a probe specific for chromosome 10 centromere.

Single copy sequences from selected clones are now being used in other cloning and mapping strategies for chromosome 10p11.2-10q11.2 including isolation of yeast artificial chromosomes (YACs) and generation of a physical map of overlapping DNA fragments by pulsed-field gel electrophoresis (PFGE).

HOW DO WE IDENTIFY THE MEN 2 GENE?

While comprehensive physical and genetic maps of the MEN 2 region will facilitate our search for the disease locus, our ability to identify that locus will be determined by the nature of mutations occurring there. The loci responsible for other inherited cancer syndromes, such as retinoblastoma, have contributed to tumourigenesis by loss of gene activity. If this mechanism also applies in MEN 2, cases of germline deletion or rearrangement like those found in retinoblastoma might be detected by using DNA probes for loci close to the disease locus to search for altered fragments by PFGE analysis. Similarly, allele loss at marker loci close to MEN 2 in tumours, indicating loss of a normal parental allele at the disease locus, might be predicted.

A summary of our results to date is shown in Table 1. We have no evidence of either germline deletions or allele losses in tumours in a sample which includes cases of MEN 2A, 2B and MTC-only MEN 2.

Table 1. Allele Loss at loci in the MEN 2 Region

Probe	Number of tumours examined	Number Informative	Losses
MEN203	40	28	0
ret	35	11	0
MEN284	27	5	0
pMCT50	30	13	0
IRBP9	31	14	0

Our results suggest several possible interpretations (Ponder et al, 1989):

1] The genetic mechanism of MEN 2 differs from that of other inherited cancer syndromes. The disease mutation might represent an activation of the MEN 2 gene, a more difficult change to detect since a simple point mutation might result in a disease allele. This type of mutation would be undetectable by the methods described above, requiring a different strategy for detection.

2] Alternatively, the MEN 2 phenotype may indeed result from loss of gene activity but hemizygous rather than homozygous loss may be sufficient for tumour formation (there is a precedent for this in familial adenomatous polyposis). In this case, allele losses in tumours would not be required for tumourigenesis.

3] Finally, our failure to detect germline or tumour specific alterations may result from a low frequency of gross DNA alterations in MEN 2, perhaps due to the proximity of the centromere which is known to suppress recombination events which we might recognize as gene rearrangement or allele losses.

Our strategy now is to improve further the physical map, which will allow a more systematic search for genetic alterations in germline and tumour DNA. In parallel we will consider alternative strategies including the identification of candidate genes which map to the pericentromeric region.

GENETIC EVENTS IN TUMOUR PROGRESSION

Secondary genetic events which may play a significant role in tumour progression have been identified in a number of human neoplasias, and will presumably occur in medullary thyroid carcinoma and pheochromocytoma also.

Our studies are at an early stage, and have concentrated on allele losses as possibly reflecting the requirement for loss of tumour suppressor genes. The results are summarized in Table 2. Allele

Table 2. Losses of Heterozygosity in MTC and Pheochromocytoma

Region	Frequency
1p	17/46
3p	3/15
11p	3/11
13q	3/10
22q	5/15
Total comparisons	4/391

losses occur frequently on chromosomes 1p, 3p, 11p, 13q, and 22 but not in other regions, suggesting the involvement of specific loci in these regions and not a generalized chromosome instability. We are currently refining the mapping of the critical intervals on these chromosomes to obtain better information on the genes potentially involved.

REFERENCES

Mathew, C.G.P., Easton, D.F., Nakamura, Y. and Ponder, B.A.J. (1991): Presymptomatic screening for multiple endocrine neoplasia type 2A with linked DNA markers. Lancet 337: 7-11.

Ponder, B.A.J., Smith, B.A., Marcus, G.M. et al (1989): Genetic events in tumourigenesis in multiple endocrine neoplasia type 2. Cancer Cells 7: 219-222.

Linkage analysis for hereditary medullary thyroid carcinoma

G.M. Lenoir[1]*, H. Sobol[2], I. Schuffenecker[1], S. Narod[1]
and the Groupe d'Etude des Tumeurs à Calcitonine (GETC)

(1) Centre International de Recherche sur le Cancer, 150, cours Albert-Thomas, 69372 Lyon Cedex 08, France.
(2) Centre Léon-Bérard, Département d'Oncologie et de Génétique, 28, rue Laënnec, 69373 Lyon Cedex 08, France

* Author for correspondence

More than 100 families with hereditary medullary thyroid carcinoma (MTC) have been identified in France. In the majority of these families, one or more members are affected with both MTC and pheochromocytoma, a situation corresponding to multiple endocrine neoplasia type 2A (MEN 2A) syndrome. Several families have also been identified in which medullary thyroid carcinoma is seen but without pheochromocytoma (MTCWP), suggesting genetic heterogeneity. Furthermore, rare cases of multiple endocrine neoplasia type 2B (MEN 2B) characterized by MTC and pheochromocytoma in combination with neuromas of the oral mucosa have been reported (Sobol et al., 1989a). The MEN 2A gene has been mapped recently to a location near the centromere of chromosome 10. We summarize here the most recent linkage data obtained from the families, drawn from the French national registry (GETC).

MATERIALS AND METHODS

Patients

Families with a history of MTC were ascertained through the records of the Groupe d'Etude des Tumeurs à Calcitonine (GETC) and through the participation of individuals interested physicians. Over 200 individuals from 33 families were studied. The diagnosis of MTC or the precursor lesion C-cell hyperplasia is based upon either a characteristic pathology report or upon an elevated serum calcitonin level, either basal or after stimulation with pentagastrin.

DNA markers and genotyping

Genomic DNA extracted directly from the blood or from Epstein-Barr virus immortalized lymphoblastoid cell lines was used for these studies.

Probes that have been used in this analysis include IRBP.H4 a 2,2 kb cDNA coding form human interstitial retinol binding protein (RBP3), the anonymous probes MCK2 (D10S15), TB10.163 (D10S22), TB14.34 (D10S34) (Sobol et al., 1989a) the centromeric probe pα 10 RP8 (D10Z1) (Narod et al., 1991), and the cDNA for mannose binding protein, probe 48-11 (Schuffenecker et al., 1991).

Lod scores

Lod scores were calculated with the linkage program using gene frequency of 1: 50 000 and published penetrance figures (Sobol et al., 1989b; Narod et al., 1991).

Results

As indicated in table 1, no recombination was seen between either D10S34 or D10Z1, or RBP3 and MEN2A. Concerning D10S22, a maximum lod score of 4.66 was obtained but with 5% recombination in male and 16% in female. For D10S15 and 48-11 the male recombination fraction was nil, and was of 7 and 9.7% respectively in female (Narod et al., 1991; Schuffenecker et al., 1991).

Combining our data and published ones, the most likely locus order for these markers is: FNRB, D10S34, D1021, RBP3-D10S15, 48-11 and D1022, but confirmation with multipoint analysis is required. The smallest interval containing MEN2A on this map is defined by D10S34 and RBP3 (Narod et al., 1991).

Linkage for the three selected syndromes

Table 2 summarizes linkage data on the three syndromes MEN 2A, MTCWP and MEN 2B. Because no recombination was found between the D10S15 and RBP3 loci in our data, we also assessed linkage between the MTC gene and the RBP3-D10S15 haplotype. In the MTCWP families a maximum lod score of 2.61 was seen with a recombination fraction of 10% (Sobol et al., 1989a). For MEN 2B a cooperative effort was required to reach a 3.75 lodscore at 4% recombination (Norum et al., 1990).

DISCUSSION

The linkage analyses described here have permitted to localize the MEN 2A locus to a small interval defined by the D10S34 and RBP3 loci. Because of the lack of recombination with the centromeric alpha satellite probe pα10RP8 (D10Z1) (Carson et al., 1990; Narod et al., 1991) we are however not yet able to determine whether MEN 2A maps on the short or on the long arm of chromosome 10. However, the high lod score with no or little recombination obtained with D10Z1, D10S34, RBP3, D10S15 indicates that (1) the precise location of the gene is likely to be resolved soon (2). These linked genetic markers will prove to be useful for genetic screening in the MTC families (Sobol et al., 1989b; Narod et al., 1989). Two newly described DNA markers MEN203 and D10S94 (Goodfellow et al., 1990) show to be also very closely linked to MEN 2A will prove valuable with respect to cloning and genetic screening. The presence of two cross-overs between MEN 2A and the candiadate gene Mannose binding protein (MBP) in these families indicates that a defect of MBP itself is not the cause of the hereditary thyroid cancer syndrome (Schuffenecker et al., 1991). The linkage data do not suggest that different genetic loci may underlie the different MTC syndrome (table 2). Epidemiologic studies of MTCWP families are still required for determining linkage parameters with better precision.

Table 1.

Lod scores for linkage between Multiple Endocrine Neoplasia type 2a and chromosome 10 loci

Locus	Maximum Lod Score	Recombination Fraction*	
		Male	Female
D10Z1	9.43	0.000	0.000
D10S34 (TB14.34)	6.27	0.000	0.000
RBP3	11.46	0.000	0.000
D10S15 (MCK2)	13.85	0.000	0.070
48-11	7.54	0.000	0.097
D10S22	4.86	0.050	0.160

*The recombination fraction is estimated to be that at which the lod score is highest.

Most likely order:

```
FNRB - D10S34 - D10Z1 - RBP/MCK2 - 48.11 - D10S22
               ↑_____↑
                    MEN 2
```

Table 2. Summary of linkage results for the three inherited forms of MTC.

SYNDROME	MEN 2A*	MTC ONLY*	MEN 2B**
Probes	RBP3-D10S15	RBP3/D10S15	D10S15
Lodscore	15.05	2.61	3.75
θ	0.00	0.10	0.04

* from Narod et al.

** from Norum et al.

REFERENCES

Carlson, N.L., et al. (1990): The mutation for medullary thyroid carcinoma with parathyroid tumors (MTC with Pts) is closely linked to the centromeric region of chromosome 10. Am. J. Hum. Genet. 47, 946-951.

Goodfellow et al. (1990): A new DNA marker (D10S94) very tightly linked to the multiple endocrine neoplasia type 2A (MEN 2A) locus. Am. J. Hum. Genet. 47, 952-956.

Narod et al. (1989): Linkage analysis of hereditary thyroid carcinoma with and without pheochromocytoma. Hum. Genet. 83, 353-358.

Narod et al. (1989): Early detection of hereditary medullary thyroid cancer with polymorphic DNA probes. Henry Ford Hosp. Med. J. 37, 106-108.

Narod et al. (1991): The gene for MEN 2A is tightly linked to the centromere of chromosome 10. Hum. Genet. (in press).

Norum et al. (1990): Linkage of the multiple endocrine neoplasia type 2B gene (MEN 2B) to chromosome 10 markers linked to MEN 2A. Genomics, 8, 313-317.

Schuffenecker, I. et al. (1991): The gene for mannose binding protein maps to chromosome 10 and is a marker for multiple endocrine neoplasia type 2. Cytogenet. Cell Genet. (in press).

Sobol, H. et al. (1989a): Hereditary medullary thyroid carcinoma: genetic analysis of three related syndromes. Henry Ford Hosp. Med. J. 37, 109-111.

Sobol, H. et al. (1989b): Screening for multiple endocrine neoplasia type 2a with DNA-polymorphism analysis. New England J. Med. 321, 996-1001.

Epidemiologic and genetic analysis of medullary thyroid carcinoma in France

Myriam Rosenberg-Bourgin, Diane Farkas, Claude Calmettes(*),
Nicole Feingold and the French GETC

INSERM U 155, Université Paris 7, 2, place Jussieu, 75251 Paris Cedex 05 and
(*) INSERM U 113, Faculté Saint-Antoine, 27, rue Chaligny, 75571 Paris Cedex 12, France

Summary. Between 1968 and 1988, 837 MTC probands have been ascertained, on clinical features, before any familial investigation, by the French GETC. Complete analysis of 156 of them showed that the goiter (82 per cent of cases) was the main clinical manifestation and that the presence of clinically palpable cervical lymph nodes (34 per cent of the cases) indicated poor prognosis.
30 per cent were hereditary forms and 59 per cent of them were MEN 2A. Pheochromocytoma was present in two-thirds of the MEN 2A cases and was most often diagnosed at the same time as MTC.
In less than one-third of studied familial forms, MTC was the only feature diagnosed in each affected member.
Estimation of the age related probability to develop hereditary MTC for a genetically predisposed individual with a biological negative screening, using 30 sibs of probands and 154 children of probands or secondary cases, confirmed the high penetrance of the disease gene,

The French Groupe d'Etude des Tumeurs à Calcitonine (GETC; Calmettes, 1984) initiated, in 1983, a national study on medullary thyroid carcinoma (MTC). Its aim was to collect a maximum of the cases diagnosed in France for better characterization of the principal features of MTC, and improved MTC screening and treatment.
A questionnaire was established by the members of the GETC. It included individual and familial demographic data, as well as MTC-related characteristics consisting of the circumstances of diagnosis, clinical features, associated syndromes, treatment, pathology and course of the disease.

The aim of this epidemiological study was especially to analyze the main characteristics of the disease for patients diagnosed on the basis of clinical features, before any familial investigation. These patients were termed MTC probands. Between 1968 and 1988, 837 MTC probands were diagnosed. The number of MTC patients diagnosed per year increased during this period, with about 34 per cent being diagnosed after the creation of the GETC.

From these data, we will define the general characteristics of the MTC probands, compare the clinically isolated cases of MTC (MTC only) to the MEN 2A forms, and the hereditary to the non hereditary types.
A prospective study in some MTC patients' families was also conducted and familial segregation analysis was performed on the hereditary forms. We will also report the preliminary results of this analysis.

I) RETROSPECTIVE STUDY ON MTC PROBANDS

MATERIAL AND METHODS

Data were collected either by the physican having in charge the patient (more than 200 of them took part in the study) or by an investigator who consulted the patient's medical record (V. Boiteau, S. Casanova, A. Chompret, and R. De Sahb).
For most of the patients, the last informations dated from less than a year. However, the classification established in September 1990 may subsequently evolve, especially for the MTC only and non hereditary groups.

The data were entered and analyzed by PIGAS software, developed by the Centre de Calcul INSERM, Villejuif. Statistical analyses were carried out using chi-square and Student t test. The actuarial method, the logrank and adjusted logrank tests were used to analyze the survival data.

RESULTS

A) General characteristics of the MTC patients

The main characteristics of the MTC patients diagnosed on clinical features are presented on table 1.

Table 1 : Characteristics of the probands'population

Number	837
Sex ratio: Males/Females	0.67
Age at M.T.C. diagnosis in years	
Mean (Standard Deviation)	46.4 (16.4)
Clinical manifestations of M.T.C. (%)	
goiter	82.1
palpable cervical lymph nodes	34.4
neck sensitivity	9.6
diarrhea	28.2
flush	25.4
Classification related to syndroms (%)	
MEN 2A	14.1
MEN 2B	5.4
MTC only	80.5

The higher proportion of females (sex ratio 0.67) was independent of the year of diagnosis.

The mean age at MTC diagnosis was 46.4 years, the same for males and females, with a range of 2 to 87. 40 per cent of the probands have been diagnosed at the age of 40.

A complete analysis of clinical features of MTC and associed tumours at the time of diagnosis was performed for 156 patients representative of the MTC proband population .

Goiter, present in 82 per cent of the cases, was the most frequent feature and the only clinical characteristic in 48 per cent of the cases.

Diarrhea and flush were both present in more than one-fourth of the cases, and often associated with goiter; diarrhea was found alone in only 3 per cent of the cases, whereas flush was the only symptom in 14 per cent.

Neck sensitivity, including painful palpation and dysphagia, was found in less than 10 per cent of the cases. Never present alone, it was always associated with goiter and/or palpable cervical lymph nodes.

No differences were noted in clinical features according to the year and the age at diagnosis, but goiter was significantly more frequent in females. On the contrary, palpable cervical lymph node and cervical lymph node metastases (present in 64 per cent of the cases) were more frequently found in males than in females.

81 per cent of the patients underwent total thyroidectomy, performed in one step for 44 per cent. Cervical lymph node

dissection was carried out in 41 per cent. Less than 8 per cent of the patients simultaneously underwent total thyroidectomy and bilateral lymph node dissection.

26 per cent of the probands died from MTC or pheochromocytoma. Females had a better survival rate than males, respectively 85 per cent and 77 per cent at 5 years.

Adjusted logrank tests showed that palpable cervical lymph node was the only factor relevant to poor prognosis.

In our population, 5.4 per cent of the MTC patients simultaneously presented a MEN 2B syndrome. In most of the other cases, screening for pheochromocytoma and/or hyperparathyroidism was undertaken and a MEN 2A form was found in 14 per cent of the cases. Among the patients with the MEN 2A form, pheochromocytoma alone was present in two-thirds of the cases and hyperparathyroidism alone very rarely (less than 5 per cent).

B) Comparison between MTC only and MEN 2A probands

The main results for 475 probands with confirmed MTC as only feature and MEN 2A syndrome are reported in table 2.

Table 2 : Comparison between MTC only and MEN 2A patients

	MTC only	MEN 2A	
N	404	71	
Age at M.T.C. diagnosis in years Mean (Standard Deviation)	47.1 (15)	38.8 (12.6)	$p<10^{-5}$
Clinical manifestations of M.T.C. (%)			
palpable cervical lymph node	55	8.5	$p<10^{-5}$
diarrhea	39	11.8	$p<10^{-2}$
Pathological features (%)			
bilateral tumors	41.8	95.3	$p<10^{-4}$
cervical lymph node metastasis	71.4	51.4	$p<0.05$

The mean age at diagnosis of MTC was significantly different for MTC only and MEN 2A: 47.7 years versus 38.8.

The MEN 2A form of MTC on the one hand and pheochromocytoma and/or hyperparathyroidism on the other were diagnosed at the same time in 42 per cent of the cases. In 32 per cent, MTC was diagnosed before, with a mean interval of 6 years. In 26 per cent, clinical diagnosis of MTC followed that of pheochromocytoma and/or hyperpathyroidism, with a mean interval of 5 years. The mean age at diagnosis of pheochromocytoma and/or hyperparathyroidism was 39.8 years, with a range of 15 to 70.

Palpable cervical lymph nodes and diarrhea were the only two clinical features significantly more frequent in MTC only patients. These observations were correlated with the fact that in these patients, MTC was diagnosed in the later stages of the disease.
Almost all the MEN 2A patients were affected with bilateral tumors. Such bilateral tumors were observed in less than half of the apparently MTC only cases.

C) Comparison between hereditary and nonhereditary forms

Familial screening of 185 probands allowed identification of 58 hereditary cases. The main results of comparisons between hereditary and nonhereditary forms are reported on table 3.

Table 3 : Comparison between hereditary and nonhereditary cases

	hereditary	apparently nonhereditary	
Nunber of cases	58	137	
MEN 2A syndrom (%)	58.6	5.2	$p<10^{-4}$
Age at M.T.C. diagnosis in years Mean (Standard Deviation)	38.3 (12.3)	47.8 (15.2)	$p<10^{-4}$
Palpable cervical lymph nodes (%)	18.0	73.9	$p<0.03$
Bilateral tumors (%)	100	29	$p<10^{-6}$

The mean age at diagnosis of MTC was significantly lower for hereditary than for nonhereditary cases, respectively 38.3 versus 47.8. This mean age remains significant lower for hereditary cases, when taking into account MTC only probands, respectively 40.3 versus 47.8.
For the probands, MEN 2A syndrome was found almost exclusively in hereditary cases.
Palpable cervical lymph node was the only clinical feature with a different distribution. However, when taking into account the MTC only probands, this difference was no longer significant.
All the hereditary cases had bilateral tumors. In apparently nonhereditary cases bilateral tumors were found in less than one-

third of the cases. This major difference between hereditary and nonhereditary probands remains important when considering the MTC only cases.

In conclusion it should be pointed out that most of the results obtained in this study are in agreement with those reported by Saad et al (1984) and Bergholm et al (1989)

II) FAMILIAL ANALYSIS

Among the families so far recorded by the G E T C, 84 families with at least two confirmed affected members and a clear clinical investigation were selected; 31% are MTC only families, 63% are MEN 2A families and 6% MEN 2B families.

A nonsignificant excess of females was observed in MEN 2A and MEN 2B forms. Statistical analysis showed that ages at diagnosis of MTC was similar to that of the general data. The 84 pedigrees are probably representative of the familial form of MTC, identified in France in recent years.

The composition of the MTC only and MEN 2A families was given in table 4.

Table 4: Number of affected members in MTC only and MEN 2A families

Number of affected members per family	Number of MTC only families	Number of MEN 2A families
2	10	19
3	6	14
4	5	4
5	2	4
6	2	3
7		5
8	1	1
11		1
12		1
17		1
Total	26	53

In 38 per cent of the cases, there are at least 4 affected members. In MTC only families the mean number of affected members was 3.5 and 4.5 in MEN 2A families. Apparently there was no distorsion of the sex ratio among the affected members.

Segregation analysis of the syndrome is complicated by the variable expression of the disease and the various biological investigations.
Here, as a first step, we considered the transmission of MTC.
It was necessary to calculate the age-related probability to develop hereditary MTC, that is the risk of MTC development for a genetically predisposed individual with normal plasma concentration of calcitonin after pentagastrin provocative stimulation (Gagel et al, 1982).
For this prospective study, data were obtained from 21 sibships having one affected parent. In these sibships, screened regularly once a year, 26 subjects converted from negative to positive. The diagnosis of MTC was confirmed by histological techniques.
The mean age at conversion was 17 years. 50 per cent of predisposed individuals were diagnosed before 14 and 90 per cent of the group had converted by age 29. In Gagel's study, 90 per cent of the group had converted by age 25.
It appears that females were diagnosed earlier than males.

From the cumulative incidence the conversion probability for an individual with a negative test at age h was calculated.
The formula: $\frac{1/2(1-p_h)}{1/2 + 1/2(1-p_h)}$ is an application of Bayes' theorem and p_h the proportion of individuals who have converted at age h.
For example, the probability to develop MTC for an individual with an affected parent and a negative test is 0.5 before the age of 5. This probability becomes 0.22 at the age of 20, 0.06 at the age of 30, and almost zero at 40.

Using this information, the members of the pedigrees were classified into four phenotypes:
-affected (MTC confirmed)
-nonaffected, but investigated before the age of 40; status was corrected by the previous calculated conversion probability
-clinically normal after the age of 40
-unknown
An affected individual was defined as a secondary case if diagnosed through a family study and as a proband if diagnosed without any familial investigation.
To perform the segregation analysis, two types of nuclear families were distinguished: the sibship of each proband (single selection) and the children of probands and secondary cases (complete selection)

Disease distribution between brothers and sisters of an affected person were obtained from 30 studied sibships, with a total of 117 investigated members.
69 clinically affected individuals were observed (no correction was necessary, all being more than 32 years old).
The segregation ratio was 69-30 / 117-30 = 0.45. The observed segregation ratio, 0.45, was not significantly different from the expected ratio for a dominant gene.

Disease transmission from one affected parent to his children was established for 57 families, including 154 children. The observed number of clinically affected individuals was 61. The estimated number of affected individuals, after correction by age, was 81.5.
The segregation ratio was: 81.5 / 154 = 0.53. Again, the observed segregation ratio was not significantly different from the expected ratio for a dominant gene.

It is clear that the postulated gene presents various phenotypical expressions in addition to incomplete penetrance in some families. However the total information takes into account each family, so that, as a first approach, the gene's penetrance could be considered as complete.
Further genetic analysis of the data will permit estimation of the proportion of sporadic cases, variation of penetrance by age, recurrence risks and possible genetic heterogeneity.
A realistic approach to segregation analysis of multigeneration pedigrees requires a complex strategy of analysis and a clear knowledge of the familial history. It is also necessary to obtain a more precise estimation of screening age-at-onset distibution for the syndrome (Easton et al, 1989)
The various factors involved in the determination of the disease require modelling. In particular, as observed in retinoblastoma and in agreement with Knudson's theory of two mutational events to induce cancer, hereditary cases of MTC are diagnosed at an earlier age and more frequently present bilateral tumors (Jackson et al, 1979). However, preliminary results of a more detailed statistical analysis of the age at diagnosis show that more than two mutational events were involved in the process of MTC tumor formation, and some of the bilateral tumors in nonhereditary cases may be due to metastasis.

REFERENCES

Bergholm U., Adami H.O., Bergström R., Johansson H., Lundell G., Telenius-Berg M., Akerström G., and the Swedish MTC Study Group (1989) Clinical Characteristics in Sporadic and Familial Medullary Thyroid Carcinoma. A Nationwide Study of 249 Patients in Sweden from 1959 through 1981. *Cancer 63:* 1196-1204.

Calmettes C. (1984) Création d'un Groupe d'Etudes des Tumeurs à Calcitonine. *Bull. Cancer 71:* 266-73.

Easton D.F.,Ponder M.A., Cummings T., Gagel R.F., Hansen H.H., Reichlin S., Tashjian AH. Jr.,Telenius-Berg M., Ponder B.A.J. and the Cancer Research Campaign Medullary Thyroid Group.(1989) The clinical and screening age-at-onset distribution for the MEN-2 syndrome. *Am. J. Hum. Genet 44:* 208-215.

Gagel R.F., Jackson. Ch. E.,Block M. A., Feldman Z.T., Reichlin S., Hamilton B.P., and Tashjian AH. Jr. (1982) Age related probability of development of hereditary medullary thyroid carcinoma *J. Pedia.*101: 941-946

Jackson. Ch. E., Block. M. A., Greenawald. K. A. and Tashjian. A. H. (1979) The Two-mutational-event theory in medullary thyroid cancer. *Am. J. Hum. Genet.*31: 704-710.

Saad M. F., Ordonez N.G., Rashid R.K., Guido J.J., Hill Stratton C. Jr., Hickey R. C and Samaan N.A. (1984) Medullary Carcinoma of the Thyroid. A Study of the Clinical Features and Prognostic Factors in 161 patients. *Medicine 63*: 319-342.

RESUME Entre 1968 et 1988, le Groupe d'Etude des Tumeurs à Calcitonine a rassemblé 837 cas de CMT recensés à partir de données cliniques et sans investigations familiales. L'étude précise de 156 d'entre eux montre que le goitre (82 pour cent des cas) est l'élément révélateur principal et que l'existence de ganglions cervicaux (34 pour cent des cas) est de mauvais pronostic.
30 pour cent de ces cas sont héréditaires et parmi eux 59 pour cent presentent une forme NEM 2A avec, dans les deux tiers des cas, un pheochromocytome diagnostiqué dans un délai de moins de 5 ans, avant pendant ou après le diagnostic de CMT.
Dans moins d'un tiers des formes familiales étudiées un CMT seul est identifié chez chacun des sujets atteints.
L'estimation de la probabilité, pour un sujet à risque, de developper un CMT, avec un screening negatif à un age donné, a permis, par l'étude de 30 fratries de probands et de 156 enfants de sujets atteints, de confirmer la très grande pénétrance du gène.

règle de discrimination manifeste. On peut cependant classer 77% des cas étudiés en utilisant 3 variables.

Plaide en faveur d'un NEM II A une tumeur sans différenciation vésiculaire, comportant des cellules fusiformes, avec une positivité à la calcitonine intéressant moins de 50% des cellules immunomarquées.

. NEM II B :

L'échantillon de population utilisable était insuffisant statistiquement familiaux n=3, apparemment sporadique n=5.

Il nous a cependant paru intéressant de comparer de 5 à 25 ans ce groupe à celui des CMT seul ou NEM II A familiaux. Dès l'âge de 5 ans des tumeurs de plus d'1cm de diamètre sont rencontrées dans les NEM II B avec métastases. Le diamètre tumoral moyen pour la même tranche d'âge dans les CMT seul et les NEM II A est de 1 à 4mm sans métastase. Au delà de l'âge de 14 ans apparaissent des formes avec métastases dans les NEM II A et CMT seul avec un diamètre moyen tumoral de 8,8mm, puis de 23mm au delà de 20 ans.

COMMENTAIRES

L'utilisation d'une analyse multifactorielle nous permet ici de retenir que les CMT bilatéraux sont prédictifs d'une affection familiale, qu'elle soit de type NEM IIA, NEM II B ou CMT seul. Le critère hyperplasie à cellules C n'est pas plus informatif.

Plus difficile est l'identification des NEM II A par rapport aux CMT seuls.

Les paramètres étudiés sont-ils insuffisants pour les discriminer ? Existe-t-il entre ces deux formes un contingent mal classé en raison de l'expression plus tardive de la maladie dans sa totalité ? Cette dernière hypothèse ne peut être exclue. Il semble que certaines formes familiales étiquetées CMT seuls, développent ultérieurement un phéochromocytome les authentifiant alors comme des NEM II A. Le groupe des NEM II B confirme son caractère d'emblée plus malin.

Au delà de l'âge de 14 ans NEM II A et CMT seuls deviennent des tumeurs agressives.

Ces données confortent et justifient les détections précoces. Il manque un paramètre morphologique, biologique ou génétique plus manifeste du risque de cancérisation de la cellule C éventuellement déjà hyperplasique.

BIBLIOGRAPHIE

1. ALBORES-SAAVEDRA J, LIVOLSI V.A, WILLIAMS E.D. Medullary Carcinoma. Seminars in Diagnostic Pathology 1985, 2 (2), 137-146
2. AL SAADI A. Ultrastructure in C cell hyperplasia in asymptomatic patients with hypercalcitoninemia and a family history of medullary thyroid carcinoma. Human Path. 1981, 12 (7), 617-622
3. De LELLIS R.A, NUNNEMACHER G, BITMANW.R, GAGEL R.F, THASHJIAN A.H, BLOUNT M, ASCP, WOLFE J.H. C-cell hyperplasia and medullary thyroid carcinoma in the rat. An immunohistochemical and ultrastrutural analysis. Laboratory Investigation 1979, 40 (2), 140-154
4. Franc B. Le cancer médullaire de la thyroïde (CMT) : Acquisitions récentes. Arch. Anat. Cytol. Path. 1989, 37, n°1-2, 29-35
5. WOLFE H.J., MELVIN K.E.W, CERVI-SKINNER S.J, AL SAADI A.A, JULIAR J.F, JACKSON C.E, TASHJIAN A.H. C-cell hyperplasia preceding medullary thyroid carcinoma. New England Journal of Medecine 1973, 289, 437-441.

RESUME

Les aspects morphologiques des formes familiales des CMT ont été analysés dans deux situations :
. sur thyroïdectomie totale lors de détection précoce biologique dans des familles déjà connues,
. sur des CMT avérés, où une analyse multifactorielle par régression logistique a pu être effectuée.
164 cas ont été utilisés, dont 80 formes familiales. Le facteur le plus prédictif discriminant formes familiales / formes sporadiques est la bilatéralité. La présence d'une importante quantité de substance amyloïde apparait péjorative. Moins performantes sont les tentatives d'identification des NEM IIA familiaux par rapport au CMT seuls familiaux. Il existe peut-être entre les deux groupes un contingent commun.

Rôle de l'anthropologie génétique (généalogie) dans le diagnostic de la forme familiale du cancer médullaire de la thyroïde

A. Chaventré[1], C. Calmettes[2], C. Houdent[3], H. Sobol[4], C. Proye[5], G. Bellis[1] and H. Allannic[6]

[1] Département d'anthropologie et de démographie génétiques, INED, 27, rue du Commandeur, 75014 Paris. [2] INSERM U 113, CHU Saint-Antoine, 75571 Paris Cedex 12. [3] CHU Rouen, 147, avenue du Maréchal-Juin, 76230 Bois-Guillaume. [4] Oncologie génétique, Centre Léon-Bérard, 69373 Lyon. [5] Hôpital C. Huriez, 59037 Lille Cedex. [6] Hôpital Sud, BP 129, 35056 Rennes Cedex, France

ABSTRACT

Genealogical surveys enable us to establish a diagnosis by locating a common factor in the genealogical family tree of different cases possessing similar histological and/or clinical characteristics; identify certain specific geographical regions prone to the disease by tracing descendants of the original muted case; increase reliability of results (lod-scores) by establishing family genealogical ties. A certain number of family ties have so far been established in France (Normandie, Maine et Loire, Vendée) and several geographical regions identified (Morbihan, Bray-Vexin, Massif Central, Ille et Vilaine, Nord).

La diversité des aspects cliniques du cancer médullaire de la thyroïde pose au praticien un certain nombre de problèmes auxquels une approche anthropologique et plus spécifiquement généalogique peut apporter certaines solutions. La distinction entre les cas sporadiques et familiaux comporte, en particulier, quelques difficultés car s'il est parfaitement établi que le mode de transmission est de type autosomal dominant, les proportions mendeliennes attendues peuvent ne pas apparaître sur les courtes séries ou les fratries réduites. Par ailleurs le gène hétérozygote se manifestera presque toujours au niveau du phénotype cependant qu'existent des variations selon l'âge. Ainsi une enquête auprès d'un proposant peut ne pas révéler le caractère familial de la pathologie selon l'importance numérique de la famille et l'âge des sujets considérés.

C'est pour répondre à ce type de difficultés qu'une méthodologie a été mise au point et développée à l'Institut National d'Etudes Démographiques, au sein du département d'anthropologie et de démographie génétiques. Celle-ci consiste, partant d'un cas index, à établir des généalogies aussi profondes et complètes que possible. Dans un premier temps il suffit d'informations telles que le nom, la date et le lieu de naissance pour obtenir les actes d'état civil que nous adressent les mairies, démarche qui a pu être entreprise après l'accord de la Commission Nationale Informatique et Liberté ainsi que celui du Comité National d'Ethique pour les sciences de la vie et de la santé. Dans un souci de confidentialité, un numéro de généalogie est attribué à chaque individu, prenant place dans un réseau d'ascendance et de descendance où sont figurés les principaux évènements démographiques le concernant : naissance, mariage(s), décès avec leurs dates et lieux. Cette procédure épistolaire peut être maintenue tant que les mairies disposent des sources nécessaires après quoi (généralement pour les périodes antérieures à 1802) les actes d'état civil sont à consulter directement auprès des centres d'archives. La réalisation de ces recherches a pu s'effectuer grace à la participation financière de l'A.R.C.[1]

---

[1] Contrat Ass. 1124.

110 familles ont fait à ce jour l'objet d'enquêtes généalogiques (celles-ci ont débuté en 1988), les proposants étant surtout originaires de régions telles que la Bretagne, la Normandie, la Picardie, le Nord-Pas-de-Calais, la Champagne-Ardennes. A un moindre degré apparaissent également le Limousin et la région Midi-Pyrénnées.

La tenue de l'état civil ancien est de qualité fort variable d'une commune à l'autre et ceci conditionne la fiabilité ainsi que la rapidité de la reconstitution généalogique. 53% des familles ont été remontées en ligne directe à 5 générations au moins ce qui nous a permis, à plusieurs reprises, de procéder à des regroupements familiaux ; ainsi deux familles normandes présentant des NEM II a ont pu être reliées auxquelles s'est ajouté un individu dont le cancer semblait initialement de type sporadique. De même des apparentements entre deux familles ont été retrouvées dans le Maine et Loire d'une part, en Vendée d'autre part. Quand les généalogies sont suffisamment profondes il est donc possible de réunir un vaste ensemble de personnes à un ancêtre commun, réalisant un "bouclage" entre sous-familles.

L'ensemble des informations recueillies est mis en forme à partir du logiciel GAO (Généalogies Assistées par Ordinateur) permettant de relier, à l'aide de "pointeurs" un individu à ses parents, son conjoint, ses frères et sœurs, ses enfants. Le programme se charge, en temps réel, d'assurer la cohérence des liens généalogiques et de tracer un arbre ascendant ou descendant. Dans ce cas, partir du couple fondateur permet de répertorier l'ensemble des individus apparentés et soumis au risque de développer un cancer.

Pour les familles normandes précédemment mentionnées nous disposons de la liste nominative des sujets à risque. Cette méthode comporte un aspect essentiellement préventif et permet au clinicien de pratiquer auprès des individus concernés les explorations pouvant mettre en évidence un CMT à un stade infraclinique. L'intérêt est en même temps de limiter le dépistage aux seuls descendants du couple fondateur, optimisant de ce fait ce que les investigations peuvent comporter du point de vue matériel et économique.

L'exploitation généalogique permet en outre de retrouver dans le temps et l'espace les trajets migratoires effectués par les ancêtres. Ainsi, nombre de familles présentent dès les trisaïeux des convergences géographiques étroites, montrant que les échanges matrimoniaux s'effectuaient entre deux ou trois villages seulement. Ces données apparaissent nettement si l'on considère les régions telles que le Morbihan où deux familles sont localisées dans le même canton, le Pays de Bray et le Vexin où se situent trois familles, le Sud du Massif Central (deux familles), l'Ille et Vilaine (cinq familles), le Nord (quatre familles). Ceci est reporté sur la figure 1.

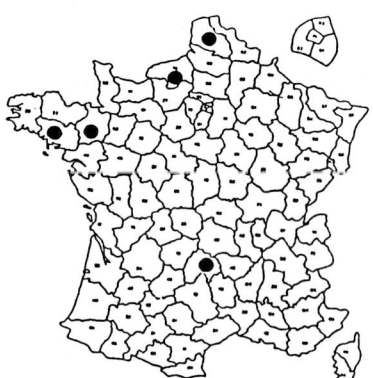

Figure 1 : origines géographiques familiales.

A l'inverse, une famille présente une dissémination importante comme en témoigne la figure 2.

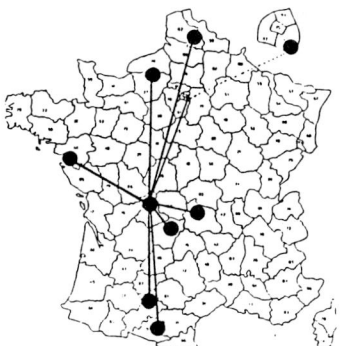

Figure 2 : dispersion de la famille 5.

Enfin les apparentements permettent d'accroître la fiabilité des études génétiques, en particulier celles concernant les études de liaison au niveau du chromosome 10.

L'ensemble de cette méthodologie permet certes de faciliter les investigations cliniques, d'en optimiser les coûts, elle permet une approche préventive du cancer médullaire de la thyroïde tout en donnant au biologiste-moléculaire des informations précieuses, elle n'en reste pas moins pour l'anthropologue et le généalogiste lourde et souvent très longue. Dans cette perspective il apparaît fondamental qu'un échange constant et soutenu s'établisse entre les différents spécialistes attachés à cette pathologie.

REFERENCES

CALMETTES C. (1984) : Problèmes posés par le cancer médullaire de la thyroïde. *Rev. Méd. Int. 5*, 279-282.
GULIANA J.M., MODIGLIANI E., GUILLAUSSEAU P.J., AUBERT P., MILHAUD G., MOUKHTAR M.S., CALMETTES C. (1989) : Détection et pronostic du cancer médullaire de la thyroïde. *Presse Méd. 18*, 521-524.
HOUDENT C., AVRONSART B., DUBUISSON M., OZENNE G., TESTARD J., CALMETTES C., CHAVENTRE A., SOBOL H., LENOIR G.M., WOLF L.M. (1990) : Cancer médullaire familial de la thyroïde. *Presse Méd. 19*, 549-552.
MATHEW C.G.P., CHIN K.S., EASTON D.F. et al. (1987) : A linked genetic marker for multiple endocrine neoplasia type 2a on chromosome 10. *Nature. 328*, 527-528.
PONDER B.A.J., EASTON D.F., MATHEW C.G.P. (1988) : Génétique du cancer médullaire de la thyroïde. *Ann. Endocrinol. 49*, 4-9.
SIMPSON N.E., KIDD K.K., GOODFELLOW P.J. et al. (1987) : Assigment of multiple endocrine neoplasia type 2a to chromosome 10 by linkage. *Nature. 328*, 528-530.
SOBOL H., NAROD S.A., NAKAMURA Y. et al. (1989) : Screening for multiple endocrine neoplasia type 2a with DNA-polymorphism analysis. *N. Engl. J. Med. 321*, 996-1001.

RESUME

Les enquêtes généalogiques permettent de faire le diagnostic de la forme familiale par rattachement de cas dispersés possédant les mêmes critères histologiques et/ou cliniques ; de localiser les aires géographiques de la maladie à partir des descendants des têtes de mutation ; d'accroître la fiabilité des résultats (lod-scores) par la jonction des branches familiales. D'ores et déjà un certain nombre d'apparentements familiaux ont été retrouvés (Normandie, Maine et Loire, Vendée) et quelques localisations géographiques effectuées (Morbihan, Bray-Vexin, Sud du Massif Central, Ille et Vilaine, Nord).

V. Multiple endocrine neoplasia type 2
V. *Néoplasie endocrinienne multiple type 2*

Men 2A pheochromocytomas : GETC French multicentric retrospective study (1960-1988)

J. Caron[1]*, V. Boiteau[1], S. Casanova[2], D. Farkas[3], M. Rosenberg-Bourgin[3], N. Feingold[3], C. Calmettes[4], E. Modigliani[2], and the GETC

[1] Service d'Endocrinologie, Hôpital Maison Blanche, 45, rue Cognacq-Jay, 51092 Reims Cedex. [2] Endocrinologie CHU Bobigny, 93009 Bobigny. [3] Epidémiologie génétique, INSERM U155, Université Paris VII, 75251 Paris Cedex 5. [4] INSERM U 113, CHU Saint-Antoine, 75571 Paris, France

* Author for correspondence

Abstract :

Main features of 106 MEN 2A Pheochromocytomas in 53 french families collected by GETC are reported.
MEN 2A Pheochromocytomas may be clinically asymptomatic (21,4 %). Urinary high metanephrines appear as the most sensitive index of tumour. Predominantly unilateral lesions suggested unilateral adrenalectomy in 33 %. Detection of pheochromocytomas preceded MTC in 39 %.

*****

The aim of this study was to analyze the main features of MEN 2A Pheochromocytomas collected by GETC (Groupe d'Etude sur les Tumeurs à Calcitonine). The study period includes 28 years which is a critical period for MEN 2A :
1 - Concept of MEN 2A and of familial screening appears in medical practice after 1970 and is not yet fully generalized,
2 - Improvement of hormonal study methods is evident : catecholamine metabolism was in the 60th mostly evaluated by fluorimetric dosage of VMA and now by HPLC dosage of each catecholamine metabolites,
3 - Improvement of morphological investigations is note-worthy, with progressive introduction of non-invasive morphological techniques : TDM, ultrasonography and MIBG Scintigraphy.
For these reasons this analysis, has araised some difficulties and results have to be considered as an historical approach of this problem, and not as the expression of new developments in this field.

I - MATERIAL :

Among 993 MTC patients screened for Adrenal Medullary Disease (AMD) and primary hyperparathyroidism, 159 MEN 2A (16 %) were identified. MEN 2A were considered as sporadic (negative familial screening) in 23 %, and familial in 77 % (53 families).

Sufficient information was obtained for further analysis in only 116 MEN 2A patients (106 patients : MTC + Pheochromocytoma ± HPT[1] ; 10 patients : MTC + HPT[1]).

Histologically proven pheochromocytomas were only considered in analysis.

II - METHODS :

Information (Diagnosis circumstances, time interval between MTC and pheochromocytoma diagnosis, clinical symptoms, hormonal pattern, morphological, surgical and histological datas), has been systematically collected through a questionnary.

III - RESULTS :

a - <u>Diagnosis circumstances</u> (Table 1) : most pheochromocytomas (58 %) have been detected through systematic investigations. In these patients, clinical symptoms of pheochromocytomas were absent or latent.

In 42 % clinical symptoms were highly suggestive of pheochromocytoma.

-Systematic detection (without patent clinical symptoms)		58 %
-before MTC surgery	27	%
-familial screening	14,6	%
-MTC follow up	13,6	%
-HPT[1] investigation	2,2	%
-Clinical symptoms of pheochromocytoma		42 %
-during a familial screening	2	%
-without any orientation towards MEN	40	%

Table 1 : MEN 2A Pheochromocytomas = DIAGNOSTIC CIRCUMSTANCES OF PHEOCHROMOCYTOMAS

b - <u>Chronological occurence of pheochromocytoma versus MTC</u> (Table 2) : simultaneous diagnosis is observed in 41,2 %, but in 58,8 % pheochromocytoma occurs before (39 %) or after (18,5 %) MTC diagnosis, mostly within 5 years.

Concomitant detection	41,2%
Non concomitant detection	58,8%
Pheo before MTC	39 %
< 1 year	11,4 %
1 << 5 years	17,54%
5 << 10 years	7 %
10 < 5 years	1,8 %
> ` years	1,8 %
MTC before héo	18,5%
< year	9,6 %
1 << years	4,4 %
5 << years	0,9 %
10 << years	1,8 %
15 << 25 years	1,8 %

Table : MEN 2A Pheochromocytomas =
CHRONOLOGICAL OCCURENCE PHEOCHROMOCYTOMA VS MTC

c - <u>Clinical symptoms</u> (Table 3):

- Asymptomatic		21,4%
- Death perioperatory	1,9%`	
sudden	6,9	8,8%
- Hypertension		57,4%
- Hypotension orthostatic		14,1%
- Hypersudation		43,2%
- Palpitations		12 %
- Headache		7 %
- Hypertension		
-only		4 %
-headache hypersudation palpitations		1,6%

Table 3 : MEN 2A Pheochromocytomas =
CLINICAL FEATURES

Asymptomatic pheochromocytomas are observed in 21,4 %. Most of them are detected through systematic screening before MTC surgery. Death is observed in 9 % and is still persistent after 1980. Death usually occurs in patient with previous suggestive symptoms of pheochromocytoma, and is induced by classical agents such angiography, surgery, labour.

Hypertension is present in 57,4 %, often associated with hypersudation (43,2 %), or palpitations (12 %). Neverthless the classical triad, hypersudation palpitations headache, has been reported in only 1,6 %.

d - <u>Hormonal pattern</u> : Diagnosis of pheochromocytoma was usually established when total urinary catecholamines, metanephrines and VMA were elevated mostly in one only 24 h urine sample. Total metanephrine increase appears as the most sensitive index of these pheochromocytomas since, high urinary levels are observed in 90 %. Total catecholamine increase (74 %), and VMA increase (71 %) are less reliable. In this series one only patient had repeated normal urinary hormonal pattern.

   e -Morphological datas (Table 4):

- No information		30 %
- Informative patients		
Adrenal TDM	(n=70)	96 % +
MIBG ScintiG	(n=45)	86 % +
U S	(n=45)	77 % +
MIBG + TDM	(n=43)	

Table 4 : MEN 2A Pheochromocytomas = MORPHOLOGICAL ASPECTS

   Adrenal CT Scan has been more often performed than MIBG scintigraphy. In this series TDM was positive in 96 % and MIBG in only 86 %.
   MIBG and TDM datas were concordant in 72 %, discordant information is reported for 10 patients. In 8/10 histology confirmed TDM datas and not MIBG.

   f - Adrenal surgery has been primarily bilateral in 39.3%, secondarily bilateral in 15 % . Mean time between the 2 surgical procedures was 4.5 years (one month and 15 years). Unilateral adrenalectomy has been performed in 33 %.

   g - Histological datas confirmed pheochromocytoma in 94 %, nodular hyperplasia was reported in 6 %.
Distant metastasis were not reported.

DISCUSSION - CONCLUSION

   Analysis of this series of 106 MEN 2A Pheochromocytomas focus on some points :

   High number of MEN 2A french families may be stressed. Neverthless screening in these 53 MEN 2A families appears not optimal since in each MEN 2A family, only 2,3 MEN 2A patients are identified. These results contrast with exhaustive reports of large european families (1,2) but focus on the high prevalence of MEN 2A families in France.

   Diagnosis of pheochromocytoma may precede MTC and this suggests that familial screening in MEN 2A family, must be simultaneously directed towards thyroid parathyroid and adrenal medullary function.

As previously reported in the litterature, clinically asymptomatic phreochromocytoma are not unfrequent in MEN 2A, so hormonal screening must be systematic, even in asymptomatic patients.

As in sporadic pheochromocytoma high urinary MN appears as the most sensitive index of histologically proven pheochromocytoma.

Predominantly unilateral adrenal lesions have suggested unilateral adrenalectomy in 33 % in this series.

Distant metastasis have not yet been reported.

*****

We want to thank all french physicians whose names are here reported for their collaboration,

Allanic, Bachelot, Baulieu, Bennet, Bernard, Berthezene, Bigorgne, Blanc, Boneu, Bonnichon, Bouchard, Chabrier, Chadenas, Charpentier, Chupin, Cloche, Cohen, Combes, Conte-Delvox, Corvol, Croisier, Delambre, Delepine, Delisle, Desbois, Doumith, Duchene, Dupond, Duprey, Feruscla, Fossati, Fouqueray, Gainet, Gardet, Gay, Gilson, Godefroy, Guillaume, Guillaumie, Guillausseau, Guliana, Houdent, Jaquet, Lalau, Leclere, Lecomte, Lefebvre, Lorcy, Luquel, Mace, Mahoudeau, Maunand, Modigliani, Mornex, Plouin, Pugeat, Putelat, Roger, Rohmer, Schaison, Siame-Mourot, Tcherdakoff, Tourniaire, Treffot, Verges, Wemeau, Wolf.

*****

1 - VASEN HFA, NIEUWENHUIJZEN-KRUSEMAN AC, and Al. (1987) : Multiple endocrine neoplasia syndrome type 2 : The value of screening and central registration. Am. J. of Medicine, 83, 847-852.
2 - TELENIUS BERG M, BERG B, and Al. (1984) : Impact of screening on prognosis in the multiple endocrine neoplasia type 2 syndromes : natural history and treatment results in 105 patients. Henry Ford Hosp. Med. J., 32,4, 225-232.

*****

Les caractéristiques des 106 phéochromocytomes issus de 53 familles françaises de MEN 2A sont rapportées.

La précession du phéochromocytome par rapport au CMT dans 39 % des cas est soulignée, ainsi que la latence clinique du phéochromocytome (21,4 % des cas).

L'élévation des métanéphrines urinaires apparait comme l'index le plus sensible de tumeur.

La surrénalectomie unilatérale est choisie dans 33 % des cas en raison de lésions strictement, ou, à prédominance unilatérale.

Hyperparathyroïdie et néoplasie endocrinienne multiple de type 2A. Aspects cliniques, biologiques et chirurgicaux

Pierre-Jean Guillausseau[1], Claudine Guillausseau-Scholer[2], Emile Sarfati[3], Philippe Chanson[1], Marie-Emilie Chauveau[1], Jean-Louis Baulieu[4], Gérard Gay[5], Jean Lubetzki[1] and the GETC

(1) Service de Médecine Interne, Hôpital Lariboisière, 75010 Paris. (2) Service de Médecine Nucléaire, Hôpital de la Pitié, 75013 Paris. (3) Service de Chirurgie, Hôpital Saint-Louis, 75010 Paris. (4) INSERM U 316 et Service de Médecine Nucléaire, Hôpital Bretonneau, 37044 Tours. (5) Service de Médecine Interne, Hôpital Saint-Nicolas, 55100 Verdun, France

RESUME

La prévalence de l'atteinte parathyroïdienne au cours des néoplasies endocriniennes de type 2a est en moyenne de 30 % avec des extrêmes de 15 à 92 %. Parfois asymptomatique, et découverte de dépistage systématique, l'hyperparathyroïdie peut révéler l'affection par une lithiase urinaire récidivante et être à l'origine de complications infectieuses. Une hypercalcémie est habituelle, avec une élévation inappropriée des concentrations de PTH immunoréactive dans tous les cas. Le recours à des tests dynamiques est inutile dans la majorité des cas. L'aspect anatomopathologique est celui d'une hyperplasie d'une ou de plusieurs glandes dans 80 % des cas. L'éxérèse systématique de trois glandes sur quatre, même macroscopiquement normales, associée à l'excision des reliquats thymiques, apparaît le geste chirurgical le plus adapté.

MOTS-CLES : Hyperparathyroïdie, néoplasie endocrinienne multiple de type 2a, hypercalcémie, lithiase urinaire, PTH, parathyroïdectomie.

Dès la description princeps faite par Sipple (1961) de la néoplasie endocrinienne multiple de type 2a (NEM 2a), l'atteinte parathyroïdienne est notée, sous forme d'une hypertrophie nodulaire. Néanmoins, cette atteinte s'efface, comme dans d'autres publications ultérieures consacrées au syndrome, derrière le carcinome médullaire thyroïdien et l'atteinte médullo-surrénalienne. Individualisée ensuite, la néoplasie endocrinienne multiple de type 2b qui associe au carcinome médullaire et au phéochromocytome un aspect marfanoïde et des neuromes muqueux semble épargner cliniquement et biologiquement les parathyroïdes. L'étude systématique réalisée par Carney et coll (1980) à la Mayo Clinic indique tout au plus une absence d'involution parathyroïdienne chez l'adulte, avec un aspect d'hyperplasie des cellules principales.

Notre propos ne s'adressera donc qu'à l'atteinte parathyroïdienne des NEM 2a.

ASPECTS EPIDEMIOLOGIQUES

Notre travail repose sur l'étude de 5 familles grâce à une collaboration s'inscrivant dans l'activité du Groupe d'Etude des Tumeurs à Calcitonine. Deux de ces familles ont leur origine en France, la description de l'une d'entre elle ayant déjà été publiée (Guillausseau et coll, 1988). Les trois autres familles sont originaires du Maghreb (respectivement régions de Bizerte de Tizi Ouzou et de Casablanca. Ces familles ont fait l'objet d'une évaluation approfondie et répétée afin de dépister les différentes atteintes, et pour quatre d'entre elles d'une détermination des marqueurs de la région péricentromérique du chromosome 10. Le diagnostic d'atteinte parathyroïdienne a reposé sur le dosage de la calcémie, de la parathormone-immunoréactive (i-PTH), le diagnostic de carcinome médullaire sur les résultats du dosage de la calcitonine plasmatique à l'état basal et/ou après stimulation par la pentagastrine, celui de phéochromocytome sur le dosage de la métadrénaline et de la normétadrénaline dans les urines de 24 heures. Dans tous les cas, le diagnostic a été confirmé par l'examen anatomo-pathologique des pièces d'exérèse, ou de l'étude nécropsique. L'étude des 5 familles a révélé l'existence de 31 cas de NEM 2a, avec un carcinome médullaire bilatéral (ou une hyperplasie nodulaire des cellules C) dans 27 cas/27 (100 %) (4 cas autopsiques sans examen cervical), un phéochromocytome dans 19 cas sur 31 (61 %), et une atteinte parathyroïdienne dans 13 cas sur 28 (46,5 %).
La prévalence de l'atteinte parathyroïdienne apparaît très variable dans la littérature (tableau 1), comprise entre 15 et 92 %. Si l'on calcule la prévalence à partir des 237 cas de NEM 2a de ce tableau, on aboutit à une valeur de 30 % (72/237).

	Familles de NEM 2a n	Cas de NEM 2a n	Atteinte parathyroïdienne n	%
Melvin et coll (1972)		12	11	92
Gagel et coll (1988)	1	22		
		34		32
Keiser et coll (1973)	1	25	16	64
Block et coll (1975) Sizemore et coll (1977)	3	63	19	30
Vasen et coll (1987)	10	87	13	15
Présente série (1990)	5	31	13/28	46,5
Total	20	237	72/237	30 (15-92 %)

Tableau 1 : Prévalence de l'atteinte parathyroïdienne dans les néoplasies endocriniennes multiples de type 2a (NEM 2a).

L'enquête épidémiologique dans le cadre du Groupe d'Etude des Tumeurs à Calcitonine indique un chiffre proche : 33/116 soit 28,4 %. Les divergences relevées entre les différentes séries ne s'expliquent pas par l'âge des patients lors de la survenue de l'atteinte parathyroïdienne. Pour des âges moyens compris entre 30 et 38 ans (tableau 2), la prévalence varie de 15 % à 92 %.

	Prévalence de l'atteinte parathyroïdienne		Age moyen (années)
Melvin et coll (1972)	92 %		38,5
Gagel et coll (1988)	0 %		11,8
Keiser et coll (1973)	64 %		34
Block et coll (1975)			
Sizemore et coll (1977)	30 %		30
Vasen et coll (1987)	15 %	A	38,6
		B	29,2
		C	13,2
Présente série	46 %		38,2

Tableau 2 : Prévalence de l'atteinte parathyroïdienne en fonction de l'âge moyen des patients atteints de néoplasie endocrinienne multiple de type 2a étudiés.

De même l'atteinte parathyroïdienne est absente dans l'étude longitudinale d'une famille par Gagel et coll (1988) où l'âge initial moyen est de 11,8 ans. Chez l'un de nos patients, âgé de 15 ans, âge moyen proche de celui des précédents, une hyperparathyroïdie a été découverte lors de l'enquête familiale initiale.
L'atteinte parathyroïdienne est synchrone ou métachrome aux autres atteintes, et ne précède le carcinome médullaire de la thyroïde qu'exceptionnellement. Le cas rapporté par Allo et coll (1983) semble à cet égard unique. Une coïncidence pourrait d'ailleurs être évoquée pour cette observation non familiale. Comme celui des autres atteintes, le mécanisme de l'atteinte parathyroïdienne des NEM 2a est inconnu, au contraire de celui des NEM 1. Le rôle d'une hyperstimulation des parathyroïdes par hypersécrétion prolongée de calcitonine est actuellement écarté par tous les auteurs.

ASPECTS CLINIQUES ET BIOLOGIQUES

L'étude de notre série de 13 cas indique que la bénignité clinique de l'atteinte parathyroïdienne n'est qu'apparente. Dans 4 cas (13 %), l'hyperparathyroïdie est la première manifestation amenant à la découverte de la NEM 2a. Dans six cas, une lithiase urinaire, bilatérale et récidivante a été mise en évidence. Dans un cas, cette lithiase a été responsable de pyélonéphrites aiguës à répétition, et d'une orchite à pyogènes, conduisant à une orchidectomie unilatérale. Chez une femme de 69 ans, l'hyperparathyroïdie et la NEM 2a ont été découvertes au stade d'insuffisance rénale sévère par néphrocalcinose. Dans un cas unique, une hypercalcémie aiguë (3,67 mM/l) a été responsable du décès du patient à l'âge de 31 ans après exérèse d'un carcinome

médullaire et d'une parathyroïde hyperplasique. Une telle évolution ne semble pas avoir été rapportée à ce jour dans la littérature. Dans 5 cas, l'hyperparathyroïdie a été découverte devant l'existence d'une hypercalcémie a ou pauci symptomatique lors du dépistage systématique. Dans 3 cas, la calcémie était dans les limites de la normale. Dans un cas le patient présentait une lithiase urinaire, dans les deux autres cas, il existait une élévation inappropriée de la PTH immunoréactive. L'âge moyen de découverte était de 48 $\pm$ 14,7 ans en cas de lithiase et de 30 $\pm$ 11 ans dans les formes sans lithiase urinaire.
La calcémie était élevée dans 10 cas sur 13, alors que la

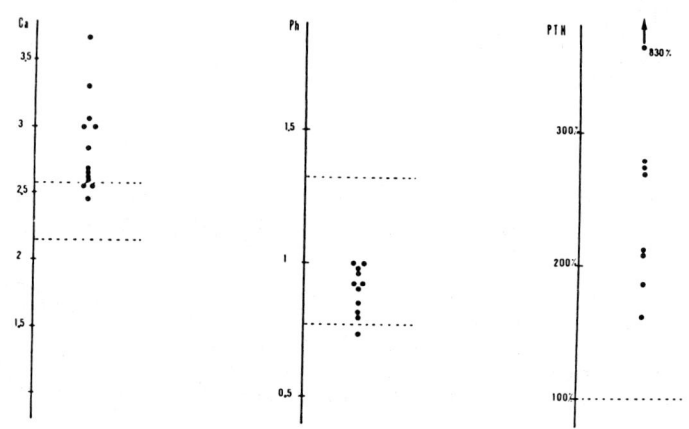

Légende fig.1 : Calcémie (mM/l), phosphorémie (mM/l), i-PTH plasmatique chez des patients atteints d'hyperparathyroïdie dans le cadre d'une néoplasie endocrinienne multiple de type 2a.
En pointillé : limites de la normale. Les résultats d'i-PTH sont exprimés en pourcentage (%) de la limite supérieure de la normale.

phosphorémie n'était basse que dans 1 cas (fig. 1). Le dosage de la PTH immunoréactive a été réalisé dans 8 cas. Exprimée en pourcentage de la limite supérieure de la normale (compte-tenu de la multiplicité des méthodes de dosage au cours du temps), elle est élevée dans 8 cas sur 8.

Le dosage du fragment C terminal 53-84 (élevé dans 4 cas sur 4) et celui du fragment intermédiaire 44-68) élevé dans 7 cas sur 7 semblent donner des résultats équivalents. Le dosage de la PTH intacte 1-84 est disponible depuis peu. Utilisé dans les deux derniers cas que nous avons étudiés, les résultats étaient normaux en valeur absolue mais "inappropriés" par rapport à la valeur élevée du calcium ionisé plasmatique contemporain. Le dosage de fragments à durée de demi-vie plus longue pourrait être plus adapté au dépistage, le dosage de la PTH 1-84 serait à réserver aux tests de freination telle la perfusion intra-veineuse de calcium proposée par Heath et coll (1976). Des études supplémentaires sont nécessaires pour préciser ces points. Nous n'avons réalisé d'épreuve de freinage que dans 3 cas. Le test utilisé comporte une détermination de l'AMPc néphrogénique (rapporté à la filtration glomérulaire) avant et après charge orale de 1 g de calcium. Une absence de freinage ou une augmentation paradoxale a été observée dans ces 3 cas.

Plusieurs observations d'hypercalcémies réversibles après exérèse d'un phéochromocytome ont été rapportées dans la littérature (Gagel et coll, 1988 ; Stewart et coll, 1985). Plusieurs hypothèses ont été proposées : effet des catécholamines sur la sécrétion de PTH ou sur la résorption osseuse ostéoclasique, sécrétion de peptide PTH-semblable. Cette dernière hypothèse a été démontrée par Heath et coll (1990) grâce à la mise en évidence de l'ARN messager de la protéine liée à la PTH (PTH-related protein) dans un phéochromocytome.

ASPECTS ANATOMO-PATHOLOGIQUES

Dans 8 cas, deux parathyroïdes ou plus étaient pathologiques (hyperplasie et/ou adénome). Dans 5 cas, une seule glande était anormale, et son exérèse a conduit à la normalisation du bilan phosphocalcique. Nous avons relevé l'existence d'une hyperplasie d'une ou plusieurs glandes dans 8 cas/13 (66 %) de 1 ou plusieurs adénomes sans hyperplasie dans 3 cas, de l'association adénome d'une glande associée à une hyperplasie dans un cas.

	Nb de cas de NEM 2a	Nb de cas d'atteinte parathyroïdienne	Hyperplasie	Adénome
Melvin et coll (1972) Gagel et coll (1988)	12	11	10	1
Keiser et coll (1973)	25	16	12	4
Block et coll (1975) Sizemore et coll (1977)	63	19	17	2
Présente série	31	13	9	4
Total	131	59	48 (81 %)	11 (19 %)

Tableau 3 : Aspects anatomo-pathologiques de l'atteinte parathyroïdienne au cours des néoplasies endocriniennes multiples de type 2a (NEM 2a).

Des valeurs comparables sont trouvées dans la littérature (tableau 3), l'hyperplasie d'une ou plusieurs glandes étant relevée en moyenne dans 81 % des cas.

TRAITEMENT

La localisation des glandes pathologiques ne relève que de l'expérience du chirurgien. Les tentatives de visualisation préopératoire sont donc inutiles. Sur le plan chirurgical, l'hyperparathyroïdie des NEM 2a pose des problèmes voisins de ceux des NEM 1. Faut-il uniquement enlever les glandes macroscopiquement pathologiques ? L'hyperplasie des NEM 2a est particulière car asymétrique, avec des glandes de grande taille et des glandes de taille normale, simulant ainsi un adénome. Pour éviter un tel écueil, il nous apparaît logique et surtout prudent de considérer qu'il s'agit dans tous les cas d'une maladie diffuse des parathyroïdes, et qu'il convient donc de faire un geste chirurgical sur les quatre glandes. De fait, n'enlevant que les glandes manifestement pathologiques, Malnaeus et coll (1986) déplorent 88 % d'hyperparathyroïdies persistantes et récidivantes et Van Heerden et coll (1983) observent 25 % d'hyperparathyroïdies persistantes. La recherche d'une glande surnuméraire doit être menée de manière systématique, avec excision des 2 résidus thymiques. L'éventualité d'une glande surnuméraire n'est pas plus fréquente dans les NEM 2a que dans la population générale. Lorsqu'elle existe une telle glande est aussi hyperplasique.

Deux gestes chirurgicaux sont possibles, la parathyroïdectomie totale avec réimplantation et la parathyroïdectomie sub-totale. Les preuves de la supériorité d'une méthode sur l'autre font défaut. Au cours de la thyroïdectomie totale pour carcinome médullaire, le chirurgien doit conserver une des glandes bien vascularisées, en la laissant en place et en la repérant. Si les quatre glandes sont dévascularisées, il convient de réaliser une réimplantation dans un muscle long supinateur.

La majorité des patients atteints de NEM 2a (soit en moyenne 70 %) n'ont pas d'hyperparathyroïdie. De fait il apparait logique, et sans inconvénient, lorsqu'au cours de la thyroïdectomie les quatre glandes apparaissent normales, d'enlever trois glandes parathyroïdes et les reliquats thymiques et de laisser une glande normale en place.

REFERENCES

Allo, M.D. & Thompson, N.W. (1983) : Hyperparathyroidism as a part of MEA I and MEA II syndromes. In Surgery of the thyroid and parathyroid glands, ed. E.L. Kaplan, pp 177-187. Edinburgh : Churchill Livingstone.

Block, M.A., Jackson, J.E. & Tashjian, A.H. (1975) : Management of parathyroid glands in surgery for medullary thyroid carcinoma Arch. Surg. 110, 617-624.

Carney, J.A., Roth, S.I., Heath, H., Sizemore, G.W. & Bayles, A.B. (1980) : The parathyroid glands in multiple endocrine neoplasia type 2b. Am. J. Pathol. 99, 387-395.

Gagel, R.F., Tashjian, A.H., Cummings, T., Papathanasopoulos, N., Kaplan, M.M., De Lellis, R.A., Wolfe, H.J. & Reichlin, S. (1988) : The clinical outcome of prospective screening for multiple endocrine neoplasia type 2a. N. Engl. J. Med. 318, 478-484.

Guillausseau, P.J., Guillausseau, C., Calmettes, C., Feingold, N., Demenais, F., Sobol, H., Gony, J., Hors, J., Schaison, G., Seret, D., Lubetzki, J., Baulieu, J.L., Guilloteau, D., Gay, G., Hamon, P., Thomas, J.L., Leclere, J., Perrier, P., Tourniaire, J. & Betuel, H. (1988) : Polyadénomatose endocrinienne de type 2a (MEN 2a). Etude clinique et génétique d'une famille. Ann. Endocrinol. (Paris) 49, 17-21.

Heath, D.A., Senior, P.V., Varley, J.M. & Beck, F. (1990) : Parathyroid-hormone-related protein in tumours associated with hypercalcaemia. Lancet i, 66-69.

Heath, H., Sizemore, G.W. & Carney, J.A. (1976) : Preoperative diagnosis of occult parathyroid hyperplasia by calcium infusion in patients with multiple endocrine neoplasia, type 2a. J. Clin. Endocrinol. Metab. 43, 428-435.

Keiser, H.R., Beaven, M.A., Doppman J., Wells S. & Buja, L.M. (1973) : Sipple's syndrome : medullary thyroid carcinoma, pheochromocytoma and parathyroid disease. Studies in a large family. Ann. Intern. Med. 78, 561-579.

Malmaeus, J., Benson, L., Johanson, H., Ljunghall, L., Rastad, J., Akerstrom, G. & Oberg, K. (1986) : Parathyroid surgery in the multiple endocrine neoplasia type 1 syndromes : choice of surgical procedure. World J. Surg. 10, 668-672.

Melvin, K.E.W., Tashjian, A.H. & Miller, H.H. (1972) : Studies in familial (medullary) thyroid carcinoma. Rec. Progr. Horm. Res. 28, 399-470.

Sipple, J.H. (1961) : The association of pheochromocytoma with carcinoma of the thyroid gland. Am. J. Med. 31, 163-166.

Sizemore, G.W., Carney, J.A. & Heath, H. (1977) : Epidemiology of medullary carcinoma of the thyroid gland : a 5-year experience (1971-1976). Surg. Clin. North America 57, 633-645.

Stewart, A.F., Hoecker, J.L., Mallette, L.E., Segre, V., Amatruda, T. T. & Vignery, A. (1985) : Hypercalcemia in pheochromocytoma. Evidence for a novel mechanism. Ann. Intern. Med. 102, 776-779.

Van Heerden, J.A., Kent, R.B., Sizemore, G.W., Grant, C.S. & Remine, W.H. (1983) : Primary hyperparathyroidism in patients with multiple endocrine neoplasia syndromes. Surgical experience. Arch. Surg. 118, 533-536.

Vasen, H.F.A., Nieuwenhuijzen Kruseman, A.C., Berkel, H., Beukers, E.K.M., Delprat, C.T., Van Doorn, R.G., Geerdink, R.A., Haak, H.R., Hackeng, W.H.L., Koppeschaar, H.P.F., Krenning E.P., Lamberts, S.W.J., Lekkerkerker, F.J.F., Michels, R.P.J., Moers, A.M.J., Pieters, G.F.F.M., Wiersinga, W.H. & Lips, C.J.M. (1987) : Multiple endocrine neoplasia syndrome type 2 : the value of screening and central registration. A study of 15 kindreds in the Netherlands. Am. J. Med. 83, 847-852.

La néoplasie endocrinienne multiple de type 2B. Etude de 25 cas apparemment sporadiques. Recherche d'éléments de pronostic

Anne Meer[*], Claude Calmettes[**][1], A. Munck[***] et le Groupe d'Etude des Tumeurs à Calcitonine (GETC)

[*] Service de Médecine Générale et Nutrition, Hôtel Dieu, Paris.
[**] INSERM U 113, CHU Saint-Antoine, 184, rue du Faubourg-Saint-Antoine, 75571 Paris Cedex 13.
[***] Service de Gastro-Entérologie, Hôpital Robert-Debré, Paris, France
[1] Auteur pour correspondance

La Néoplasie Endocrinienne Multiple type 2B (NEM 2B) associe en particulier un cancer médullaire de la thyroïde (CMT), un phéochromocytome (Phéo), un syndrome dysmorphique marfanoïde et une neurofibromatose diffuse atteignant l'ensemble du tube digestif et l'appareil ophtalmique.

En France, le GETC a recensé actuellement 29 cas de NEM 2b apparemment sporadiques. Nous en avons étudié 25 et recherché à leur propos d'éventuels éléments pronostiques.

L'âge moyen de diagnostic de la maladie est de 16,9 ans (de 2 mois à 57 ans dont 52 % avant 16 ans. L'élément ayant conduit au diagnostic est :
  * le CMT dans 18 cas (72 %)
  * Le phéochromocytome dans 3 cas (12 %)
  * La présence de neuromes buccolabiaux dans 1 cas (4 %)
  * L'existence d'une pseudo-obstruction intestinale chronique néonatale (communément appelé pseudosyndrome de Hirschsprung) dans 3 cas (12 %).

- Le CMT et/ou hyperplasie des cellules C étaient présents dans 100 % des cas avec un âge moyen de diagnostic de 17,25 ans (2 à 57 ans).

- Le phéochromocytome a été retrouvé chez 10 patients soit 40 % avec un âge moyen de diagnostic de 23,9 ans (13 à 30 ans).
Il est bilatéral dans 5 cas, unilatéral dans 3 cas et de topographie non précisée dans 2 cas.
Il est exclusivement surrénalien et toujours bénin.
Les symptômes ayant permis le diagnostic sont soit absents, soit frustes (HTA dans 2 cas, malaise et céphalées dans 2 cas).

La fréquence des différents éléments de la la neurofibromatose est difficile à évaluer, les observations n'étant pas toujours suffisamment précises :

* La neurofibromatose oculaire a été affirmée dans 9 cas, éliminée dans 7, les autres cas étant insuffisamment documentés.
* La neurofibromatose buccale est fréquente et retrouvée chez 21 patients soit 84 % des 25 patients.
* L'atteinte intestinale a été montrée chez 8 patients sur 20 ayant subi soit une biopsie de muqueuse rectale, soit une intervention chirurgicale, soit une autopsie.
* 3 sujets avaient une pseudo-obstruction intestinale chronique.

L'âge d'apparition de la neurofibromatose ne peut être évalué, les données dont nous disposons étant incomplètes sur ce sujet.

Les seuls 2 cas de rémission concernent 2 patients porteurs d'une simple hyperplasie pathologique des cellules C :
1°) un enfant dont le diagnostic de MEN 2B a été porté à l'âge de 2 mois à l'occasion d'une pseudo-obstruction intestinale chronique. Cet enfant a été thyroïdectomisé à l'âge de 8 ans devant un test à la pentagastrine devenant pathologique. Il est en rémission depuis 10 ans.
2°) un patient porteur d'un phéochromocytome dont la maladie a été découverte à l'âge de 16 ans. Le recul n'est actuellement que de 1 an.

Dans tous les autres cas, la calcitoninémie reste élevée, soit immédiatement après la thyroïdectomie, soit s'élève secondairement.

Des métastases sont localisées chez 18 patients :
- 18 métastases ganglionnaires
- 6 métastases hépatiques
- 11 métastases pulmonaires
- 5 métastases osseuses

3 sujets n'ont pas de métastases décelables, les 4 derniers ont des dossiers incomplets ne permettant pas de conclure.

Le décès est survenu chez 12 patients (1 seul perdu de vue). Il est toujours dû au cancer thyroïdien avec un âge moyen de 26,8 ans (12-58 ans) et un délai après le diagnostic de 5 ans en moyenne. Actuellement 12 patients sont vivants avec un recul par rapport au diagnostic de :
- moins de 3 ans dans 3 cas
- de 3 à 10 ans dans 3 cas
- et plus de 10 ans (10-18) dans 6 cas, remettant en cause le pronostic très péjoratif à court terme du CMT dans les MEN 2B.

La recherche d'éléments prédictifs d'une évolution plus favorable nous a donc paru intéressante.

Le seul élément pronostic qui a pu être retenu est la présence d'un phéochromocytome. En effet, il n'y a pas de différence évolutive en fonction du sexe des patients, ni de la présence ou non de métastases. La valeur des taux de calcitoninémie ne peut être prise en compte, les méthodes de dosage utilisées étant non comparables d'un patient à l'autre. Cette différence évolutive existe par contre entre sujets porteurs de phéochromocytome ou non.

L'âge de diagnostic est plus tardif 20,5 ans (13-30 ans) contre 14,5 ans (2 mois à 57 ans) (p<0,02*) et l'âge de décès plus élevé 32,2 ans (26-37) contre 19,3 ans (12-28 ans) (p<0,02*) si on les compare aux sujets n'ayant pas de phéochromocytome ; la durée de survie après le diagnostic de NEM 2B étant de 9,75 ans pour les 5 patients décédés avec Phéo contre 3,14 ans pour les 7 patients décédés sans Phéo.

On peut donc penser que le phéochromocytome apparaît chez des sujets dont le CMT aurait une moindre agressivité laissant le temps à la tumeur surrénalienne de se développer.

La présence d'un phéochromocytome pourrait être considérée comme "marqueur" d'une forme de NEM 2B de meilleur pronostic. Du fait de la rareté de la maladie, cette étude est restée limitée à 25 cas ; son interprétation reste donc difficile.

* Méthode non paramétrique de MANN Whitney ou WILCOXON.

ROUND TABLE : screening diagnosis and treatment of pheochromocytomas associated with MTC

Participants : J.L. Baulieu[1], C. Calmettes[2], J. Caron[3], J.L. Dupont[4], J.F. Henry[5], R. Mornex[6], G. Opocher[7], P.F. Plouin[8], C. Proye[9] and F. Raue[10]

[1] INSERM U 316 et Médecine Nucléaire, CHRU Bretonneau, 37044 Tours Cedex, France. [2] INSERM U 113, Faculté de Médecine Saint-Antoine, 75571 Paris Cedex 12, France. [3] Département d'Anthropologie et de Démographie Génétiques, Hôpital de Maison Blanche, 51092 Reims Cedex, France. [4] Service de Médecine Interne, Hôpital Jean-Minjoz, 25000 Besançon, France. [5] Unité de Chirurgie Endocrinienne, CHU de la Timone, 13385 Marseille Cedex 05, France. [6] INSERM U 197, Faculté de Médecine Alexis Carrel, 69372 Lyon Cedex 08, France. [7] Institute of Semeiotica Medica, University of Padova, 35128 Padova, Italy. [8] Département d'Hypertension, Hôpital Broussais, 75674 Paris, France. [9] Service de Chirurgie Générale et Endocrinienne, Hôpital Huriez, 59037 Lille Cedex, France. [10] Department of Internal Medicine I, University of Heidelberg, 69000 Heidelberg, Germany

Five questions were submitted for discussion :
MEN 2A pheochromocytomas
1. Screening who ?
2. Screening why ?
3. Screening methods
4. Natural evolution of AMD early stages
5. Surgery

1 - Which patients have to be screened for Adrenal Medullary Disease (AMD) ?

Consensus exists around the fact that all patients with thyroid disease and abnormal CT function must be screened systematically for AMD before thyroïd surgery since pheochromocytoma may be asymptomatic, to surgically cure pheochromocytoma before MTC surgery and so prevent cardio-vascular attacks during thyroïd surgery.

In MEN 2A families question is araised whether screening of pheochromocytoma must be proposed to all members together with PG test or only to the members with abnormal CT function ; the keypoint is around the possibility that pheochromocytoma may precede MTC.

Dr RAUE (HEIDELBERG) reported his experience of the large variability in expression of MEN 2 Pheochromocytomas. Pheochromocytoma may occur before (till 20 years) or after (11 years) MTC.

Dr CALMETTES (PARIS) reported 6 MEN 2 patients with overt pheochromocytomas, normal basal CT levels and increased CT response to PG. She stressed that PG test must be performed in every patient with sporadic pheochromocytoma.

Pr PLOUIN (PARIS) said that in his experience, PG test had always been negative when performed in apparently sporadic pheochromocytoma.

Pr HENRY (MARSEILLE) suggested that MEN 2 would be specifically evoked when pheochromocytoma is multinodular or associated with hyperplasia.

It has been stressed that some pheochromocytomas may secrete CT and Dr CALMETTE suggested that PG test be repeated in this situation after adrenal surgery.

Question has been araised whether in MEN 2A families, pheochromocytomas may occur together with negative PG test. Dr NEUMANN (FREIBURG) reported 2 cases with multiple pheochromyctomas and negative PG test.

Synthesis : It clearly appeared, in the first part of this round table that in MEN 2A families, pheochromocytoma may precede MTC, but more information is necessary as to the possible coexistence of pheochromocytoma and negative PG test in MEN 2A patients.

2 - Risk of pheochromocytoma :
Vital risk of large pheochromocytomas has been extensively documented in the litterature, so discussion was oriented towards risk of clinically asymptomatic pheochromocytomas and of early stages of adrenal medullary disease.
Pr MORNEX (LYON) emphasized that clinically asymptomatic pheochromocytomas were observed with the same prevalence (25 %)in sporadic than in MEN 2 pheochromocytomas.
Pr PLOUIN stressed that in his experience, 24 hour semi continuous monitoring of arterial pressure even in apparently normotensive patients always showed brief hypertensive peaks, and he suggested that this monitoring be performed for analysis of adrenal medullary tumours.
Pergravidic or per surgical vital risk in patients with apparently asymptomatic pheochromocytoma has been stressed by Prs MORNEX, NEUMANN,and PROYE and primary adrenal surgery appeared as imperative for adrenal medullary tumour.

At the opposite risk of very early stage of Adrenal Medullary Disease which have been recently individualized, have not yet been well documented. Most participants estimated that when urinary catecholamine and metabolites were in the normal range without any detectable tumour in patients with an only high MIBG adrenal uptake, vital risk was probably absent.

Synthesis : Hormonaly active and CT scan detectable tumours even if clinically asymptomatic may induce complications and must be surgically cured, *at the opposite* more information are required to confirm that medullary adrenal hyperplasia is harmless.

3 - Screening methods :
Pr MORNEX (LYON) showed preliminary results of plasma metanephrine dosage in pheochromocytoma. He demonstrated that plasma metanephrines evaluation was more sensitive than plasma catecholamines for detection of pheochromocytomas.He also reported in asymptomatic patients with MEN 2A pheochromocytomas, high urinary and plasma metanephrines levels.
Pr PLOUIN (PARIS) said that simultaneous determination of arterial pressure by 24 h semi continuous monitoring together with urinary catecholamines increased sensitivity of hormonal detection : in patients with suspected pheochromocytoma coexistence of normal urinary catecholamines, with permanent or paroxystic hypertension allowed exclusion of pheochromocytoma. At the opposite pheochromocytoma may not be eliminated in patients with normal urinary catecholamines pattern and normal 24 h arterial pressure. It was suggested to substitute systematic 24 h urine collection three successive days by simultaneous determination of urinary catecholamines and automatic monitoring of arterial pressure.

Pr NEUMANN (FRIBOURG) showed that plasma chromogranin A was elevated in pheochromocytoma and focused on his experience in Von Hippel Lindau familial screening. He described correlation between plasma CgA levels and tumour weight. Sensitivity of plasma CgA determination for detection of early adrenal medullary disease without adrenal tumour was anyway not evaluated.

Pr BAULIEU (TOURS - F) presented MIBG scintigraphy as a potential tracer of adrenal medullary hyperplasia and suggested for this purpose quantification of MIBG accumulation (adrenal/peripheral ratio $< 1,3$ = normal - $1,3 << 3,$ = medullary adrenal hyperplasia - > 3 = pheochromocytoma.)

Synthesis : Urinary metanephrines and perhaps plasma metanephrines are the most sensitive index of pheochromocytomas with detectable tumour (> 1 cm). Simultaneous determination of arterial pressure improved interpretation of hormonal results. Diagnosis of early stages of adrenal medullary disease requires more information: high bilateral adrenal MIBG uptake is a potential tracer of medullary adrenal hyperplasia which deserves further evaluation. Sensitivity of other tracers have to be evaluated (chromogranin A plasma metanephrines or adrenaline).

4 - Natural evolution of AMD early stage still appears as an unsolved problem, which is poorly documented except in some reports of unilaterally adrenalectomized MEN 2A patients.

It appears useful to recognize the factors which influence progression of the adrenal medullary disease. This would greatly contribute to the management of early stages of AMD whithout franK detectable tumour.

5 - Surgery :
Divergent opinions are reported in the litterature as the optimal surgical procedure for MEN 2 Adrenal Medullary disease. Consensus exist for bilateral adrenalectomy in bilateral adrenal tumours. But controversy persist in patients with apparently unilateral tumour. Some authors perform resection of the only morphologically abnormal adrenal gland and this opinion was supported by experience of most participants. Pre or per surgery high MIBG uptake, palpation or macroscopic appearance of the apparently normal controlateral adrenal, has suggested in some patients, systematic bilateral adrenalectomy.
The managment of this apparently normal controlateral adrenal gland implies further discussion.

VI. Therapeutic means
VI. *Moyens thérapeutiques*

Prognostic factors in medullary thyroid carcinoma (MTC) : a study based on 207 patients treated at the Institut Gustave Roussy

C. Parmentier[*], P. Gardet, F. de Vathaire, J.P. Travagli, B. Caillou[*] and M. Schlumberger[*]

INSERM U 66[*] and Institut Gustave-Roussy, 94800 Villejuif, France

INTRODUCTION

Due to the rarity of Medullary Thyroid Carcinoma (MTC), prognostic factors have not been widely studied and only two multivariate analyses have been published so far (Gardet et al, 1984, SAAD et al, 1984). The aim of the present study was to identify independent prognostic factors by using multivariate analysis and then prognostic groups in order to provide guidelines for treatment protocols and follow-up.

PATIENTS

Between 1945 and 1989, 207 patients with MTC were seen at Institut Gustave Roussy, Villejuif. One hundred ninety patients had a clinical disease. An enquiry with pentagastrin stimulation tests was performed in the family of 112 of them. The disease was classified i) as familial in 25 patients when at least two members of the family were affected and as isolated (in 15) or as part of a Multiple Endocrine Neoplasia IIa (MENIIa in 10) when a pheochromocytoma had been found in the family .ii) as MENIIb in 11 patients. iii) as sporadic in the other 154 patients. Seventeen subjects had a disease found by a pentagastrin test performed during a familial enquiry. On January 1st, 1990, 29 patients were lost to follow-up, 106 were alive and seventy two patients died, 55 from MTC, 8 from an intercurrent disease and 19 from an unknown cause. Mean follow-up of alive patients was 6.8 years (range 1-36 years).

Feature	Sporadic	Familial isolated	MENIIa	Pg	MENIIb
Number	154	15	10	17	11
Age at diagnosis (mean)	43.7	37.2	30.5	28.7	16.4
(range)	(13-80)	(19-51)	(13-62)	(11-61)	(2-37)
Sex (M/F)	75/79	5/10	5/5	6/11	4/7
Thyroid tumor	143 (97%)	15	10	0	7 (70 %)
Palpable lymph nodes	93 (68%)	3 (23%)	1 (14%)	0	8 (73 %)
Distant metastases	35 (24%)	1(7%)	0	0	3 (30%)
Pheochromocytoma	0	0	7	1	4
Hyperparathyroidism	0	0	1	0	0
Neuromatosis	0	0	0	0	9
Dysmorphy	0	0	0	0	11
Survival 5 yr (±2SD)	72% ±8%	100%	90 % ± 19%	100 %	71 % ±28 %
10 yr (±2SD)	55% ±10%	88% ±24%	90 % ± 19%	100 %	59% ±32%

Table 1 : Clinical characteristics at presentation of the 207 patients treated at IGR for a MTC.
Pg : pretumoral disease discovered by a pentagastrin test.

NATURAL HISTORY

Tumor

Tumor size was available from clinical, scintigraphic or histological reports for 188 patients. Its diameter was ≤ 10 mm in 32, ranged 11-40 mm in 92, 41-60 mm in 20 and was greater than 60 mm in 44 patients. Tumor size was strongly related to vascular invasion and capsular effraction, to isthmus involvement, existence of clinical lymph nodes and of distant metastases.

Lymph nodes

Clinical lymph nodes, which were histologically involved, were present initially in 105 patients and in none of the 17 patients whose disease was discovered by a pentagastrin test.
Lymph node dissection was performed in 156 patients (105 with palpable lymph nodes and 51 without). Involvement of at least one site was found in 138 (88%), in all of those with clinical lymph nodes and in 66 % of those without clinical lymph nodes.
Lymph node metastases were found in the paratracheal groove in 79 %, in the lower third of the jugulo-carotid chain in 67 % and in the upper two thirds of the jugulo-carotid chain in 90 %. The antero-superior mediastinum was dissected in 23 patients with an involvement of the paratracheal groove and was found to be involved in 73 %. The spinal chain was dissected in 13 patients with palpable spinal nodes and was involved in 23 % .Ninety six per cent of the patients (26/27) with an involvement of the paratracheal chain also had an involvement of the lower third of the jugulo-carotid chain. The opposite was true for 68 % of the patients (26/38). Furthermore, 98 % of the patients (44/45) with an involvement of the upper two thirds of the jugulo-carotid chain also had an involvement of its lower third, the opposite being true in 68 % of the cases (44/69).
These data clearly show that lymph node involvement is frequently present. All sites are involved simultaneously in a large number of patients.From a practical point of view, this should dictate a bilateral lymph node dissection in all patients, including the paratracheal groove and the jugulo-carotid chain. This should be performed systematically even if no lymph node is palpable in the neck.
The occurrence of local relapses and of distant mestastases is strongly related to lymph node involvement. It must be noted that none of the 15 patients without paratracheal involvement relapsed or developed distant metastases. The existence of clinical lymph nodes further increased the risk of developing distant metastases over non palpable lymph node metastases ($p < 0.01$).

Distant metastases

Distant metastases were present initially in 39 (21 %) patients with a clinical tumor and were discovered during the follow-up in 37 other patients. None of the 17 subjects in whom the disease was discovered by a pentagastrin test developed a local relapse or distant metastases.
At their discovery, they were located in one site in 40 patients (liver in 10, lung in 13, bone in 17), in 2 sites in 15 patients (liver and lung in 6, liver and bone in 9) and in 3 sites (liver, lung and bone) in 21 patients. There is no indication that one of these sites is preferentially involved before the other two. However, the involvement of one site dramatically increased the risk of subsequent involvement of other sites (by a factor 7 to 10).

Survival rates

Overall survival rate (± 2SD) after initial treatment of the 190 patients with a clinical disease was 87 % (± 5%) at 2 years, 75 % (± 7%) at 5 years, 60 % (± 9%) at 10 years and 36 % (± 13%) at 20 years. Cancer related deaths were due to distant metastases and not to local invasion. In those 151 patients without initial distant metastases, it was 84 % (±7%) at 5 years, 70 % (±9%) at 10 years, 42 % (±15%) at 20 years. In these patients, disease free survival was 48 % (±9%) at 5 years,

37 % (±9%) at 10 years and 18 % (±11%) at 20 years. Survival after the discovery of distant metastases was 51 % (±13%) at 1 year, 43 % (±13%) at 2 years, 26 % (±13%) at 5 years and 10 % (±16%) at 10 years.
None of the 17 patients in whom the disease was dicovered by a Pg died from the disease with a follow up of 1 to 9 years.

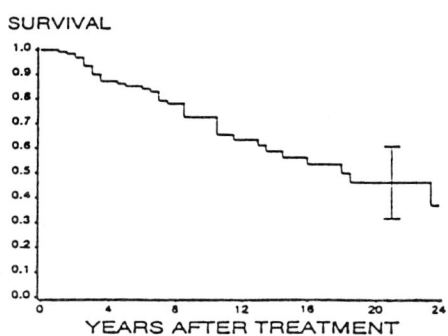

SURVIVAL CURVE IN 207 MTC PATIENTS

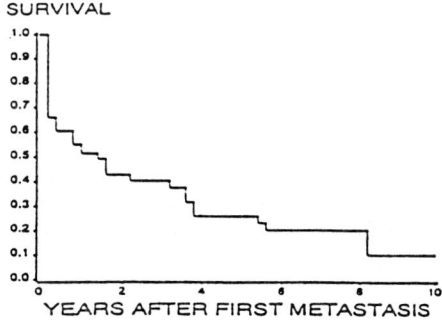

SURVIVAL CURVE IN PATIENTS WITH METASTASES AT DIAGNOSIS

PROGNOSTIC FACTORS

Univariate analysis (table 2).
An univariate analysis showed that several factors significantly influenced the overall survival rates. These were clinical (age, sex, tumor size, palpable lymph nodes, distant metastases), histological (vascular invasion, capsular effraction) and biological (post-operative basal CT level).

	n	SURVIVAL Death (n)	p value
Age (yr)			
≤ 30	54	12	
31-50	105	36	$< 10^{-4}$
51-70	41	18	
> 71	7	6	
Sex			
M	95	34	0.10
F	112	38	
Tumor size (mm)			
≤ 10	32	5	
11-40	92	25	
41-60	20	10	0.08
> 60	44	15	
N+ cl			
no	79	7	$<10^{-4}$
yes	105	56	
Distant Metastases			
no	156	39	$<10^{-4}$
yes	39	23	
Capsular effraction			
no	69	9	0.001
yes	37	17	
Vascular invasion			
no	36	3	0.08
yes	40	15	
Post-operative CT			
normal	48	1	0.001
abnormal	114	35	

Table 2 : Univariate analysis of prognostic factors at initial treatment in the 207 MTC patients.

Multivariate analysis (table 3).
A multivariate analysis was carried out using Cox's proportional hazard regression model by taking into account all clinical and histological factors which were found to be significant in univariate analysis. The 17 patients in whom the disease was discovered by a pentagastrin test were excluded from this analysis.
It appeared that only four factors were independently significant for survival : age of the patient at initial treatment, size of the tumor, presence of clinical lymph node metastases, and presence of distant metastases (table 3).
Based on these 4 prognostic factors, three groups of patients could be designed (Fig.), in whom survival rates at 5,10 and 15 years were significantly different. This should guide the initial therapeutic modalities : in group 1 where all prognostic factors were favourable (age ≤ 30 years, tumor size < 40 mm, absence of clinical lymph nodes and absence of distant metastases), initial therapy should have a curative aim and include surgery as complete as possible, followed by external radiotherapy if CT level remains elevated post-operatively. In group 2 in whom all

prognostic factors except one were favourable and who had no distant metastases, relapse rate and mortality due to MTC were elevated : initial therapy should be aimed to decrease the risk of relapse and be followed by a strict follow-up. Group 3 included the other patients for whom new therapeutic modalities should be developed.

Factor	Relative risk of death		p-value
	RR	(95 % CI)	
Age at first treatment (years)			
31-50 vs ≤ 30	1.9	(0.71 - 5.1)	
51-70 vs ≤ 30	5.5	(1.8-17)	< 0.001
71 or + vs ≤30	8.0	(2.1-30)	
Clinical lymph node			
Yes vs No	4.7	(1.6-14)	0.005
Initial Metastasis			
Yes vs No	11.2	(5.0-25)	0.001
Tumor size			
Risk per cm^2	1.01	(0.99-1.02)	0.118

Table 3 : Survival analysis : Cox's proportional hazards regression analysis in 190 patients with clinical disease.

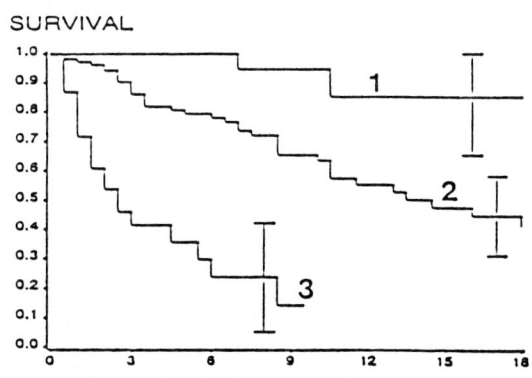

SURVIVAL CURVES ACCORDING TO PROGNOSTIC FACTORS IN 207 MTC PATIENTS

YEARS AFTER DIAGNOSIS

M- 1 - Age < 45, Size < 40 mm, clinical lymph nodes -
M- 2 - Age > 45, Size > 40 mm, clinical lymph nodes +
M+ 3 - Metastases at diagnostic time.

CONCLUSIONS

1 - The pattern of lymph node invasion justifies systematic lymph node dissection.
2 - Distant metastases are often multiple with involvement of multiple sites. They are predictive of a bad prognosis.
3 - In the absence of distant metastases, mulivariate analysis shows that age, tumor size and clinical lymph node metastases are the only independent prognostic factors. When combined, 3 risk groups can be defined. Patients can then be treated on an individualized risk basis.

REFERENCES

GARDET P., ROUGIER Ph., LAPLANCHE A., DELISLE M.J., CAILLOU B., SCHLUMBERGER M., TRAVAGLI J.P., PARMENTIER C. (1984). Non associated sporadic Medullary Thyroid Carcinoma. Prognostic factors and surgical treatment. In Bull. Cancer (Paris), 71,pp 188-191.
SAAD M.F., ORDONEZ N.G., RASHID R.K., GUIDO J.J., HILL C.S., HICKEY R.C., SAMAAN N.A. (1984). A study of the clinical features and prognostic factors in 161 patients. In Medicine 63,pp 319-342.

Cancer médullaire de la thyroïde : moyens thérapeutiques, chirurgie de première intention

C. Proye(*), T. Marmousez(*), et L'Association Française de Chirurgie Endocrinienne et le Groupe Français d'Etude des Tumeurs à Calcitonine

(*) *Clinique Chirurgicale Adultes Est, Service de Chirurgie Générale et Endocrinienne, CHU de Lille, Hôpital Huriez, place de Verdun, 59037 Lille Cedex, France*

SUMMARY

15% at least of "seemingly sporadic" medullary thyroid carcinomas (MTC) are actually of familial origin. Therefore the diagnosis of sporadic MTC is only provisional, and total thyroidectomy is mandatory for any case of MTC, as familial cases are always multicentric. Nodal metastasis are extremely common, as confirmed by a national survey covering 259 cases (168 sporadic MTC, 41 familial MTC, 50 occult MTC diagnosed by screening via a positive pentagastrin stimulation test), with a 54% node involvement rate, gross invasion being 39% and additional microscopic invasion 15%. Gross nodal, involvement rate reached 52% in sporadic cases, 41% in familial cases and 2% in occult cases, with an additional microscopic invasion rate of 16%, 32% and 6% respectively. Thus, a bilateral neck dissection procedure is mandatory, at least central neck dissection. Frozen sections of those central nodes are mandatory, and, if positive, indicate lateral neck dissection. Mediastinal node clearance via sternal split should not be routinely performed, but only in the case with documented invasion of the most caudally located cervical nodes.

Le diagnostic de cancer médullaire de la thyroïde (CMT) étant posé, avant d'en envisager le traitement il faut respecter 3 préambules fondamentaux.
1) Prévenir le coordonnateur régional du groupe d'étude des tumeurs à calcitonine (GETC) pour
- savoir si le cancer est familial
- éventuellement initier une enquête familiale à partir du propositus. En effet 15% des CMT apparemment sporadiques sont authentiquement familiaux selon PONDER.
2) Rechercher chez le propositus un possible phéochromocytome par la clinique, la biologie, l'imagerie médicale, éventuellement la scintigraphie à la MIBG.
3) Vérifier la calcémie et la parathormonémie.
Si l'existence d'un phéochromocytome est prouvée, il faut d'abord traiter le ou les phéochromocytomes avant la cervicotomie.
La cervicotomie initiale constitue une opportunité unique, "l'occasion dorée" de guérir le patient. La qualité de l'acte chirurgical est un facteur essentiel du pronostic mais n'est pas le seul.
Interviennent comme éléments de pronostic favorable
- la découverte du CMT au stade infra-clinique occulte impalpable (5, 6, 7, 8, 20)
- le type étiologique, le CMT familial sans contexte de polyendocrinopathie de type II étant le meilleur pronostic que toute autre variété (10)
- l'euploïdie appréciée sur la pièce opératoire
Interviennent comme éléments de pronostic défavorable

- l'existence d'une ou plusieurs tumeurs palpables (9, 18)
- la survenue du CMT dans un contexte de polyendocrinopathie de type IIb
- l'aneuploïdie (1, 3, 12)
- et, jugé sur la pièce de thyroïdectomie, la faible immuno-réactivité de la tumeur à la calcitonine (3)

Il est heureux qu'une première intervention manquée ne compromette pas définitivement le pronostic. Si le geste thyroïdien initial a été correct, une reprise ganglionnaire peut réussir à négativer le test à la Pentagastrine comme l'a bien montré TISSELL (23, 24), infirmant les conclusions pessimistes de JACKSON (13), et confirmant l'optimisme mesuré exprimé par NORTON (15) dans de tels cas.
Le protocole chirurgical que nous recommandons se fonde sur les données de la littérature et les résultats d'une enquête rétrospective menée par l'Association Française de chirurgie endocrinienne (AFCE) à propos de 286 cas opérés (14). Il accorde une place prééminente à l'examen histologique extemporané des ganglions des compartiments centraux et latéraux du cou, dont nous considérons les résultats comme fondamentaux pour la définition de la tactique chirurgicale devant tout cancer thyroïdien différencié (17).
Ce protocole est le suivant

```
                        THYROIDECTOMIE TOTALE
            ←                                       →
CURAGE CERVICAL CENTRAL    TOUJOURS      CURAGE MEDIASTINAL SUPERIEUR
     ↓ +        ←      EXTEMPORANE      →     + ↓
                       GANGLIONNAIRE
CURAGE LATERAL DU COU                    CURAGE MEDIASTINAL PAR STERNOTOMIE

PARATHYROIDECTOMIE ?   ───────────────→          ECLECTIQUE
```

Comment le légitimer ?

I - LA THYROIDECTOMIE DOIT TOUJOURS ETRE TOTALE

Dans les cas familiaux, la bilatéralité de l'hyperplasie à cellules C est constante, et la bilatéralité tumorale pratiquement constante. Or, les formes supposées sporadiques peuvent être relatrices d'une forme familiale, tandis qu'une forme authentiquement sporadique peut être authentiquement multicentrique. En témoignent les pourcentages de bilatéralité tumorale relevés par RUSSELL dans l'expérience de la Mayo Clinic (18) : bilatéralité tumorale constatée dans 88% des MEN 2a, 93% des MEN 2b, 20% des cas sporadiques.

II - UN GESTE GANGLIONNAIRE DOIT TOUJOURS ACCOMPAGNER LA THYROIDECTOMIE TOTALE

1) Car l'envahissement ganglionnaire cervical est très fréquent dans le CMT

Pour RUSSELL (18) il est de 41% dans les CMT cliniquement palpables, 60% dans les CMT sporadiques, 60% dans les CMT des MEN 2b, soit 75% de toutes les pièces de curage. Pour SAMAAN (19) il est de 65% dans les CMT sporadiques, 40% dans les CMT des MEN 2a, 80% dans les CMT des MEN 2b. Dans l'enquête que nous avons conduite pour l'Association Française de chirurgie endocrinienne (AFCE) en 1989 parmi 286 cas recensés, 259 ont bénéficié d'un curage ganglionnaire cervical. Les ganglions étaient histologiquement envahis dans 54% des cas : envahissement macroscopiquement évident dans 39% des cas, et purement microscopique dans 15% des cas.

2) Car l'envahissement ganglionnaire cervical est très précoce et peut s'observer même dans les cancers infra-cliniques

Dans l'enquête de l'AFCE (14) 6% des CMT infra-cliniques occultes détectés par la positivité du test à la Pentagastrine réalisé dans le cadre d'une enquête familiale, 6% des cas présentaient un envahissement ganglionnaire microscopique, sans anomalie macroscopique des ganglions. Dans le cadre des MEN 2a GAGEL (11) et TELENIUS-BERG (22) ont décrit des envahissements ganglionnaires quand la tumeur était d'un diamètre inférieur à 5mm. Dans les CMT du diagnostic infraclinique, DUH (9) retrouve 40% d'envahissement ganglionnaire cervical et WELLS (27) 4%.

3) Le curage ganglionnaire cervical doit être systèmatique

En effet il ne faut pas se contenter de curage de nécessité, réalisé uniquement en cas d'envahissement ganglionnaire macroscopiquement évident. La maladie est alors déjà au stade dépassé et les résultats en sont médiocres (18) avec 30% de réintervention pour récidive locale et 8% seulement de survivants sans récidive avec un recul moyen de 5 ans (extrême 3-23 ans).

4) Le curage ganglionnaire bilatéral du compartiment central du cou constitue le minimum indispensable dans tous les cas

Ce curage, véritable cellulo-lymphadénectomie, "éviscère", à l'exclusion des éléments nobles nerveux, tout le tissu compris entre les 2 gaines jugulo-carotidiennes latéralement, l'os hyoïde en bas, et la face antérieure des vaisseaux brachio-céphaliques dans le médiastin, accessible par voie cervicale. Il emporte également les coulées thymiques.

a) Il assure la guérison biologique, et donc l'éradication de tout le tissu extra-thyroïdien possiblement envahi, en cas de cancer infraclinique détecté par test à la Pentagastrine comme le confirme l'expérience de TISSEL (24). De l'expérience de cet auteur il apparaît que la rémanence d'une adénopathie d'un diamètre de 3mm suffirait à positiver la thyro-calcitonine basale. WELLS (26) arrive aux mêmes conclusions et l'on peut comprendre de ses travaux qu'un ganglion envahi de la taille d'une parathyroïde normale (6x3x2mm) suffit à positiver le test à la Pentagastrine post-opératoire.

b) Il n'est peut être pas suffisant dans tous les cas de CMT familial infraclinique.

En effet NORTON et WELLS (16), après réalisation d'une thyroïdectomie totale avec curage cervical central chez 34 patients porteurs de CMT de MEN 2a de diagnostic "biochimique" c'est à dire avec cancer impalpable et élévation de la calcitonine basale ou stimulée, retrouvent dans 6 cas une positivité du test à la Pentagastrine post-opératoire. Un patient sur six reste donc porteur de tissu sécrétant, vraissemblablement adénopathie cervicale latérale.

c) Il doit être étendu loin vers le haut et vers le bas.
En effet SPAY (21) a observé des récidives ganglionnaires hautes sous maxillaires et pré-trachéales.

d) Il ne mérite pas pour autant d'être poursuivi systèmatiquement en direction caudale par une sternotomie systèmatique.
La technique de cette sternotomie a été bien décrite par SARRAZIN (20). Mais les résultats de TISSEL (23) montrent bien qu'un évidement mené soigneusement par voie cervicale pure peut suffir à assurer la guérison biologique de la maladie.

5) La réalisation d'un curage cervical latéral jugulo-carotidien et spinal doit être éclectique

En effet le curage central peut suffir à guérir la plupart des formes infracliniques.
Mais l'analyse des résultats de la littérature (6, 9, 24) fait recommander comme impérative la réalisation par première intention d'un curage jugulo-carotidien spinal et sus-claviculaire dans les circonstances suivantes :
- si la tumeur est palpable (24), des 2 côtés en cas de CMT de MEN 2, du côté de la lésion en cas de CMT sporadique.
- si l'examen extemporané des ganglions jugulo-carotidiens moyens prélevés en cours d'intervention est positif (6)
- si la tumeur palpable mesure plus de 2cm car dans ce cas l'envahissement ganglionnaire latéral atteint le taux de 60%
- et également si les ganglions prélevés lors du curage central sont envahis (9). Pour notre part, nous serions tentés de considérer également l'existence de métastases viscérales comme une indication à la réalisation d'un curage latéral, pour diminuer le volume de tumeur sécrétante et favoriser l'effet des thérapeutiques non chirurgicales sur ces métastases distales.

La définition de ces indications fait apparaître l'importance cruciale de l'examen histologique extemporané des ganglions cervicaux prélevés par curage central ou par adénectomie (ou picking) jugulo-carotidien moyen qui doit être systèmatique.
De la positivité de cet examen extemporané dépend directement l'indication de curage latéral au cours de la chirurgie de première intention du CMT (6).

III - TRAITEMENT CHIRURGICAL DE L'HYPERCALCEMIE DES CMT

Bien que systématiquement recherchée, l'hypercalcémie reste relativement rare lors de la présentation initiale des CMT. Hypercalcémie ne signifie pas hyperparathyroïdie. Un phéochromocytome peut être hypercalcémiant, qu'il soit malin ou bénin. Dans la première éventualité il peut déterminer une hypercalcémie par sécrétion ectopique de PTH related peptide, dans les 2 éventualités, l'action osseuse des catécholamines peut expliquer l'hypercalcémie. Donc, dans tous les cas d'hypercalcémie associée à un CMT et à un phéochromocytome synchrone, l'exérèse du phéochromocytome, toujours indiquée avant la cervicotomie, peut normaliser la calcémie.

Reste le problème de l'hyperparathyroïdie associée dans le cadre des MEN 2, qui est relativement rare ou dont la fréquence va diminuant eu égard à la plus grande précocité du diagnostic. NORTON (16) retrouvait 60% d'hyperparathyroïdiens parmi les CMT familiaux en 1973, 17% seulement en 1989. La normo calcémie n'exclut pas l'hyperparathyroïdie sous-jacente.

Mais l'hyperparathyroïdie reste le dernier souci au cours d'une cervicotomie pour CMT familial (4, 6). Elle est souvent discrète et asymptomatique. Le risque de la thyroïdectomie totale avec curage latéral est plutôt celui de dévascularisation des parathyroïdes et il serait catastrophique de substituer à un hyperparathyroïdisme asymptomatique un hypoparathyroïdisme invalidant. Nous recommandons lors de la réalisation du curage, le respect des artères thyroïdiennes supérieures qui vascularisent les parathyroïdes supérieures tandis que les parathyroïdes inférieures tomberont presque toujours avec la pièce de curage pré-trachéal ou seront réimplantées. Il ne faut pas effectuer de parathyroïdectomie totale, même avec auto-transplantation, ou subtotale de principe. Seule est indiquée l'exérèse des glandes macroscopiquement augmentées de volume et ceci même chez les patients normo calcémiques. Les autres glandes de taille normale doivent simplement être marquées par clip ou tout autre moyen et une partie du parenchyme parathyroïdien réséqué sera cryo-préservée pour implantation ultérieure en cas d'hypoparathyroïdisme iatrogène.

IV - CONDITIONS DE REALISATION DE L'INTERVENTION PREMIERE POUR CMT

La philosophie générale du traitement chirurgical du CMT a évolué. De plus en plus les chirurgiens sont confrontés à des patients très particuliers issus du dépistage familial. Il s'agit souvent de patients jeunes, voire d'enfants, présentant une maladie infraclinique pour lesquels existe une "obligation de résultat". Le chirurgien doit donc naviguer entre 2 écueils, d'une part le souci de réaliser un geste carcinologiquement maximal dans les cas "patents" sachant que l'espoir de guérison est extrêmement ténu et, d'autre part, la nécessité de réaliser un geste suffisant dans les cas infracliniques, sans compromettre une guérison possible par des séquelles invalidantes récurrentielles et surtout parathyroïdiennes. Ce but reste difficile à atteindre et dans notre pratique personnelle si nous ne déplorons que 3% de fistule chyleuse rapidement tarie, et si la morbidité parathyroïdienne définitive est nulle (au prix de 15% d'hypoparathyroïdie transitoire) nous déplorons encore 20% d'atteinte récurrentielle unilatérale permanente.

V - PROBLEMES PARTICULIERS

Nous ne ferons qu'évoquer
1) La possibilité d'un thrombus veineux néoplasique cave supérieur
Cette éventualité rencontrée par BARBIER (2) légitime une sternotomie de première intention pour thrombectomie.

2) Le contrôle de la qualité de l'exerèse par détection isotopique per-opératoire comme l'ont suggéré UDELSMAN et ses collaborateurs (25), en marquant les tissus pathologiques par l'acide dimercaptosuccinique.

3) L'intérêt éventuel de l'administration post-opératoire d'iode 131 pour stériliser "par contiguité" d'éventuels reliquats carcinomateux médullaires au contact de reliquats de tissu authentiquement thyroïdien.

** L'étude française multicentrique a pu être réalisée grâce aux observations des patients opérés par les chirurgiens dont les noms suivent : Prof. Bacourt(Neuilly-sur-Seine), Prof. Blondeau (Paris), Prof. Canonni (Marseille), Prof. Charleux (Paris), Prof. Dubost (Paris), Prof. Henry (Marseille), Prof. Mellière (Créteil), Prof. Norlinger (Paris), Prof. Peix (Lyon), Prof. Proye (Lille), Prof. Reynier (Paris), Dr Rodier (Strasbourg), Dr Travagli (Villejuif), Membres du GETC et/ou de l'AFCE. Nous leur adressons tous nos remerciements.

BIBLIOGRAPHIE

1 - BACKDAHL (M), TALLROTH (E), AVER (G). (1985)
   Prognostic value of nuclear DNA content in medullary thyroid carcinoma.
   World J. - 9 - 980-987

2 - BARBIER (J), KRAIMPS (JL), BABIN (Ph), CARRETIER (M), JARDEL (P). (1986)
   L'envahissement jugulo-cave dans le cancer médullaire de la thyroïde.
   Chirurgie - 112 - 633-637

3 - BERGHOLM (U), ADAMI (HO), BERGSTROM (R), BACKDAHL (M), AKERSTROM (G). (1990)
   Long-term survival in sporadic and familial medullary thyroid carcinoma with special reference to clinical characteristics as prognostic factors
   Acta Chir. Scand. - 156 - 37-46

4 - BLOCK (MA), JACKSON (CE), TASCHJIAN (AH). (1975)
   Management of parathyroid glands in surgery for medullary thyroid carcinoma
   Arch. Surg. - 110 - 617-624

5 - BLOCK (MA), JACKSON (CE), TASCHJIAN (AH). (1978
   Management of occult medullary thyroid carcinoma.
   Arch. Surg. - 113 - 368-372

6 - BRUNT (LM), WELLS (SA) Jr. (1987)
   Advances in the diagnosis and treatment of medullary thyroid carcinoma.
   Surg. Clin. North. Amer. - 67 - 263-279

7 - CALMETTES (C), for the French Medullary Study Group. (1989)
   Multiple Endocrine Neoplasia Type II : Clinical, Biological and Epidemiological Feactures.
   Horm. Research - 32 - 41-46

8 - CANCE (WG), WELLS (SA) Jr. (1985)
   Multiple endocrine neoplasia type II a.
   Curr. Probl. Surg. - 22 - 1-56

9 - DUH (QY), SANCHO (JJ), GREENSPAN (FS), HUNT (TK), GALANTE (M),
   DE LORIMIER (AA), COMTE (FA), CLARK (OH). (1989)
   Medullary thyroid carcinoma : the need for early diagnosis and total thyroïdectomy.
   Arch. Surg. - 124 - 1206-1210

10 - FARNDON (JR), LEIGHT (GS), DILLEY (WG) et al. (1986)
   Familial medullary thyroid carcinoma without associated endocrinopathies : a distinct clinical entity.
   Br. J. Surg. - 73 - 278-281

11 - GAGEL (RF), MELVIN (KEW), TASHJIAN (AH) Jr et al (1975)
   Natural history of the familial medullary thyroid carcinoma - pheochromocytoma syndrome and the identification of preneoplastic stages by screening studies : a five-year report.
   Trans. Ass. Am. Physicians - 88 - 177

12 - HAY (ID), RYAN (JJ), GRANT (CS), BERGSTRATH (EJ), VAN HEERDEN (JA), GOELLNER (JR). (1990).
Prognostic significance of non diploid DNA determined by flow cytometry in sporadic and familial medullary thyroid carcinoma.
Surgery - 108 (in press)

13 - JACKSON (CE), TALPOS (GB), KAMBOURIS (A), YOTT (JB), TASHJIAN Jr (AH), BLOCK (MA). (1983)
The clinical course after definitive operation for medullary carcinoma.
Surgery - 94 - 995-1001

14 - MARMOUSEZ (T), MELLIERE (D), PROYE (C) et CALMETTES (Mme C.) (1990)
Actualisation de la prise en charge des cancers medullaires de la thyroïde.
Lyon Chir. - 86 - 104-107

15 - NORTON (JA), DOPPMAN (JL), BRENNAN (MF). (1980)
Localization and resection of clinically inapparent medullary carcinoma of the thyroid.
Surgery - 87 - 616-622

16 - NORTON (JA), WELLS (SA) Jr. (1990)
Medullary thyroid carcinoma and multiple endocrine neoplasia Type 2 Syndromes in Surgical Endocrinology
ed. S.R. FRIESEN and NW THOMPSON pp 359-375 Philadelphia - JB LIPPINCOTT Company

17 - PROYE (C), GONTIER (A), QUIEVREUX (JL), CARNAILLE (B), CAMP (D), Mme LECOMTE-HOUCKE (M). (1990)
Décision de curage ganglionnaire en chirurgie du cancer thyroïdien. Apport de l'examen extemporané des ganglions sus-claviculaires externes.
Chirurgie - (à paraître)

18 - RUSSELL (CF), VAN HEERDEN (JA), SIZEMORE (GW), EDIS (AJ), TAYLOR (WF), REMINE (WH), CARNEY (JA). (1983)
The surgical management of medullary thyroid carcinoma
Ann. Surg. - 197 - 42-48

19 - SAMAAN (N), SCHULTZ (PN), HICKEY (RC). (1988)
Medullary Thyroid Carcinoma : Prognosis of Familial versus sporadic disease and the role of radiotherapy.
Journ. Clin. End. Metab. - 67 - 801-805

20 - SARRAZIN (R), ROUX (JF), DYON (JF). (1990)
Curage cervico-médiastinal dans les cancers médullaires de la thyroïde.
Lyon Chir. - 86 - 108-112

21 - SPAY (G), CROCHET (E), BERGER-DUTRIEUX (N), VUILLARD (P), BOUCHET (A), SOUSTELLE (J). (1983)
La présence d'adénopathies jugulo-carotidiennes dans le cancer médullaire du corps thyroïde.
Chirurgie - 109 - 656-660

22 - TELENIUS-BERG (M), BERG (B), HAMBERGER (B) et al. (1984)
Impact of screening on prognosis in the multiple endocrine neoplasia type 2. Syndromes : Natural history and treatment results in 105 patients.
Henry Ford Hosp. Med. J. - 32 - 225

23 - TISSEL (LE), JANSSON (S). (1988)
Recent results of reoperative surgery in medullary carcinoma of the thyroid.
Wien. Klin. Wochens. - 11 - 347-348

24 - TISSEL (LE), HANSON (G), JANSSON (S), SALANDER (H). (1986)
Reoperation in the treatment of asymptomatic metastasizing medullary thyroid carcinoma.
Surgery - 99 - 60-66
25 - UDELSMAN (R), MOJIMINIVI (O.A.), SOPERS (NDW), BULEY (ID), SHEPSTONE (BJ), DUDLEY (NE). (1989)
Medullary carcinoma of the thyroid : management of persistent hypercalcitoninemia utilizing [99^m Tc] (V) dimercaptosuccinic acid scintigraphy.
Br. J. Surg. - 76 - 1278-1281
26 - WELLS (SA) Jr., BAYLIN (SB), GANN (DS), FARRELL (RE), DILLEY (WG), PREISSIG (SH), MARSTON LINEHAN (W), COOPER (CW). (1978)
Medullary thyroid carcinoma : Relationship of method of diagnosis to pathologic staging
Ann. Surg. - 188 - 377-383
27 - WELLS (SA) Jr., BAYLIN (SB), LEIGHT (GS) et al (1982)
The importance of early diagnosis in patients with hereditary medullary thyroid carcinoma.
Ann. Surg. - 195 - 595-599

RESUME

15% au moins des cas "apparemment sporadiques" de cancer médullaire de la thyroïde (CMT) sont en fait des cas familiaux. Le diagnostic de CMT sporadique ne doit donc être qu'un diagnostic provisoire, et l'indication de thyroïdectomie totale pour tout CMT est absolument impérative, eu égard à la multi-focalité constante des cas familiaux. D'autre part l'extrême lymphophilie du CMT se confirme au terme d'une enquête nationale portant sur 259 cas (168 CMT sporadiques, 41 CMT familiaux, 50 CMT occultes détectés par test à la Pentagastrine) avec une fréquence d'envahissement ganglionnaire globale de 54%, macroscopique de 39% et purement microscopique de 15%. L'envahissement macroscopique est de 52% pour les CMT sporadiques, 41% pour les CMT familiaux et 2% pour les CMT occultes détectés par test à la Pentagastrine, tandis que l'envahissement microscopique sans envahissement macroscopique évident est respectivement de 16% pour les CMT sporadiques, 32% pour les CMT familiaux et 6% pour les CMT occultes. D'où la nécessité absolue d'un geste ganglionnaire complémentaire bilatéral. Ce geste ganglionnaire doit être au minimum une cellulo-lymphadénectomie du compartiment central du cou entre les gaines vasculo-nerveuses latéralement, l'os hyoïde en haut et les vaisseaux médiastinaux supérieurs en bas. L'examen extemporané des ganglions de ce compartiment central est indispensable, et sa positivité doit conduire à élargir le curage en dehors de l'axe jugulo-carotidien, emportant la totalité des chaînes jugulo-carotidiennes et spinales. Le curage médiastinal par sternotomie est indiqué si les ganglions cervicaux inférieurs sont envahis, mais non de principe.

Medullary thyroid carcinoma : surgery for persistent disease

Guy Andry and Pierre Dor

Institut Jules Bordet, Tumor Center de l'Université Libre de Bruxelles, rue Héger-Bordet 1, B1000 Bruxelles, Belgique

Summary :
Adequate surgery is the prerequisite to potentially curative treatment for the patient for whom the diagnosis of medullary thyroid carcinoma (MTC) has been established. Chemotherapy and radiotherapy are largely ineffective (Lynn 1981, Saad 1984, Samaan 1988) although the latter has been reported to be of some interest (Rougier 1983, Schlumberger 1991 in the present issue).
The minimal operation for MTC is a total thyroidectomy and central neck compartment clearance (i.e. removal of lymph nodes from bilateral paratracheal and pretracheal areas, from the hyoid bone down to the innominate vessels in the antero superior mediastinum).
In case of clinically suspicious nodes in the lateral neck, a modified radical neck dissection should be performed, preserving the spinal accessory nerve, the internal jugular vein and the sternocleidomastoid muscle. These three structures should be sacrificed, in our opinion, if there is a risk of capsular rupture, i.e. for metastatic lymph nodes exceeding 2 cm in diameter.
Ipsilateral prophylactic modified lateral neck dissection should be advocated for any unilateral sporadic primary exceeding 4 cm in diameter or spreading beyond the thyroid capsule. Bilateral prophylactic modified neck dissections would be advocated for hereditary tumors (Tisell 1989).
The question as to whether a meticulous microdissection (with lenses) should be performed is debatable (Tisell 1989, Bühr 1990).
After adequate operation on the neck, persistent high immuno-assayed calcitonin (iCT) levels in the serum after pentagastrin injection, in the absence of localizable foci of tumor by radionuclide tracers (Hoefnagel 1988), may lead the clinician to attempt further localization by selective catheterization and blood sampling for iCT measurements (Gautvic 1989, Norton 1980, Ben Mrad 1989, Buhr 1990).

INTRODUCTION

Persistent disease is a common clinical situation for two main reasons : 1) Many patients with medullary thyroid carcinoma are still referred to tumor centers when the diagnosis has already been established after subtotal surgery performed on the thyroid and/or on lymph nodes of the neck (Russel 1982 ; Quan-Yang Duh 1989 ; Bühr 1990); 2) The incidence of occult lymph node micrometastases has been reported to be as high as 90% (Tisell 1989) and standard surgery has not been unanimously determined yet.
In the present article, we will try to define the extent of surgery advocated for persistent disease and estimate the results expected both for tumor clearance and for complications.

DEFINITION OF PERSISTENT DISEASE

Persistent disease is usually detected by the presence of a residual elevated level of immuno-assayed calcitonin (iCT) in the peripheral blood (either basal level or after pentagastrin i.v. test). This secretion of calcitonin comes from foci of disease, often occult, that the clinician should look for

1. in remnants of thyroid after a subtotal thyroidectomy
2. in lymph nodes of the central neck compartment
3. in lymph nodes of the lateral neck compartment(s)
4. in distant metastases.

A variety of clinical situations may arise from different combinations of the afore-mentioned possibilities. If the disease is still confined into the first three localizations, it should get under control of surgery, at least theoritically.

REVIEW OF CURRENT LITERATURE ON THE EXTENT OF SURGERY FOR MTC

Total thyroidectomy should be performed in every case because the possibility of an hereditary type of MTC cannot be excluded before operation (Freier 1977; Block 1978; Russell 1982; Jackson 1983; Saad 1984; Sizemore 1987; Tisell 1989) ; a thorough microscopic examination of the surgical specimen by the pathologist is necessary to rule out the possibility of bilateral lesions (occult foci of MTC, or micronodular hyperplasia, or even only C-cell hyperplasia).

Central neck lymph node dissection is mandatory in order to stage the disease as well as to avoid a recurrence in an area where salvage surgery is difficult if not impossible (Block 1978; Clarck, O.H. 1989). This should include lymphatic tissues from the hyoid bone to the innominate vessels and laterally to the jugular veins (delphian, subisthmic, tracheosophageal and superior mediastinal nodes).

Lateral neck lymph node dissection
Although generally recommended for clinically suspicious nodes (Freier 1977; Block 1978; Russell 1982; Rougier 1983; Saad 1984; Sizemore 1987) lateral neck dissection(s) for undetectable nodes are still a matter of debate : some authors have emphasized the relative uselessness of reoperations on the neck of patients with persistent supranormal iCT levels (Freier 1977; Block 1978; Russell 1982; Jackson 1983; Saad 1984; Thompson 1978) whereas other surgical teams have reported encouraging results in terms of tumor clearance after reoperations for such patients (Norton 1980; Tisell 1986; Buhr 1990).

Table I summarizes the results of reoperations on the neck in terms of iCT levels.

TABLE I : REOPERATIONS FOR PERSISTENT MTC

	Patients	Reoperations	iCT after pentagastrin		
	n	n	-	+	+++
Norton 1980	7	7	1	5	1
Tisell 1986	11	17	4	4	3
Bühr 1990	11	11	2	7	2

- : normalization of iCT;
+ : reduced iCT stimulation;
+++ : no change.

Tisell (1986 and 1989) and Bühr (1990) have described and recommended a so-called microscopic modified neck dissection, aimed at removing all microscopic lymph node metastases with magnifying lenses. This procedure, tailorized on the initial clinical situation, may last 6 to 12 hours (depending on the necessity of doing one or both sides of the neck). Bühr et al (1990) reported their complications after 11 reoperations of that type : 3 temporary lymphatic fistulae, 2 recurrent nerve paralysis (which improved later), three Horner's triad (which resolved incompletely), two temporary weakness of the arm and two hypoparathyroidism. Tisell et al (1989) reported the following percentages (of lymph node involvement in the neck) :
- 1) when the primary is palpable : 90%
- 2) for hereditary palpable forms : 88% (bilaterality)
- 3) for hereditary non palpable forms : 27%.

Based on these observations, Tisell's (1989) recommendations for the lateral compartment of the neck are :
- for unilateral, palpable, sporadic primary
    ⟶ ipsilateral modified neck dissection

- for bilateral, hereditary, even non palpable primaries
    ⟶ bilateral modified neck dissections
(modified neck i.e. : preserving the spinal nerve, the internal jugular vein and the sternocleidomastoid muscle).

Tisell (1989) also emphasized that venous sampling by selective catheterization in order to localize persistent disease should be reserved for cases with elevated iCT after an adequate primary operation had been performed. He also admitted the uselessness of new reoperations for large primaries with palpable nodes after a total thyroidectomy plus central and ipsilateral neck dissection because the incidence of distant metastases may explain residual elevated iCT level in these cases. Corroborating this latter assertion, the results of Gautvik (1989) suggested that the majority of the patients with MTC have early occult hepatic metastases : 13 out of 13 thyroidectomized patients showed elevated iCT values in the hepatic vein after pentagastrin stimulation; peak values in the hepatic veins were higher and occured sooner than in the peripheral or jugular veins. For only 3 of those 13 patients were hepatic metastases confirmed by computerized tomography, which suggested occult hepatic disease in 10 other patients.

Block (1978), Vanheerden (1978), Thompson (1978) have suggested that abnormal postoperative iCT may not necessarily be predictive of a worse outcome because minute foci of metastatic medullary thyroid carcinoma could remain quiescent for prolonged periods of time. Saad (1984) reported that there was no difference in adjusted survival rates between patients with normal and abnormal postoperative serum iCT levels (basal or post pentagastrin test) in 161 MTC patients followed from 1 month to 28,8 years (median 6,1 years).

Sizemore (1987) reported that familial non-MEN or MEN2a MTC appear to have long term survivorship, even with metastases. He suggested that, for those patients, with unchanging or moderately changing iCT concentrations, vigorous attempt to localize, reoperate, or treat tumor with present avaiable modalities may not be useful. However, emphasizing the need of an individualized therapy for each patient, he thought that a logical approach to persistent MTC in MEN2b and sporadic disease would be microdissection as done by Tisell, followed by external radiation.

CONCLUSIONS

Based on the various experiences reported so far, it is difficult to advocate a standardized treatment for persistent MTC.
Ideally, surgery should include totalization of thyroidectomy and a central neck compartment clearance, through a collar incision. A modified radical lateral neck dissection should be performed to remove any clinically suspicious nodes. A classical radical neck dissection being reserved for those cases with overt lymph nodes, exceeding 2 cm in diameter.
The question arise as to whether prophylactic modified lateral neck dissection(s) should be avocated for undetectable nodes
- ipsilateraly for sporadic cases with a palpable primary
- bilateraly for every hereditary cases.
Also questionnable are the necessity and the feasibility of a so-called meticulous neck dissection (with lenses), with prophylactic intend.
In our opinion, the surgical attitude should take into account the main prognostic factors : age and sex of the patient, size of the primary, presence of clinically involved nodes (Saad 1984; Sizemore 1987; Schröder 1988).

REFERENCES

Ben Mrad, M.D., Gardet P., et al., (1989) : Value of venous catheterization and calcitonin studies in the treatment and management of clinically inapparent medullary thyroid carcinoma. Cancer, vol. 63 : 133-138.
Block, M.A., Jackson, C.E., et al., (1978) : Management of Occult Medullary Thyroid Carcinoma. Arch. Surg., vol. 113 : 368-372.
Bühr, H.J., Lehnert, T., et al., (1990) : New operative strategy in the treatment of metastasizing medullary carcinoma of the thyroid. Eur. J. of Surg. Onc., 16 : 366-369.
Clark, O.H., (1989) : Personnal communication in discussion, Arch. Surg., vol. 124 : 1210.
Freier, D.T., Thompson, N.W., et al., (1977) : Dilemmas in the early diagnosis and treatment of multiple endocrine adenomatosis, type II. Surgery, vol. 82, 3 : 407-413.
Gautvik, K.M., Talle, K., et al., (1989) : Early Liver Metastases in Patients With Medullary Carcinoma of the Thyroid Gland. Cancer, vol. 63 : 175-180.
Hoefnagel, C.A., Delprat, C.C., et al., (1988) : New radionuclide tracers for the diagnosis and therapy of medullary thyroid carcinoma. Clin. Nuclear Med., vol. 13 : 159-165.
Jackson, C.E., Talpos, G.B., et al., (1983) : The clinical course after definitive operation for medullary thyroid carcinoma. Surgery, vol. 94, 6 : 995-1001.
Lynn, J., Gamvros, O.I., et al., (1981) : Medullary carcinoma of the thyroid. World J. Surg., 5 : 27-32.
Norton, J.A., Doppman, J.L., et al., (1980) : Localization and resection of clinically inapparent medullary carcinoma of the thyroid. Surgery, vol. 87, 6 : 616-622.
Quan-Yang Duh, Sancho, J.J., et al., (1989) : Medullary thyroid carcinoma : the need for early diagnosis and total thyroidectomy. Arch. Surg., vol. 124 : 1206-1210.
Rougier, P., Parmentier, C., et al., (1983) : Medullary thyroid carcinoma : pronostic factors and treatment. Int. J. Radiation Oncology Biol. Phys., vol. 9 : 161-169.
Russell, C.F., Van Heerden, J.A., et al., (1983) : The surgical management of medullary thyroid carcinoma. Surgery, vol. 197, 1 : 42-48.
Saad, M.F., Ordonez, N.G., et al., (1984) : Medullary carcinoma of the thyroid. Medicine, vol. 63, 6 : 319-342.
Schlumberger, M., Gardet, P., et al., (1991) : External radiotherapy and chemotherapy in MTC patients. In Medullary Thyroid Carcinoma, 1st European Congress. Paris, nov. 15-17, 1990. Oral communication # 43 and in the present issue.
Schröder, S., Böcker, W., et al., (1988) : Prognostic factors in medullary thyroid carcinomas. Cancer, vol. 61 : 806-816.
Sizemore, G.W. (1987) : Medullary carcinoma of the thyroid gland. Seminars in Oncology, vol. 14, 3 : 306-314.
Thompson, N.W., (1978) Personnal communication in discussion, Arch. Surg., vol. 113 : 371-372.
Tisell, L.E., Hanson, G., et al., (1989) : Surgical treatment of medullary carcinoma of the thyroid. In : multiple endocrine neoplasia type 2. Hormone and metab. research. suppl. series, vol. n° 21, ed. E.F. Pfeiffer & G.M. Reaven, Thieme, pp 29-31. Stuttgart - New-York.
Tisell, L.E., Göran Hansson, Ph.D., et al., (1986) : Reoperation in the treatment of asymptomatic metastasizing medullary thyroid carcinoma. Surgery, vol. 99, 1 : 60-66.
Vanheerden, J.A. (1978) Personnal communication in discussion, Arch. Surg., vol. 3 : 371.

RESUME

Une chirurgie adéquate est indispensable pour espérer obtenir une guérison chez le patient atteint d'un cancer médullaire thyroïdien (CMT). La chimiothérapie et la radiothérapie sont peu efficaces (Lynn 1981; Saad 1984; Samaan 1988) bien que la dernière modalité ait montré quelques résultats intéressants (Rougier 1983; Schlumberger 1991 dans le présent ouvrage).

L'intervention minimale pour le CMT consiste en une thyroïdectomie totale avec curage ganglionnaire du compartiment central du cou (c-à-d exérèse des ganglions lymphatiques des deux gouttières paratrachéales et aire prétrachéale, depuis l'hyoïde jusqu'aux vaisseaux innominés dans le médiastin antéro-supérieur).

En cas de ganglion suspect dans la partie latérale du cou, un évidement du cou modifié doit être réalisé, préservant le nerf spinal, la veine jugulaire interne et le muscle sternocleïdomastoïdien. Ces trois structures devraient être sacrifiées, à notre avis, s'il y a un risque de rupture capsulaire ganglionnaire, c-à-d pour des adénopathies d'un diamètre excédant 2 cm.

Un évidement homolatéral modifié du cou devrait être proposé, de manière prophylactique, pour tout CMT unilatéral sporadique de plus de 4 cm de diamètre ou s'il y a effraction de la capsule thyroïdienne par la tumeur. Des évidements bilatéraux, modifiés, du cou seraient conseillés pour les formes CMT héréditaires (Tisell 1989).

Après une chirurgie adéquate sur les aires cervico-faciales, des taux élevés de calcitonine circulante (iCT) provoqués par l'injection de pentagastrine, pourraient amener le clinicien à effectuer des cathétérismes endoveineux avec prélèvements sanguins sélectifs pour tenter de localiser des foyers de CMT occultes, passés inaperçus aux techniques scintigraphiques récentes préconisées par Hoefnagel (1988).

External radiotherapy and chemotherapy in MTC patients

M. Schlumberger(*), P. Gardet, F. de Vathaire, D. Sarrazin, J.P. Travagli and C. Parmentier(*)

INSERM U 66 and * Institut Gustave-Roussy, 94800 Villejuif, France

External Radiotherapy to the neck.

Surgery still remains the basic treatment for medullary thyroid carcinoma (MTC). Although external radiotherapy (RT) has been used for a number of years (Williams et al, 1966, Melvin et al, 1972, Chong et al, 1975, Halnan, 1975, Steinfeld, 1977, Simpson et al, 1982, Tubiana et al, 1985, Samaan et al, 1988), its role in the treatment of MTC continues to be controversial.
There are at least three reasons for current doubts and controversy. Firstly, the growth rate of MTC is often slow, requiring a long follow-up in order to evaluate the results of any treatment modality. Secondly, in all series, there is no suitable control group. The effectiveness of post-operative radiotherapy is therefore difficult to assess after macroscopically complete excision of the neoplastic tissue present in the neck. Furthermore MTC is relatively radioresistant and radiotherapy can only be effective when doses of 50 Gy or over are delivered to the neoplastic tissue. In most centers, doses have varied over the last three decades avoiding any conclusion. Thirdly, the interpretation of the results should take into account the completeness of surgical excision and known prognostic factors, including the initial presence of distant metastases, since they strongly influence the course of the disease.
Data obtained in the series of MTC patients treated at Villejuif, clearly show that external RT to the neck is useful in MTC patients without distant metastases in whom the CT level remains elevated post-operatively, even if surgery appeared to have been macroscopically complete.

Patients and methods

From 1943 to 1989, 207 patients with MTC were treated at IGR. One hundred ninety patients had a clinical disease at presentation, 98 of whom were irradiated with external beam therapy (table 1).

INITIAL TREATMENT	SURGICAL EXCISION			LYMPH NODES				DISTANT METASTASES	
	COMPLETE	DUBIOUS	INCOMPLETE	N-	N+	N+cl	X	-	+
SURGERY	41	35	13	16	24	27	22	70	19
SURGERY + RT	23	41	28	4	15	70	3	77	15
RT only	0	0	6	1	0	5	0	4	2
NO TREATMENT	0	0	3	0	0	3	0	0	3

Table 1 : clinical characteristics at presentation and therapeutic procedures performed in the 190 MTC patients with a clinical disease. Incomplete : macroscopically incomplete or impossible. RT : external radiotherapy. N+cl : palpable lymph nodes. X : no lymph node dissection or negative biopsy.

The surgical protocol included a total thyroidectomy with bilateral dissection of the jugulocarotid chain and of the paratracheal groove (Travagli et al, 1984). Surgical excision of neoplastic tissue was considered as complete, dubious or macroscopically incomplete or impossible according to surgical report.

External radiotherapy to the neck was undertaken within 2-3 months after surgery.

Patients are irradiated with high energy radiation (Sarrazin et al, 1984). The target volume should include the thyroid bed, the neck lymph nodes and the upper part of the mediastinum. The average tumor dose is 50 Gy in 25 fractions over 5 weeks. A boost of 5 to 10 Gy is often delivered to any palpable residual tumor. Patients are irradiated with a direct anterior field shaped by lead blocks to protect the lungs and the larynx and with a posterior field limited to the upper mediastinum. The respective doses delivered with these two fields should be adapted according to the anteroposterior diameter of the upper thorax. The choice is based on a study of the dose distribution carried out in a saggital plane or in several transverse planes. Another technique uses a single anterior electron field of appropriate energy. Whatever the technique, assiduous attention must be paid to avoid doses in excess of 40 Gy to the spinal cord, since higher doses can induce non recoverable transverse myelitis.

Results

For the whole series of 181 patients with clinical disease who underwent surgery, the relapse free survival and survival rates of the 92 patients treated by external RT were identical to those of the 89 patients treated by surgery alone.

External radiotherapy had no significant effect on survival in two subgroups of patients : i) in those without lymph node involvement in whom adequate primary surgery provides the best chance for cure as shown by the post-operative normalization of CT levels. ii) in patients with distant metastases because they are likely to die from these metastases.

However, external radiotherapy appeared to be effective in other subsets of patients, in terms both of survival and of local control. This was studied in the 145 patients without initial distant metastases who underwent surgery (table 2).

	Local Control (± 2SD) %		RFS (± 2 SD) %		Survival (± 2 SD) %	
	5 yr	10 yr	5 yr	10 yr	5 yr	10 yr
Surgery alone (n = 68)	71 (± 12)	46 (± 16)	56 (±12)	41 (± 13)	87 (±9)	78 (±12)
Prophylactic RT (n = 59)	84 (± 10)	71(± 14)	49 (±13)	39 (±14)	83 (±10)	75 (±13)
RT after incomplete surgery (n = 18)	67 (± 24)	67 (± 24)	22 (±20)	15 (± 9)	88 (±16)	53 (±26)

Table 2 : Local control, relapse free survival (RFS) and overall survival in 145 MTC patients treated by surgery alone or combined with post-operative radiotherapy.

Prophylactic irradiation. This group includes 59 patients in whom excision appeared macroscopically complete but who were given RT for various reasons : extensive lymph node involvement, upper mediastinal involvement or invasion of neighboring tissues.Total survival and relapse free survival after RT were very close to those of the 68 patients treated by surgery alone. This is not surprising since irradiation was used in patients in whom excision had been difficult and whose prognosis appeared to be less favorable. However the rate of local control was significantly higher than after surgery alone, demonstrating that RT is highly effective for tumor control.

Post-operative RT after incomplete surgery. This group includes 18 patients in whom pathologic tissue was still macroscopically remaining after surgery. The local control, TS and RFS are given in Table 2 and clearly show that RT can control macroscopic tumor masses.

Clinical lymph nodes. In patients with clinical lymph nodes, 5 year survival rates (± 2sd) after surgery alone, prophylactic radiotherapy and radiotherapy after incomplete surgery were 36 % (± 28 %), 81 % ((± 13 %) and 61 % (± 27 %), respectively.
In fact, the completeness of surgical excision depends on the extent of lymph node involvement. Palpable lymph node metastases were present in 19 % of the patients treated by surgery alone, in 83 % of those irradiated after macroscopically complete surgery and in 88 % of those irradiated after incomplete (or impossible) surgery.

Post-operative CT level. Post-operatively, CT level should be used as a guide for external radiotherapy (table 3).

Post-operative CT level	Clinical lymph nodes		External RT		Neck Relapse
Normal (n= 31)	Yes	7	Yes	5	0
			No	2	0
	No	24	Yes	2	0
			No	22	1
Abnormal (n=66)	Yes	45	Yes	37	9
			No	8	7
	No	21	Yes	7	0
			No	14	8

Table 3 : Neck relapse according to post-operative basal CT level, clinical lymph nodes and external radiotherapy to the neck. CT level was measured within 1 to 3 months after surgery, in 97 patients without initial distant metastases.

Only one relapse occurred in the 31 patients who normalized their basal CT level, 7 of whom were irradiated. A relapse occurred in 24 of the 66 patients in whom CT level remained elevated in the absence of distant metastases, in 9 of the 44 patients who were irradiated and in 15 of the 22 who were not irradiated (p = 0.001).Indeed, CT level normalized post-operatively in 53 % of the 45 patients without palpable lymph nodes and in 13 % of the 52 with palpable lymph nodes.
Whatever the completeness of surgical excision according to surgical report, CT level should be measured post-operatively as it appears to be the most reliable indicator of the presence of neoplastic tissue. In fact it normalized in 44 % of patients treated by surgery alone, in 17 % of those irradiated after macroscopically complete surgery and in none of those irradiated after incomplete (or impossible) surgery.

Discussion

It has been claimed that external RT is ineffective in MTC patients and that it may even worsen long term prognosis. This type of conclusion was drawn from analysis of MTC patients without taking into account known prognostic indicators. In fact in all series, irradiated patients were those with larger tumor, with extensive lymph node involvement or unsatisfactory surgical excision, all

factors which strongly influence the course of the disease, i.e. the relapse rate, the occurence of distant metastases and death rate from thyroid carcinoma. This probably explains the poor results reported in most series of irradiated patients, especially when these were compared with non irradiated patients who had more favorable prognostic indicators.
Indeed in the present study, in the whole series of patients, survival after RT was not better than after surgery alone.Furthermore, relapse free survival and total survival were similar after prophylactic radiotherapy and after surgery alone. However, prophylactic RT is highly effective for local control of the tumor. When using other criteria to select patients for external RT, it appears that it should not be given to all patients,but is effective in at least two subsets of patients : i) in those with macroscopic residual tumor in the neck after impossible or incomplete surgery in whom a stabilization or a slow decrease in tumor size and in serum marker levels is frequently obtained(Simpson et al, 1982, Tubiana et al, 1985). ii) in patients without known distant metastases, when excision of neoplastic tissue appeared to have been macroscopically complete, and in whom CT level remains elevated post-operatively. In these patients, a complete work-up is warranted before irradiation and should include a bone scintigraphy, ultra-sounds, CT or MRI scans and in the absence of demonstrable distant metastases, venous sampling catheterization. If limited neoplastic foci are found in the neck, further surgery should be decided. It frequently allows for a subsequent decrease in CT level but failed to normalize it in the majority of patients (Ben Mrad et al, 1989). A detectable CT level should then indicate external RT. In fact surgery and radiotherapy should be associated since they are complementary : surgery can excise the gross masses and irradiation can eradicate subclinical disease, as indicated by elevated CT levels. This frequently occurs in patients with clinical lymph nodes since these large neoplastic masses frequently present capsular effraction and involvement of muscles or other organs. In these patients, CT level appears to be a more reliable criterion of the completeness of surgical excision of neoplastic tissue than the surgical report. CT level is measured 5 days after surgery and again 1 to 3 months later, before the start of irradiation. CT level may fluctuate but fails to normalize if it remains elevated a few days after surgery.
A few decades ago, post-operative RT was not frequently used because the prevailing view was that one should wait for recurrence in order to have something tangible to irradiate. When it was recognized that higher doses are required to eradicate gross masses than subclinical disease, prophylactic irradiation of clinically uninvolved areas at risk of containing occult deposits was advocated. This method should be used in MTC patients as favorable clinical results can now be produced.
In contrast, it should not be performed in patients who normalize their CT level after surgery since they are likely to be free of disease and their risk of relapse is very low. In those with initial distant metastases, the indication of external radiotherapy to the neck should be weighed up since these patients are likely to die from distant metastases but may be useful to avoid tumor progression in the neck.
The acute side effects of radiation include skin erythema and radiation laryngitis in the latter part of the treatment. Dysphagia may require local analgesia but rarely hospitalisation for nutrition. Laryngeal oedema may be responsible of hoarseness and in patients with a laryngeal nerve palsy, it may require a tracheotomy. Mucositis may be complicated by a superimposed infection requiring appropriate care. These effects commonly subside completely within 2-4 weeks after the completion of therapy. Delayed side effects include skin changes (hypo or hyperpigmentation, skin atrophy), oedema of subcutis and soft tissues in cases with prior extensive surgery, decrease in saliva flow. Permanent changes in laryngeal, tracheal and oesophagal function are uncommon. Brachial plexopathy and obstruction of carotid artery have been observed in patients who received doses higher than 60 Gy (Tubiana et al, 1985). Transverse myelitis should be avoided by limitation of the dose to the spinal cord.

Treatment of metastatic disease

Few trials of systemic treatment have been reported on an adequate number of MTC patients. Furthermore in many reports, MTC patients are mixed with other histological types of thyroid tumors or with other neuroendocrine tumors.This is due to the rarity of the disease and to the fact

that only patients with progressive distant metastases were included in such trials. In fact, the response rate to any of the drugs already tested is poor and toxicity may be high. On the other hand, long survivals have been observed in some MTC patients with distant metastases, even in the absence of systemic treatment.
In these patients, symptomatic treatment should be used, when needed, for instance to counteract diarrhea.
Distant metastases are generally multiple at discovery with the involvement of multiple sites.
Surgery should be considered for bone metastases in patients with orthopedic or neurological complications or in those at high risk of such complications. Surgery should also be considered in those with a single or a few lung, liver or brain metastases. However involvement of the liver and of the lungs is generally diffuse and large metastases are very often associated with small diffuse metastases which may not be detected pre-operatively by conventional means.
External radiotherapy is mandatory for bone metastases not amenable to surgery especially when they are located in the vertebral column, near the base of the skull or in sites where a pathological fracture would result in a serious disability. It induces rapid relief of bone pain and a slow recalcification of bone metastases. Embolization of bone metastases, particularly in the vertebral column, is frequently effective on bone pain and can be repeated. External radiotherapy may also be indicated in patients with brain metastases. In these patients, standard irradiation protocols are used.
Treatment with radioactive iodine of MTC patients with distant metastases or with a disease confined to the neck has not been shown to be effective in clinical settings (Saad et al,1983). In fact, radioactive iodine should not affect C cells directly as they do not take up circulating iodine. Uptake of Iodine 131 - MIBG by the neoplastic tissue is generally far too low to enable the delivery of a significant radiation dose after the administration of a therapeutic dose of this agent (Baulieu et al, 1987). Similarly, studies with radiolabeled monoclonal antibodies directed againt CEA (Parmentier et al, 1984) or CT (Manil et al, 1989) have shown low and heterogeneous concentrations of these antibodies in neoplastic tissue that make them, up to now, unsuitable for therapy.

Chemotherapy

The only reliable criteria to assess the efficiency of drugs should be the measurements of tumor masses according to the W.H.O. (Miller et al, 1981). Tumor marker levels may be misleading and should not be used alone as reliable criteria of tumor response.

Single agent.
- Doxorubicin is the most widely used drug in metastatic MTC patients. When used as a single agent at high dosage (45 to 75 mg/m^2 every 3 to 4 weeks), the tumor response rate was not as high as initially thought (Gottlieb and Hill, 1974) and probably only 20 % of patients can be expected to respond (Husain et al, 1978, Pacini et al, 1984, Droz et al, 1985, Shimaoka et al, 1985, Hoskin and Harmer, 1987). Furthermore, all responses were partial and only lasted a few months. Analogues of anthracyclines such as aclacinomycin-A (Samonigg et al, 1987), 4' epi-doxorubicin (Shimaoka, 1988) do not seem to be more effective. Mitoxantrone (16 mg/m^2/4wk) given to 9 MTC patients produced only one transient partial response (Schlumberger and Parmentier, 1989).
- Cisplatin was shown to have some activity in MTC when sufficiently high doses are given (75-100 mg/m2/4wk), with a response rate around 15 % (Droz and al, 1985, Hoskin and Harmer, 1987).
- The pathologic similarities of MTC with APUD tumors at other sites, led to the use of drugs which have shown some efficiency in these tumors. Etoposide (100 to 150 mg/m^2 x 3 every 3-4 weeks) has been given to 7 patients and 4 partial responses were observed (Kelsen et al, 1987, Hoskin and Harmer, 1987). A phase II trial with this drug is currently in progress inside the GETC group. Only anecdotal reports are available concerning the use of Streptozotocin and DTIC in MTC patients (Weiss, 1978, Kessinger, 1983).

Combination chemotherapy

Doxorubicin has been combined with a variety of other antineoplastic agents (such as Bleomycin, Vincristin, Cyclophosphamide, Streptozotocin) for the treatment of metastatic MTC (Frame et al, 1988). The overall response rate appeared to be similar to that obtained with doxorubicin alone. Doxorubicin and Cisplatin were given in combination with an overall response rate similar to that obtained with doxorubicin alone, but with greater toxicity (Droz et al, 1985, Shimaoka et al, 1985, Sridhar et al, 1985, Williams et al, 1986).

In pilot studies, 5FU and DTIC produced two partial responses in two patients (Petursson, 1988) and alternating 5FU - DTIC with 5FU - STZ produced two partial responses in 5 patients (Schlumberger et Parmentier, 1990a).

In conclusion, drugs which have shown some efficiency in other neuroendocrine tumors, should be tested as single agents in MTC patients, preferably in cooperative phase II trials in which MTC patients are not mixed with other histologic types of thyroid carcinoma nor with other endocrine tumors. It would thus be possible to pinpoint drugs able to achieve a higher response rate than doxorubicin and they would then be used in combination protocols.

Biomodulators

Interferon α2a was given to 9 patients at two dosages and for periods of time ranging from 1 to 3 months (Schlumberger and Parmentier, 1990b) : 1×10^6 U/day alone in 5 patients, 3×10^6 U/day alone in 8 patients, and in combination with a weekly administration of doxorubicin (15 mg) in 3 patients. No effect on tumor masses was observed. In only 1 patient CT and CEA levels decreased by more than 50 %. A partial relief of diarrhea (> 50 %) was observed in 4 patients, but lasted for only 3 to 8 weeks.

No data is so far available concerning the use of Interleukin 2 in MTC patients.

In conclusion, local control can be achieved in most patients by surgery alone or in combination with external radiotherapy when surgical excision has been incomplete or impossible. Most cancer related deaths are due to distant mestastases and efforts should be made towards an earlier diagnosis of this disease and effective treatment of distant metastases.

REFERENCES

BAULIEU J.L., GUILLOTEAU D., DELISLE M.J., PERDRISOT R., GARDET P., DELEPINE N., BAULIEU F., DUPONT J.L., TALBOT J.N., COUTRIS G., CALMETTES C. (1987). Radio iodinated meta iodobenzylguanidine uptake in medullary thyroid cancer. A french cooperative study. In Cancer 60, pp 2189-2194.

BEN MRAD M.D., GARDET P., ROCHE A., ROUGIER P., CALMETTES C., MOTTE P., PARMENTIER C. (1989). Value of venous catheterization and calcitonin studies in the treatment and management of clinically apparent medullary thyroid carcinoma. In Cancer 63, pp 133-138.

CHONG G.C., BEAHRS O.H., SIZEMORE G.W., WOOLNER L.H. (1975). Medullary carcinoma of the thyroid gland. In Cancer 35, pp 695-704.

DROZ J.P., SCHLUMBERGER M., ROUGIER P., CAILLOU B., GODEFROY W., GARDET P., PARMENTIER C. (1985). Phase II trials of chemotherapy with Adriamycin, Cisplatin and their combination in thyroid cancers. A review of 44 cases. In Thyroid Cancer. JAFFIOL C., MILHAUD G. (Eds.), Amsterdam Elsevier Science Pub, pp 203-208.

FRAME J., KELSEN D., KEMENY N., CHENG E., NIEDZWIECKI D., HEELAN R., LIPPERMANN R. (1988). A phase II trial of Streptozotocin and Adriamycin in advanced APUD tumors. In Am. J. Clin. Oncol. 11, pp 490-495.

GOTTLIEB J.A., HILL C.S. (1974). Chemotherapy of thyroid cancer with Adriamycin. In New Engl. J. Med. 290, pp 193-197.

HALNAN K.E. (1975). The non surgical treatment of thyroid cancer. In Br. J. Surg. 62, pp 769-771
HOSKIN P.J., HARMER C. (1987). Chemotherapy for thyroid cancer. In Radiotherapy and Oncology 10, pp 187-194.
HUSAIN M., ALSEVER R.N., LOCK J.P., GEORGE W.F., KATZ F.H. (1978). Failure of medullary carcinoma to respond to doxorubicin therapy. In Hormone Res. 9, pp 22-25.
KELSEN D., FIORE J., HEELAN R., CHENG E., MAGILL G. (1987). Phase II trial of Etoposide in APUD tumors. In Cancer Treat. Rep. 71, pp 305-308.
KESSINGER A., FOLEY J.F., LEMON H.H. (1983). Therapy of malignant apud cell tumors : effectiveness of DTIC. In Cancer 51, pp 790-794.
MANIL L., BOUDET F., MOTTE P., GARDET P., SACCAVINI J.C., LUMBROSO J.D., SCHLUMBERGER M., CAILLOU B., BAZIN J.P., RICARD M., BELLET D., BOHUON C., TUBIANA M., DI PAOLA R., PARMENTIER C. (1989). Positive anticalcitonin immunoscintigraphy in patients with medullary thyroid carcinoma. In Cancer Res. 49, pp 5480-5485.
MELVIN KEW, TASHJIAN A.H., MILLER H.H. (1972). Sudies in familial (medullary) thyroid carcinoma. In Recent. Prog. Horm. Res. 28, pp 399-470.
MILLER A.B., MOOGSTRATEN B., STAQUET M., WINKLER A. (1981). Reporting results of cancer treatment. In Cancer 47, pp 207-214.
PACINI F., VITTI P., MARTINO E., GIANI C., BAMBINI G., PINCHERA A., BASCHIERI L. (1984). Treatment of refractory thyroid cancer with Adriamycin. In Drugs Exptl. Clin. Res. 12 : pp 911-914.
PARMENTIER C., LUMBROSO J., SCHLUMBERGER M., GARDET P., MACH J.P., BERCHE C., ROUGIER P., CAILLOU B., TUBIANA M. (1984). Immunoscintigraphie avec tomographie d'émission dans les cancers de la thyroïde. In Ann. Méd. Int. (Paris) 135, pp 345-350.
PETURSSON S.R. (1988). Metastatic medullary thyroid carcinoma : complete response to combination chemotherapy with Dacarbazine and 5 Fluorouracil. In Cancer 62, pp 1899-1903.
SAAD M.F., GUIDO J.J., SAMAAN N.A. (1983). Radioactive iodine in the treatment of medullary carcinoma of the thyroid. In J. Clin. Endocrinol. Metab. 57, pp 124-128.
SAMAAN N.A., SCHULTZ P.N., HICKEY R.C. (1988). Medullary thyroid carcinoma : prognosis of familial versus sporadic disease and the role of radiotherapy. In J. Clin. Endocrinol. Metab. 67, pp 801-805.
SAMONIGG H., HOSSFELD D.K., SPEHN J., FILL H., LEB G. (1988). Aclarubicin in advanced thyroid cancer : a phase II study. In Eur. J. Cancer Clin. Oncol. 21, pp 1271-1275.
SARRAZIN D., FONTAINE F., ROUGIER P., GARDET P., SCHLUMBERGER M., TRAVAGLI J.P., BOUNIK H., PARMENTIER C., TUBIANA M. (1984). Place de la radiothérapie dans le traitement des cancers médullaires de la thyroïde. Bull. Cancer (Paris) 71, pp 200-208.
SCHLUMBERGER M., PARMENTIER C. (1989). Phase II evaluation of Mitoxantrone in advanced non anaplastic thyroid cancer. In Bull Cancer (Paris) 76, pp 403-406.
SCHLUMBERGER M., PARMENTIER C. (1990a). Unpublished data.
SCHLUMBERGER M., PARMENTIER C. (1990b). Unpublished data.
SHIMAOKA K, SCHOENFELD D.A., DE WYS W.D., CREECH R.H., DE CONTI R. (1985). A randomized trial of Doxorubicin versus Doxorubicin plus Cisplatin in patients with advanced thyroid carcinoma. In Cancer 56, pp 2155-2160.
SHIMAOKA K. (1988). There is a benefit from chemotherapy for thyroid carcinoma. In Prog. Surg. 19, pp 163-180.
SIMPSON W.J., PALMER J.A., ROSEN I.B., MUSTARD R.A. (1982). Management of medullary carcinoma of the thyroid. In Am J. Surg. 144, pp 420-422.
SRIDHAR K.S., HOLLAND J.F., BROWN J.C., COHEN J.M., OHNUMA T. (1985). Doxorubicin plus Cisplatin in the treatment of Apudomas. In Cancer 55, pp 2634-2637.
STEINFELD A.D. (1977). The role of radiation therapy in medullary carcinoma of the thyroid. In Radiology 123, pp 745-746.

TRAVAGLI J.P., GARDET P., BLAZQUEZ D., ROUGIER P., SCHLUMBERGER M., CAILLOU B., PARMENTIER C. (1984). Traitement chirurgical du cancer médullaire de la thyroïde. Bull. Cancer (Paris) 71, pp 192-194.
TUBIANA M., HADDAD E., SCHLUMBERGER M., HILL C., ROUGIER P., SARRAZIN D. (1985). External radiotherapy in thyroid cancers. In Cancer 55, pp 2062-2071.
WEISS R.B. (1978). Failure of Streptozotocin in rare hormonally active malignancies. In Cancer Treat. Rep. 62, pp 847-849.
WILLIAMS E.D., BROWN C.L., DONIACH I. (1966). Pathological and clinical findings in a series of 67 cases of medullary carcinoma of the thyroid. In J. Clin. Path. 19, pp 103-113.
WILLIAMS S.D., BIRCH R., EINHORN L.H. (1986). Phase II evaluation of Doxorubicin plus Cisplatin in advanced thyroid cancer : a souhteastern Cancer Study Group Trial. In Cancer Treat Rep. 70, pp 405-407.

Therapy of medullary thyroid carcinoma using I-131 MIBG and radiolabelled monoclonal antibodies

C.A. Hoefnagel, R.A. Valdés Olmos and C.C. Delprat

Department of Nuclear Medicine, The Netherlands Cancer Institute, Plesmanlaan 121, 1066 CX Amsterdam, The Netherlands

Introduction
Therapy of widespread MTC is difficult and the prognosis is poor. Another systemic treatment modality would therefore be a welcome addition to the therapeutic spectrum of this disease. In recent years several radiopharmaceuticals have become available, offering new possibilities for the diagnosis and therapy of MTC (Hoefnagel, 1988a). For the diagnosis and follow-up ^{201}Tl-chloride and ^{99m}Tc(V)-DMSA are the tracers of choice (Clarke, 1988; Hoefnagel, 1988a). Imaging with ^{131}I-MIBG and ^{131}I anti-CEA or anti-Calcitonin antibodies or fragments is less sensitive but very specific. These tracers can be used to evaluate their potential therapeutic use. Although ^{131}I-therapy (as iodide) of MTC has been described, ^{131}I-NaI concentration in MTC is an exceptional finding. Three tracers discussed here have the potential to direct ^{131}I to the MTC cell, either via the metabolic (MIBG) or the immunological (antibodies) route.

^{131}I-Meta-iodobenzylguanidine(MIBG)
^{131}I-MIBG, which has been successfully applied for the diagnosis and treatment of pheochromocytoma and neuroblastoma, may be used in tumors which derive from the neural crest and possess an active uptake-1 mechanism at the cell membrane and storage vesicles in the cytoplasm. Although ^{131}I-MIBG scintigraphy is a very reliable test for pheochromocytoma and neuroblastoma with sensitivities around 90%, the cumulative reported data on the diagnostic use of ^{131}I-MIBG in 178 MTC patients indicate that only 36% of medullary cancers concentrate MIBG, showing a preponderance of familial MTC cases (Baulieu, 1987; Hoefnagel 1988a). Due to the low sensitivity of this test in MTC, ^{131}I-MIBG imaging should not be used for the initial diagnosis of MTC, nor can it be relied on to exclude disease. However, once the diagnosis of medullary carcinoma has been established, it is worthwhile to investigate if the tumor concentrates ^{131}I-MIBG, as this may provide an alternative systemic treatment modality for some patients.

The basis for therapy is a good concentration of ^{131}I-MIBG in and long retention by the tumor. Worldwide around 300 patients with neural crest tumors have been reported to have been treated with ^{131}I-MIBG. At The Netherlands Cancer Institute 233 therapeutic doses of ^{131}I-MIBG have been administered to 77 patients. Most of these (54) were children with neuroblastoma, 17 had carcinoid, 4 malignant pheochromocytoma and 2 MTC.
The procedure is the following: 3.7-7.4 GBq (100-200 mCi) ^{131}I-MIBG with a high specific activity is infused intravenously over 4 hours; the patient is admitted to the hospital's isolation facilities (usually 5-6 days, dependent on local legislation) and uses KI orally for two weeks to protect the thyroid from free ^{131}I (unless a thyroidectomy has been performed). Post therapeutic total body scintigrams are made daily and regions of interest are drawn over the whole body, tumor localizations and background areas to be compared with a standard dose for dosimetry. Tumor uptake and whole body retention are expressed as a percentage of the administered dose and curves of the biological behaviour of MIBG are generated (Fig. 1).
29 of 48 evaluated neuroblastoma patients (60%) have thus attained objective remission of disease. Except for the temporary inconvenience of isolation, the treatment is well tolerated and side effects are mild, provided the bone marrow is not invaded by tumor (Hoefnagel, 1988b).

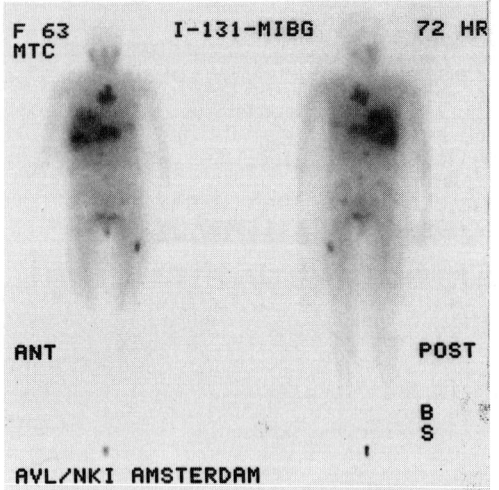
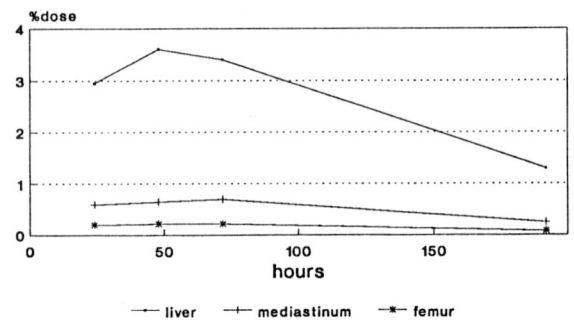

Fig. 1. I-131-MIBG therapy 7.4 GBq

To date 14 patients with MTC have been reported to have received therapeutic amounts of ^{131}I-MIBG. A 15th patient is being treated in Cuba.

In 1984 ^{131}I-MIBG therapy was given a 77-year-old man at our institute, who had inoperable MTC with lymph node metastasis in the neck showing intense ^{131}I-MIBG uptake: 3.2% dose at 48 hours after injection. MIBG imaging also revealed liver metastases which were clinically unsuspected. It was attempted to treat the tumor mass in the neck, which had been progressive during the previous months, with 3.7 GBq (100 mCi) of ^{131}I-MIBG, but after the first dose this therapy was discontinued, because the patient disapproved of further isolation. After this treatment, however, the tumor mass did shrink and the patient's condition remained stable for 3 years (Hoefnagel, 1987).

More recently ^{131}I-MIBG treatment was given to a second patient, a 63 year old female with widespread metastases in the mediastinum, liver, abdomen and left femur and extremely high calcitonin levels in serum. The patient complained of pain and frequent diarrhea. Between July 1989 and now she has received four 7.4 GBq (200 mCi) doses at 2-6 months intervals. The maximum tumor uptake in the liver metastases reached 3.6 %dose. Fig. 1 shows the total body scintigram 72 hours post therapy together with the curves representing tumor activity over time. Although the patient has not attained an objective remission, the disease appears to be arrested (no change) and the patient is relieved of symptoms and is in a good general condition.

Guerra(1987) has treated 3 patients with MTC metastatic to the lungs, liver and bone with ^{131}I-MIBG: in 2 patients no effect was observed and disease progressed, but the third attained partial remission of mediastinal and liver metastases.

Troncone(1990) integrated ^{131}I-MIBG therapy in a total treatment protocol involving total thyroidectomy + lymph node dissection + [131]I ablation or external beam radiotherapy + ^{131}I-MIBG therapy. Two patients were reported to have a complete response after this combined treatment, although calcitonin levels have not returned to normal; a third patient had a partial response of cervical lymph node metastases and stabilization of bone metastases together with relief of pain, and in a 4th patient with widespread bone metastases there was no change except for temporary pain relief. Because of the combined treatment in this study, it is not clear to which extent ^{131}I-MIBG contributed to the observed response.

Clarke(1989/1990) reported about ^{131}I-MIBG therapy in 4 patients with symptomatic, metastatic MTC. Two patients with skeletal metastases had no objective remission but did experience palliation, i.e. relief of pain and diarrhea. Two other patients with disabling dyspnea due to widespread lung metastases had meaningful palliation and dramatic improvement of the general condition, although no objective tumor regression was achieved. More recently a 5th patient was also relieved of symptoms by ^{131}I-MIBG therapy. In two of these patients the serum calcitonin levels diminished by more than 50%.

Adding up these treatment results in a total of 14 patients (Tabel 1), ^{131}I-MIBG therapy induced 2 complete responses ("integrated" therapy), 3 partial remissions, more than 50% decrease in calcitonin levels in at least 3 and palliation in 8 patients with metastatic MTC. Although according to conventional oncological criteria of objective response these results may seem to be poor, it must be emphasized that the palliation provided to these patients, for whom there is little other therapy, may be very meaningful.

Results of I-131 MIBG therapy
medullary thyroid carcinoma

Author	patients	OBJECTIVE RESPONSE			SUBJECTIVE palliation
		CR	PR	50% decrease tumormarkers	
Hoefnagel (1985/89)	2	-	1	-	1
Guerra (1987)	3	-	1	-	-
Troncone (1990)	4	2*	1*	1	2
Clarke (1989/90)	5	-	-	2	5
Total	14	2*	3	3	8

* "integrated" therapy   Tabel 1.

Radiolabelled monoclonal antibodies

During the past decade, hybridoma techniques have facilitated the preparation of a variety of monoclonal antibodies directed to antigens present on malignant cells, for diagnostic purposes. Tumor imaging using radiolabelled monoclonal antibodies directed against well-defined tumor products has proven to be feasible.
Parallel to monitoring serum levels of calcitonin and CEA as a marker of MTC and demonstrating the calcitonin and CEA production by MTC-cells with indirect immunoperoxidase staining techniques, radiolabelled antibodies raised against these products can be used for radioimmunoscintigraphy. Adding up published reports of imaging using radiolabelled anti-CEA antibodies or F(ab')2 fragments in MTC patients (44 cases) an overall sensitivity of around 60% is obtained.
In addition Manil et al. (1987) have reported positive results in patients using a cocktail of 3 anti-calcitonin monoclonal F(ab')2 fragments labelled with ^{123}I or ^{111}In, detecting both primary tumors and bone and lymph node metastases in 4 patients prior to surgery.
The specificity of these procedures is high, but only few cases show enough accumulation of the tracer at tumor sites to consider the therapeutic use of this radiopharmaceutical. Fig. 2 demonstrates a case showing the highest tumor uptake in our series of 15 MTC patients, using ^{131}I-anti CEA F(ab')2 fragments: radioimmunoscintigraphy revealed metastases in the suprarenal and sacroiliac region, and showed more tumor uptake than the ^{201}Tl scan, i.e. 0.26% and 0.64% respectively at 96 hours after administration (Zanin, 1990).

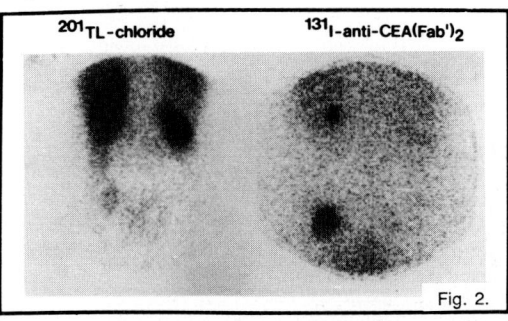

Fig. 2.

^{186}Re-Pentavalent DMSA

The successful use of ^{99m}Tc-Pentavalent DMSA for the detection of MTC has led the group at Guy's Hospital, London to substitute ^{99m}Tc by ^{186}Re, a beta emitter with a physical halflife of 3.8 days. Like ^{131}I this Rhenium isotope also emits gammas (137 KeV) enabling scintigraphic imaging and dosimetry.
Clarke et al (1990) have performed a tracer study using ^{186}Re(V)-DMSA in a patient with MTC to evaluate the potential therapeutic role of this agent. The whole body distribution was found to be identical with that of ^{99m}Tc(V)-DMSA, but the radiation dose to the kidney was relatively high, probably due to ^{186}Re(III)-DMSA in the solution. If this can be eliminated by pharmacological modification, ^{186}Re(V)-DMSA may soon prove to be useful in the therapy of metastatic MTC.

It is concluded that progress is being made in the contribution of nuclear medicine to the detection and treatment of medullary thyroid carcinoma. Preliminary experience with radionuclide therapy of metastatic MTC indicates, that objective response can be attained and that the palliative effect of such treatment is meaningful. The advantages of this approach are, that the treatment is systemic, noninvasive and well tolerated, and that patients can be selected on the basis of tracer studies. Further studies on pharmacokinetics and dosimetry are required to establish the true therapeutic feasibility of the individual radiopharmaceuticals.

References

Baulieu J-L, Guilloteau D, Delisle M-J, et al (1987): Radioiodinated Meta-iodobenzylguanidine uptake in medullary thyroid cancer. A French cooperative study. Cancer 60, 2189-2194.

Clarke SEM, Lazarus CR, Wraight P, et al (1988): Pentavalent ^{99m}Tc-DMSA, ^{131}I-MIBG and ^{99m}Tc-MDP - an evaluation of three imaging techniques in patients with medullary carcinoma of the thyroid. J Nucl Med 29, 33-38.

Clarke SEM (1989/1990): personal communication.

Clarke SEM, Blower P, Allen SJ, et al (1990): Re-186-V-DMSA: A new radiopharmaceutical for therapy of medullary carcinoma of the thyroid. Eur J Nucl Med 16, S70.

Guerra U, Terzi A, Pizzocaro C. et al (1987): ^{99m}Tc(V)-DMSA and *I MIBG in diagnostic and therapeutic strategy of the medullary thyroid carcinoma. Nuclear Medicine 26, 163-164.

Hoefnagel CA, Voûte PA, de Kraker J, et al (1987): Radionuclide diagnosis and therapy of neural crest tumors using Iodine-131 Metaiodobenzylguanidine. J Nucl Med 28, 308-314.

Hoefnagel CA, Delprat CC, Zanin D, et al (1988a): New radionuclide tracers fot the diagnosis and therapy of medullary thyroid carcinoma. Clin Nucl Med 13, 159-165.

Hoefnagel CA, Voûte PA, de Kraker J, et al (1988b): Side effects of I-131-MIBG therapy of neural crest tumors. J Nucl Med 29, 798.

Manil L, Boudet F, Motte P, et al (1987): Anticalcitonin(CT) monoclonalF(ab')2 for immunoscintigraphy(IS) of medullary thyroid carcinoma(MTC). Nuclear Medicine 26, 50.

Troncone L, Rufini V, Montemaggi P, et al (1990): The diagnostic and therapeutic utility of radioiodinated metaiodobenzylguanidine (MIBG). 5 years of experience. Eur J Nucl Med 16, 325-335.

Zanin DEA, van Dongen A, Hoefnagel CA, et al (1990): Radioimmunoscintigraphy using Iodine 131-anti-CEA monoclonal antibodies and Thallium-201 scintigraphy in medullary thyroid carcinoma: a case report. J Nucl Med 31.

VII. Physician's strategy for the management of medullary thyroid carcinoma

VII. *Stratégie du clinicien devant un cancer médullaire de la thyroïde*

Strategy for the diagnosis and the follow-up
Stratégie de diagnostic et de suivi

ROUND TABLE : Strategy of diagnosis and follow-up of medullary thyroid carcinoma

E. Modigliani[1], M. Weissel[2], B.M. Goslings[3], P.J. Guillausseau[4], B. Busnardo[5]

[1] Service d'endocrinologie, Université Paris XIII, Hôpital Avicenne, 93009 Bobigny, France.
[2] 2 Medizinische Univ. Klinik, Garnisongasse 13, A 1090, Wien, Austria.
[3] Endocrinology, Academisch Ziekenhuis Leiden, Postbus 9600, 2300 RC Leiden, The Netherlands.
[4] Hôpital Lariboisière, Université Paris VII, 75010 Paris, France.
[5] Istituto di semeiotica medica, Universita di Padova, via Ospedale Civile, 105 Padova, Italy

3 major topics have been discussed in this round table : atypical and biological presentation, place of recent CT assay for diagnosis and follow up, and post operative management.

1. ATYPICAL CLINICAL ASPECTS

These are important to be borne in mind in spite of the fact that the majority of MTC cases are diagnosed in patients with cold thyroid nodules or by screening of family members of patients with MTC or C-cell hyperplasia.

Three case reports with atypical aspects of MTC were presented. They were chosen because of an unusual first presentation of the disease.

First case

E. MODIGLIANI briefly summarizes the case of a patient in whom CEA serum levels were measured because of abdominal pain. The elevated CEA level led to extensive radiologic examination, which was negative , as was explorative laporotomy. The presence of a lymph node in the left low jugular region was misinterpreted at first. Its biopsy finally led to diagnosis of MTC, however, only by immunohistochemical analysis, revealing positivity for CT and CEA. Total thyroidectomy revealed a MTC of 7 mm diameter.

M. WEISSEL points out that in some CEA kit descriptions, MTC is not even mentioned as a possible reason for elevated serum levels.

This case illustrates that elevated CEA should lead to determination of CT serum concentrations even in patients who present only with abdominal symptoms.

Second case

This case, presented also by E. MODIGLIANI, concerns a 56 years old patient suffering from unilateral and apparently sporadic pheochromocytoma. Routine screening for MTC by a PG-test revealed a normal basal CT but a pathologically elevated CT levels after PG. This was confirmed by a new test 6 months later. Total thyroidectomy was therefore performed which revealed medullary microcarcinoma in both lobes.

Hence, routine screening for MTC (with PG tests) has to be done even in apparently sporadic pheochromocytoma regardless of the age of the patient.

Third case

F. LABAT MOLEUR and O. CHABRE report on a patient with lichen amyloidoisis associated with familial MTC. This only recently appreciated syndrome (the presented case is the third in the literature) consists of pruritous lesions situated in the interscapular region of patients with MTC in MEN II A families. In conventional histology these lesions may be misinterpreted as nevrodermitis. Only electron microscopy detects the characteristic amyloid deposits, even if immunochemistry is negative for CT. These cutaneous lesions may be encountered in other members of the family 20 to 30 years before the discovery of MTC. R. PUTELAT has also observed a MEN II A family with such lesions.

Pruritous skin lesions especially in the interscapular region are therefore now accepted as a symptom that may be associated with familial MTC.

2. RECENTLY DEVELOPED CALCITONIN ASSAYS AND THEIR ROLE IN PRE-OPERATIVE DECISION-MAKING

M. Weissel comments briefly his own results with simultaneous determination of CT serum concentrations by 4 kits (2 IRMA assays, 1 new RIA and an old classical RIA); Measurements were performed in a MEN II A family (2 affected, 8 unaffected), in 10 athyreotic patients operated for non-medullary thyroid cancer and in 4 normal subjects. Affected patients have been correctly diagnosed with all 4 methods by measurement of peak levels after PG. The old RIA had, however, an overlap of basal CT between normals and MTC patients.

J.C. BIGORGNE summarizes results of PG tests in normals with the CIS-IRMA assay : 37 of the 38 normal subjects investigated had a CT peak after PG of $<$30 pg/ml. He compares thereafter results of preoperative abnormal PG tests with histologic lesions found at surgery : in 32 patients tested by family screening because of 1 or more known MTC in the family, the following results were obtained : a) 15 patients had an elevation of $>$ 100 pg CT/ml after PG : 14 had MTC at surgery, 1 had lymphocytic thyroiditis and a papillary carcinoma ; b) 13 tested persons had peak CT levels between $>$ 50 and $<$ 100 pg/ml : micro-MTC was found in 7, C-cellhyperplasia in 6 ; c) the last 4 subjects had a peak between 30 and 50 pg/ml : 2 had C-cell hyperplasia, 2 had cancer.

A. BONEU reports similar results but stresses the importance of repeating PG tests in apparently unaffected family members : in 2 patients with histologically proven MTC, only the second PG test performed 6 months after the first one gave the pathological result that led to surgery.

Therefore consensus with the new CIS IRMA seems to be the following : Basal CT of $>$ 40 pg/ml and/or peak CT (3' after PG) of $>$ 100 pg/ml are absolutely indicative for MTC.

C. CALMETTES asks the audience whether anyone is aware of cases of MTC with elevated basal CT but no increase after PG. The answer is negative. M. SCHLUMBERGER reports 2 cases with neuroendocrine tumors with such a hormonal profile.

3. GENERAL POST-OPERATIVE STRATEGY

Surgical strategy was reviewed on friday : total thyroidectomy with bilateral central dissection has the general agreement.

B. NIEDERLE presents the results of the series of his group : if recurrent lymph nodes are not invaded, prognosis seems to be excellent. If lymph nodes are positive, a modified neck dissection is indicated : 30 % of these patients will have involvement of the upper mediastinum. He stresses, moreover, the importance of total thyroidectomy : in a small series of 9 patients with apparently limited MTC and negative lymph nodes, in whom for these reasons only subtotal thyroidectomy and no central dissection was performed, 5 developed local recurrence within 4 years.
J.F. DAVID insists about the possibility that invaded lymph nodes may appear macroscopically normal. He performs systematically bilateral functional jugular dissection, basing on his experience that if the cancer is more than 7 mm in diameter, microscopic lymph node metastases are found in 22 % of cases.

M. WEISSEL proposes a POST-OPERATIVE STRATEGY, depending on the extent of disease at first surgery. He suggests 3 possibilities :

1) Total thyroidectomy performed, lymph nodes negative :
4 weeks after surgery : clinical examination and determination of basal serum levels of CT and CEA

- if basal CT is normal : clinical follow up 3 months later with a CT provocative test (PG-tests are the most often used by the audience)
- if basal and peak CT are normal, repeat clinical examination and PG-test every 6 months until 5 years post-operatively

- if basal or stimulated CT is elevated (after surgery or during follow up) : try to localize wherefrom it is elevated. If you are unsuccessful, repeat follow up 3 months later with extensive search for metastases.

2) Total thyroidectomy performed, lymph nodes positive but removed :
This patient is more at risk to have worse prognosis. Therefore the first provocative CT test should be performed already 4 weeks after surgery together with determination of basal CEA and CT.

- If CT is abnormal, means of localization are multiple :
    - echography of neck, liver, adrenals
    - CT scan of neck, thorax, liver, adrenals and bone
    - bone scintigraphy
    - radioactive imagery with DMSA, Th201, MIBG, immunoscintigraphy
- If a local recurrence or a single metastasis is localized, surgery is the treatment of choice.

- If basal and stimulated CT is normal, repeat follow-up every 3 months the first year with PG-tests every 6 months.

3) Total thyroidectomy performed but removal of MTC only palliative and/or distant metastases present :

Different treatment modalities (with little success) may be offered :
- surgical removal of resectable metastases
- external radiotherapy of the neck or/and the metastasis
- chemotherapy
- somatostatin analogues

The following points of this general scheme of strategy were discussed :

3A : POST-OPERATIVE CALCITONIN (CT) DETERMINATIONS :

We tried to reach consensus on two questions :

a) what is the best time for measurement ?

B. BUSNARDO comments about the usefulness of CT assays 24 hours post-operatively. He suggests that CT concentrations determined at this point represent a useful prognosis index. He separates his patients in 3 groups :
- in 9 patients, basal CT was elevated. Metastases developed in all 6 months later
- in 7 patients with normal post-operative CT levels, there was no increase 6 months later
- very few patients had elevated CT levels post-operatively with normal levels 6 months later.

J. FISCHER contradicts this assumption vigorously, claiming that very high pre-operative CT levels make 24-hour post-operative values useless because of the biological half-life of CT.

C. CALMETTES advocates to perform measurement of basal CT and CEA 6 - 8 weeks after surgery, since the half-life of CEA is much longer than that of CT. In her patients with normal CT 6 weeks post-op, she observed only 1 case of recurrence with elevated CT 6 months later.

M. SCHLUMBERGER reports on the experience of his institution (Gustave Roussy Institute) : 31 patients had measurement of basal CT (by CIS IRMA) 5 days after surgery. So far there was only one recurrence of disease in the patients who had normal CT levels at this time point.

b) what is a normal post operative CT level ?

It is not easy to answer this question, indeed. Absolute concentration ranges cannot be given, since assays and methods used in the different countries are not uniform. It is, moreover, conceivable that "normal" results obtained by the hitherto used old classical RIAs turn out to be pathological when measured by the new monoclonal IRMA techniques.

Basal CT measured by the new technique may be sufficient to predict recurrence or - if elevated - to indicate extensive localizing investigations. Normal basal levels measured by these techniques indicate indeed that even if tumoral tissue is still present (as evidenced by abnormal CT peak after PG), it must be so small that it can not be localized by any imaging technique.

3B WHICH TECHNIQUES ARE USEFUL FOR POST OPERATIVE LOCALIZATION OF LOCAL OR DISTANT METASTASES ? :

We did not have time to discuss this topic in detail, although the strategy of investigation is very important in terms of cost versus benefit (S CLARKE). Everyone agrees that very expensive and numerous imaging techniques are not worthwile when CT is only moderately elevated.

1. Scanning with Radio Nuclides :
- 131-I does not seem to have any interest. 1 observation of B. BROUSSOUX showed a positive radioiodine scanning in a lymph node metastasis, but such cases are very rare. In general 131-I is of no diagnostic and therapeutic use after total thyroidectomy in MTC patients.
- MIBG scanning is not sensitive enough - at least when standard doses are used.
- Thallium is not specific
- DMSA imaging is a cheap method which is more competitive, according to S. CLARKE
- Anti CEA imaging seems of promising value when indium III-Fab of monoclonal antibodies are used (D. SANDROCK). A. GARCIA ALMEIGERAS has shown, however, that reproducibility is not very good, possibly because of development of endogenous antibodies against the tracer. It seems that this method is of doubtful benefit with respect to its high cost, especially if the investigation is not focused on a particular region, or if metastases are too small.

2. Echography and Tomodensitometry
are more useful in local recurrence if this is not too small

3. Selective venous catetherization
K. FRANK RAUE presents promising data obtained with this method : 18 patients were studied prospectively by catheterization and measurement of basal CT. The sensitivity was 89 %, whereas that of tomodensitometry was 38 % and that of echography 28 %. The demonstration of a concentration gradient by this method seems to be the best way of localizing the tumor precisely.

P.J. GUILLAUSSEAU stresses in the discussion the importance of the investigation of a gradient of CT concentration in the hepatic region also. If such a gradient (which is indicative for small hepatic metastases) exists, surgical ablation of positive cervical lymph nodes will not be followed by a fall in CT.

In the lively discussion on this method, numerous remarks are made : H. DRALLE points out that the catheter must be very close to the lesion in order to obtain a gradient. G.F.W. SCHEUMANN believes that it must be very difficult technically to perform catheterization after extensive surgery (with removal of the jugular veins !). B. BUSNARDO wonders how the sensitivity of radio nuclide imaging would be in the study of K FRANK RAUE (this method was not applied in the study).

Some authors (K.M. GAUTVIK) suggest to combine catheterization with a PG test. In the experience of K. FRANK RAUE, this seems unnecessary. P. ANDRY comments GAUTWIK'S data, where only PG stimulation revealed the concentration gradient at the hepatic region in some patients with liver metastases. M. WEISSEL points out that he would refuse as a patient a PG test during selective venous catheterization of the neck, because of the unpleasant side effects of both procedures.

It is concluded that selective venous catheterization with measurement of basal CT is a promising technique in patients with post operatively elevated CT levels and small tumoral mass. It is, however, too early to propose it as the first investigation method in such patients, as suggested by R. MORNEX and P.J. GUILLAUSSEAU : this procedure requires trained specialists.

4. MANAGEMENT OF PATIENTS WITH POST-OP. ELEVATED CT AND/OR CEA WITHOUT LOCALISABLE METASTASES

Although we did not have time to discuss this topic, the following points seem to have achieved consensus :

1. if basal CT levels are normal as measured by the new IRMA methods or if PG-stimulated are >300 pg/ml, no treatment is recommended. The best thing to do is to continue clinical and biochemical follow up regularly.

2. if basal CT levels are elevated but tumor mass not localized, even after extensive investigation, no clear recommendation can be given : although, some clinicians advocate for systemical application of radiotherapy and/or chemotherapy, many others refuse this, because of the poor success and the potential harmfulness of these treatment modalities (B. BUSNARDO). Prospective studies will indicate the place for selective venous sampling in this instance.

3. Even in the presence of distant metastases (lung, liver) the survival of some patients may be long without real clinical discomfort. Therefore, the following strategy is suggested in such patients :
- consider the spontaneous evolution, on an individual basis, for each patient (eg moderate and stable elevation of CT without frank elevation of CEA indicates a relatively good prognosis)
- ask the pathologist for more prognostic histologic arguments : eg a high level of CT immunostaining in the tumor with homogenous and strong staining together with a DNA content with high euploidy is now accepted as a good sign for slow evolution of the disease. Other histologic parameters were reviewed on friday by B. FRANC but seem to be of less prognostic value.
- apply aggressive treatment in evolutive cases only.

This strategy is only a suggestion. It is clear that it depends on the availability of better treatments in the future. Treatment with somatostatin agonists (SMS 201.995) does not appear very promising so far. Perhaps local irradiation by 131-I-MIBG or by labeled somatostatin receptors will give better results. Technical problems inherent to these methods, however, do not allow yet their wide-spread use.

Strategy in familial forms

Stratégie dans les formes familiales

Early detection of inherited MTC

P. Gardet[1], M. Schlumberger[1], B. Caillou[1], J.P. Travagli[1], H. Sobol[2], D. Bellet[1], G. Lenoir[2] and C. Parmentier[1]

[1] Institut Gustave-Roussy and (*) INSERM U 66, 94805 Villejuif Cedex, France. [2] Centre International de la Recherche sur le Cancer, 69008 Lyon Cedex, France

When medullary thyroid carcinoma (MTC) is detected at a preclinical stage, it is curable. Detection has been facilitated by the use of new techniques for calcitonin (CT) measurement (MOTTE et al, 1988) and linkage study analysis (SOBOL et al, 1989). However, the significance of CT levels after pentagastrin administration was recently questioned due to the frequency of low but significant responses obtained by a more sensitive IRMA method (GUILLOTEAU et al, 1990). In addition, immunohistochemistry has revealed the presence of C cell hyperplasia in thyroid tissue adjacent to follicular tumors (ALBORES-SAAVEDRA et al, 1988). Thus, this study was undertaken to provide practical guidance for the screening and treatment of MTC relatives.

Subjects and methods

From 1984 to 1989, 191 subjects from 59 families were explored at IGR. The subjects were related to at least one MTC patient. At presentation the subjects were assigned to one of two groups: 69 to group 1 because at least two MTC patients had already been operated in the family and 122 to group 2 because only one MTC patient was known in the family. Thirty eight patients who were to be operated for various thyroid diseases of follicular origin were included in the present study as controls.
The exploration included CT level measurements, before, then two and five minutes after administration of pentagastrin (0.5 µg/kg, I.V.). An IRMA kit using monoclonal antibodies was used (Cis Bioindustries, Gif sur Yvette, France) with a basal CT normal range of < 10 pg/ml (MOTTE et al, 1988). Using polymorphic DNA markers (IRPB and MCK2 probes), genetic linkage study, which estimates the risk of an individual being a gene carrier, was performed in subjects from group 1 who were to be operated (SOBOL et al, 1989). Surgery included a total thyroidectomy and bilateral lymph node dissection (TRAVAGLI et al, 1984). Immunohistochemistry using monoclonal antibodies directed against CT was performed on serial sections of thyroid glands and lymph nodes.

Results

CT level was detectable after pentagastrin stimulation in 24 subjects from group 1 and in 25 from group 2 (table 1). It was above 100 pg/ml in 9 subjects from group 1 and in 2 from group 2. These

subjects were referred to surgery. Five other subjects with stimulated CT levels ranging from 34-76 pg/ml also underwent surgery (2 from group 1 and 3 from group 2).
A stimulated CT level of > 100 pg/ml was associated with bilateral tumor foci in 9 patients and with C cell hyperplasia in 8 patients from group 1. C cell hyperplasia alone was found in the other 7 subjects.
After surgery all subjects had an undetectable stimulated CT level ; they are considered to be cured. Genetic linkage study was informative in 7 subjects from group 1. The pre-operative stimulated CT level was > 100 pg/ml in 5, and less than that in 2 of them. Four subjects who had a high risk of being a gene carrier (85-98 %) presented also bilateral tumor foci. Two subjects with a low risk had only C cell hyperplasia. One subject with bilateral tumoral foci had a recombination. Thus, one could not estimate the probability of whether or not this subject might be a gene carrier.
Of the 38 controls subjects, 5 had a detectable CT level after pentagastrin stimulation ranging from 13-42 pg/ml. Twenty two underwent surgery and C cell hyperplasia was found in 6 patients. It was present in all 4 patients who had a detectable CT level after pentagastrin stimulation and in 2 of the 18 whose CT remained undetectable after pentagastrin stimulation.

	n	1st degree		2nd degree	
		Pg +	Pg -	Pg +	Pg -
Group 1	69	20	23	4	22
Group 2	122	22	83	3	14

Table 1 : Pentagastrin stimulation test of 191 subjects included in the study.

Discussion

The present data show that even low but detectable CT levels after pentagastrin stimulation announce a C cell hyperplasia and furthermore, that this can be observed in conditions other than Multiple Endocrine Neoplasia type IIa (MEN IIa) or inherited MTC without pheochromocytoma (MTCWP). This stresses the importance of genetic linkage studies in familial MTC's and leads to some practical considerations.
In subjects from group 1 where at least two MTC patients have already been operated in the family, four situations can be individualized.
Situation 1 : subjects with a CT level above 100 pg/ml after pentagastrin stimulation and whose genetic linkage studies indicate a high risk of being a gene carrier. Such subjects should undergo surgery. In fact, in 4 such patients, bilateral tumor foci and bilateral C cell hyperplasia were found by immunohistochemistry.
Situation 2 : subjects with a CT level above 100 pg/ml after pentagastrin stimulation but whose genetic linkage studies are not informative. Such subjects should also undergo surgery. Four such subjects underwent surgery. Bilateral tumor foci were found in all and were associated with C cell hyperplasia in 3 of them.
Situation 3 : subjects whose CT level remains below 100 pg/ml after pentagastrin stimulation and whose genetic linkage studies show a low risk of being a gene carrier. In two such patients only C cell hyperplasia was found at surgery.For these subjects surgery can be postponed. They should be followed biologically every two or three years till the age of 40.
Situation 4 : subjects whose CT level remains undetectable after stimulation and whose genetic linkage studies show a high risk of being a gene carrier. For these, surgery can be postponed. These subjects should be followed with a yearly pentagastrin stimulation test at least till the age of 40 to see whether or not they will develop the disease. The biological and genetic screening should

also be applied to all their children since these subjects transmit the genetic defect. It seems safe to perform surgery only when stimulated CT level reaches 100 pg/ml or more.

In subjects from Group 2 where only one MTC patient is known in the family and linkage studies cannot be carried out, two situations can be individualized.
Situation 1 : subjects with a CT level after pentagastrin stimulation higher than 100 pg/ml should undergo surgery. If neoplastic foci are found, the disease should be considered as inherited and a genetic linkage study should be performed for them associated to a biological screening for all their first degree relatives.
If C cell hyperplasia without neoplastic foci is found, a familial disease should be suspected. However, C cell hyperplasia has been found in 35 % of patients who underwent surgery for various conditions of follicular origin (ALBORES-SAAVEDRA et al, 1988). In the present study, C cell hyperplasia was discovered in all 4 control patients who had a detectable CT level after pentagastrin stimulation and in 11 % of the controls with an undetectable stimulated CT level. Therefore a biological screening is warranted for all their first degree relatives. Whether or not the disease is familial in these cases remains questionable.
Situation 2 : subjects with a CT level after pentagastrin stimulation detectable, but below 100 pg/ml, should be followed with a yearly pentagastrin stimulation test and surgery can be postponed. In these cases, it appears safe to follow all first degree relatives with pentagastrin stimulation testing.

Conclusion

At least all first degree relatives of MTC patients should undergo CT determinations following pentagastrin stimulation. Subjects with stimulated CT levels above 100 pg/ml should undergo surgery. For subjects whith a relatively low but significant (<100 pg/ml) CT level after pentagastrin stimulation, DNA testing may be performed in families with at least two known MTC's. When DNA testing is informative, it indicates a careful follow-up for these subjects and their first degree relatives. The significance of C cell hyperplasia, when not associated with tumor foci remains questionable and needs further study. DNA testing may also be useful in this situation by indicating the risk of an individual being a gene carrier and therefore the need for screening the children. Finally, the number of subjects where DNA testing was not informative and the existence of recombinants underline the need of finding new probes.

References

1 - ALBORES-SAAVEDRA J., MONFORTE H. et al (1988). C. cell hyperplasia in thyroid tissue adjacent to follicular cell tumors. In Human Pathology, 19, pp 795-799.

2 - GUILLOTEAU D., PERDRISOT R., CALMETTES C. et al (1990). Diagnosis of medullary carcinoma of the thyroid (MTC) by calcitonin assay using monoclonal antibodies : criteria for the pentagastrin stimulation test in hereditary MTC. In J.Clin. Endocrinol. Metab. 71, pp 1064-1067.

3 - MOTTE P., VAUZELLE P. GARDET P. et al (1988). Construction and clinical validation of a sensitive and specific assay for serum mature calcitonin using monoclonal anti-peptide antibodies. In Clin. Chim. Acta, 174, pp 35-54.

4 - SOBOL H., NAROD S.A. et al (1989). The screening for multiple endocrine neoplasia type 2 A by DNA polymorphism analysis. In New Engl. J. Med., 321, pp 996 -1001.

5 - TRAVAGLI J.P., GARDET P. et al (1984). Surgical treatment of medullary thyroid carcinoma. In Bull. Cancer (Paris), 71, pp 192-195.

Strategy for an approach to familial medullary thyroid cancer. Practical, psychological and genetic aspects of screening

H.F.A. Vasen(*) and C.J.M. Lips(**)

* Foundation for the Detection of Hereditary Tumours, c/o University Hospital Leiden, Rijnsburgerweg 10, building no. 50, 2333 AA Leiden, The Netherlands.
** University Hospital Utrecht, Heidelberglaan 100, 3584 CX Utrecht, The Netherlands

INTRODUCTION

There are three recent reports of studies performed to assess the effect of screening, one study covering 105 patients (Telenius-Berg et al., 1984) one study dealing with 15 kindreds from our group (Vasen et al., 1987) and a study on a very extended family with a follow-up of 18 years (Gagel et al., 1988). All of these studies confirmed the value of screening conclusively. The next problem is, how an early detection programme should be instituted, nation wide, for all of the affected families.

NATIONAL REGISTRY

This led us to establish a National Registry in 1985 in The Netherlands with the following aims: (1) To improve the surveillance of family members. (2) To guarantee the continuity of periodic examination. (3) To serve general practitioners and specialists by advising them about matters related to diagnosis, treatment, and screening procedures. (4) To collect data as a basis for research.

The registry collects personal data, screening results, diagnoses, and treatment results of patients as well as personal data and screening results of all first-degree relatives. Unlike registration centres in other countries the design of the Dutch registry does not include screening of the families. The periodic examination is performed in hospitals all over the country. To improve surveillance in families with hereditary cancer, the genealogic studies are done by genetic field workers (social workers) connected with the registry. To guarantee the continuity of periodic examination the families' specialists are regularly sent a reminder (computerized) to screen family members who are at risk, and each specialist informs the registry about the screening results and the data of the next examination.

The general practitioner of each relative is informed by the Foundation when any member of a family is listed in its registration system. When the registry was established, information about the organization and its functions was presented to the medical community in lectures and publications and these led to the referral of the majority of the families known to suffer from the MEN-2 syndrome in The Netherlands.

PRIVACY ASPECTS

Due to the obviously confidential nature of the medical data, the utmost care is taken to protect the privacy of the persons about whom information has been received. Written informal consent is required before registration can take place. Furthermore, it was decided to keep personal information separate form medical reports. Information is only given to third parties with consent of the family members involved. Each registered person has carefully defined rights, including the right of correction or removal of his or her data from the registry. A supervisory committee including a lawyer, two patients, and a clergyman, was formed to make certain that these rules are adhered to.

PSYCHOLOGICAL ASPECTS

There are few data in the literature on the psychological consequenses of surveillance of families predisposed to hereditary cancer. There is one report on "*the experience and needs of MEN-2 patients and their families*" (Cleiren et al., 1989). The main questions underlying that study were: (1) Are the family members satisfied with the medical information provided by the specialist and general practitioner? (2) What was the reason for any dissatisfaction. (3) What forms of contact would the family members prefer? The results showed that the majority of family members were satisfied with the information given by the specialists, but only a minority about the information provided by the general practitioner. The main reason for dissatisfaction was the delay in reporting the results of the calcitonin test. Furthermore, it came out that there was a need for contact with fellow sufferers. This led to the establishment of a patients' organization in The Netherlands.
More studies are needed to assess the psychological problems of relatives at risk of hereditary cancer.

GENETIC ASPECTS

At present, highly reliable genetic markers with a recombination rate of less than 1 per cent are available. The question is, therefore, should the screening programme be changed? Our original programme is shown in Table 1.
If a DNA test shows that a family member has a high risk of developing the disease, but the calcitonin test is still normal, this is likely to lead to more intensive screening rather than to prophylactic surgery. If the calcitonin test becomes abnormal, surgery is indicated.

Table 1. Introduction of DNA tests: change of screening programme

	Test	age limits (years)	Interval (years)
MTC	calcitonin test	5* - 20	1
		20 - 40	2
PHEO	VMA, (Nor) Adrenalin,	5* - 20	1
	metanefrines	20 - 40	2
	24 hr urine		

* MEN-2B ≥ 1 yr

The most straightforward use of DNA prediction in the MEN-2 syndrome at present, is to exclude family members from risk, and so from the necessity of screening. Important factors to be taken into consideration with respect to stopping screening are anxiety of the family members about developing the disease and anxiety of their specialists. As a result, most specialists will continue the periodic examinations but lengthen the interval between examinations.
With respect to the implementation of the DNA tests, close cooperation between the specialist and the clinical geneticist is very important. The specialists follow the families for many years, have extensive experience with all aspects of the disease, and perform the periodic examination. The clinical geneticist is the expert in counseling and interpretation of the DNA test. At present,

most MEN-2 families are referred directly to the DNA lab. In the future, the families should be referred to the DNA lab via the clinical geneticist, who should discuss the result of the genetic test with the families.
Because of the severe impact of genetic studies, much attention should be paid to providing information to patients. Information provided before the test should include the following: (1) Concerning the MEN-2 syndrome: the clinical manifestations, the genetic aspects, the availability of treatment, and the prognosis should be discussed. (2) Information about the test should include: How the test is done; mention of the need for blood samples from other relatives, and the limitations of the test, and it should be stated clearly that a positive result of the test does not give information about the age at diagnosis. (3) Possible consequences for the individual, spouse, and/or companion, for example, socio-economic consequences (employment, insurance) which cannot be overseen at present, should be discussed. (4) Furthermore, the family members should be informed about the availability of psychological support.
Finally, some guidelines on the delivery of the results include: (1) The results should be discussed as soon as possible after completion of the test. (2) The relatives should have the right to decide not to know the results. (3) Sufficient time should be allowed for discussion of the results. (4) The specialist and general practitioner of the relative in question should be informed as soon as possible after the results have been reported.

REFERENCES

Cleiren, M.P.H.O., Oskam, W., Lips, C.J.M. (1989): Living with a hereditary form of cancer: Experiences and needs of MEN-2 patients and their families. *Henri Ford Hosp. Med. J.* 37, 164-166.

Gagel, R.F., Tashjan, A.H., Cummings, T., et al. (1988): The clinical outcome of prospective screening for multiple endocrine neoplasia type 2A. A 18-year experience. *N. Engl. J. Med.* 318, 478-484.

Telenius-Berg, M., Berg, B., Hamberger, B., Tibblin, S., Ysander, L., Welonder, G. (1984): Impact of screening on prognosis in the multiple endocrine neoplasia type 2 syndrome: natural history and treatment results in 105 patients. *Henri Ford Hosp. Med. J.* 32, 225-232.

Vasen, H.F.A., Nieuwenhuyzen Kruseman, A.C., Berkel, J., et al. (1987): The MEN-2 syndrome: The value of screening and central registration. A study of fifteen kindreds in The Netherlands. *Am. J. Med.* 83:847-852.

Genetic screening for hereditary medullary thyroid carcinoma (MTC)

H. Sobol[1]*, S. Narod[2], I. Schuffenecker[2], G.M. Lenoir[2] and the Groupe d'Etude des Tumeurs à Calcitonine (GETC)

[1] *Département d'Oncologie et de Génétique, Centre Léon-Bérard, 28, rue Laënnec, 69373 Lyon Cedex 08, France.*
[2] *Centre International de Recherche sur le Cancer, 150, cours Albert-Thomas, 69372 Lyon Cedex 08, France*

* Author for correspondence

INTRODUCTION

Familial forms of MTC are inherited as a dominant genetic trait with a high penetrance. Three subgroups are distinguishable: MEN 2A (MTC, pheochromocytoma, parathyroid involvement); MTC ONLY where the adrenal tumor does not appear and MEN 2B (MTC, pheochromocytoma, marfanoid appearance, neuromas of the lips and the buccal cavity, visceral ganglioneuromatosis).

Using DNA polymorphism (RFLP's), the genetic defect of the three syndromes has been mapped in the pericentromeric region of chromosome 10. The data do not suggest that different genetic loci may underlie the different clinical presentations (Sobol et al., 1989a; Narod et al., 1989; Norum et al., 1990).

SCREENING GENE CARRIERS IN INHERITED MTC WITH DNA MARKERS

Genetic linkage provides a new means for detecting the carrier state of MTC, prior to the onset of symptomatic disease. We have performed DNA analysis on 19 MEN 2A, 13 MTC ONLY and 1 MEN 2B families, using a number of polymorphic probes flanking the centromere of chromosome 10. MTC cases for these studies were ascertained through the records of the GETC (Calmettes, 1984). Blood samples from 110 families were collected (table 1). We present the screening by MTC subgroup(s) and discuss the limits of DNA tests.

MEN 2A

Because numerous families and extensive pedigrees were available, MEN 2A was the first inherited MTC syndrome mapped, and DNA screening proposed (Mathew et al., 1987; Sobol et al., 1989b); theoritical example is presented in figure 1. In family 5 (figure 2), the allele B of RBP3 probe has been transmitted with the susceptibility gene. All the affected members of generation V are candidates for genetic counselling. By tracing the transmission of allele B through the family, it will be possible to identify future at-risk individuals. On the contrary, family members homozygous AA for the markers have a very low risk to be gene carriers (< 2%). In family 58 (figure 2), it is possible to ascertain that susceptibility gene is located on the same chromosome as allele B in the mother (I2) because the son II2 is affected. We were able to predict that the five years old girl II2 was at risk because she shared the B allele. Two years later, a pentagastrin test (Pg) has been found positive, validating by conventional screening the results of RFLP's testing. But in practice, the small family size and the lack of informative mating may affect the power of RFLP's analysis. In family 5 (figure 2), because both parents are heterozygous AB (IV6, IV7), it is not possible to determine whether or not individual V6 is a gene carrier. In such a case, we have to use other markers. If no probe is informative, screening is based only on a conventional endocrine challenge. DNA screening is now feasible in most French MEN 2A families. This approach can permit to concentrate screening efforts on individuals considered to be at risk.

Table 1. Families and individual collected for MTC studies

Syndrome	Nb Families	Nb individuals collected
MEN 2A	54	494
MTCWP	34	329
MEN 2B	22	54
TOTAL	110	877

MTC ONLY

Several large families have been reported in which MTC has been observed in the absence of pheochromocytoma. MTC tends to be less aggressive and appears to be reduced. In our series, the only recombinant observed with D10S15 (MCK2) a thight linked marker was in a small MTC ONLY family (Figure 3) (Narod et al., 1989). But the individual III1 was not recombinant with probe D10S34 on the opposite side of the gene (Gardet et al., 1991a). This example shows a clear advantage to have informative flanking markers in calculating a recurrence risk. In the hypothetical pedigree in Figure 4, the child of generation III has inherited both linked markers. Barring a double crossover (an extremely rare event), the child will have inherited the disease gene as well. Based on current map distances, the risk is above 99% (Lenoir et al., 1991).

Because genetic heterogeneity cannot be excluded, in particular in family of small size, we propose to apply DNA screening in well documented MTC ONLY pedigrees. This method will be of valuable help to identify apparently healthy gene carriers greater than 40 years old who are generally excluded from Pg testing. For instance, in family 52 a member had a Pg conversion at age 50. Until now, linkage analyses were performed using MEN 2A penetrance data, DNA test will be of valuable help to establish penetrance curve for this clinical presentation.

Theorical tree: I

                  II

                  III

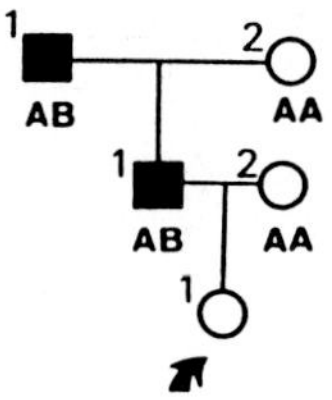

```
    1        2
    ■────────○
    AB       AA
        │
        1        2
        ■────────○
        AB       AA
            │
            1
            ○
            ↗
```

1st degree relative of an
affected member

1) Without DNA testing:
    Mendelien risk with   With a negative PG test
    a dominant autosomal   it becomes of 33%
    trait = 50%   at age 15

2) With RFLP analysis:
    (recombination fraction θ is considered to be 0.02)
  and genotype AA: With negative PG test: 1%
    this risk becomes of: 2%
  and genotype AB: with negative PG test: 96%
    this risk becomes of: 98%

Fig. 1 Affected family members are represented by solid circles (females) or solid squares (males). In the above example A and B are the two different alleles of the marker. For this hypothetical counselling situation, the pre-test likelihood for being a carrier was calculated by using age-specific penetrance curves for MTC with and without Pg test (the clinical penetrance is 0% at age 15 but 50% with Pgtest, and applying Bayes theorem (Sobol <u>et al.</u>, 1989b).

MEN 2B

The availability of only a few pedigrees with more than one living case makes linkage studies difficult (Norum <u>et al.</u>, 1990; Sobol <u>et al.</u>, 1989a). Furthermore, cases without a family history have been reported. Even the application of RFLP's method will be considerably reduced, in multiplex families it could be precious. This form generally carries an earlier age of tumor onset and MTC is very aggressive. The precise identification of a gene carrier could permit a preventive measure by thyroidectomy. Until the genetic defect will be cloned, DNA tests will not be used in other situations mainly in de novo mution cases.

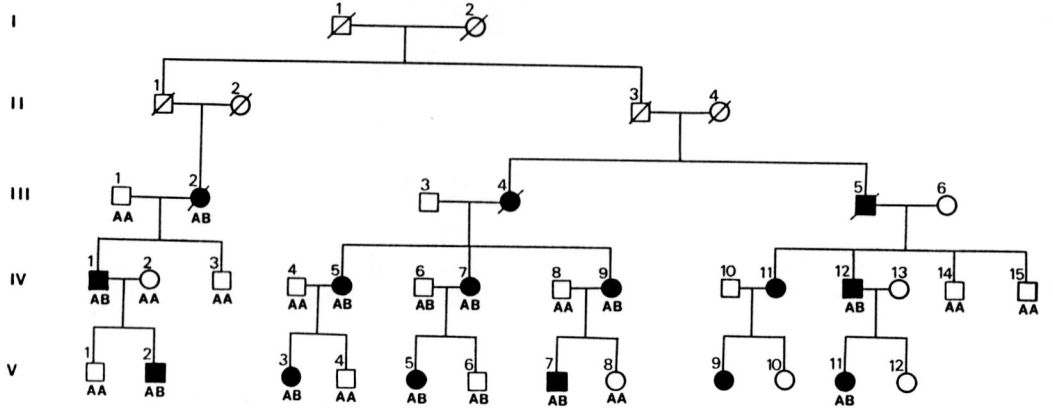

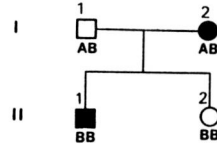

Fig. 2 Selected pedigrees of families with MEN2A to represent situations in which genetic counselling is possible or limited.

With the goal of generalizing DNA screening, we are testing first degree relative healthy members with chromosome 10 markers. 110 subjects from 35 families have been analysed with one of the three following probes: RBP3, D10S15 and D10S34. Probes were informative in 56 members: 13 have a high risk to be a gene carrier and 40 are at low risk.

PERSPECTIVES

The RFLP's method is useful to identify people at risk for the disease, who can then be followed closely for the onset of neoplastic changes with conventional endocrine methods, and to exclude for the burden of further screening those considered to be at very low risk. To validate the sequence proposed in the decisional tree (Figure 5) (Sobol, 1990), a feasability study is undertaken by our multidisciplinary group.

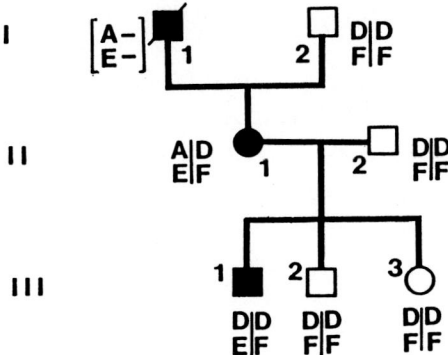

Fig. 3 Family 3 of MTC only type. This pedigree illustrates recombination between flanking markers. The upper letters represent D10S15 (MCK2), the lower represent D10S34 (TB1434). Because patient III1 inherited the D allele unliked to the disease from his mother and the E allele which is associated to the disease, we can conclude to a recombination between these two markers.

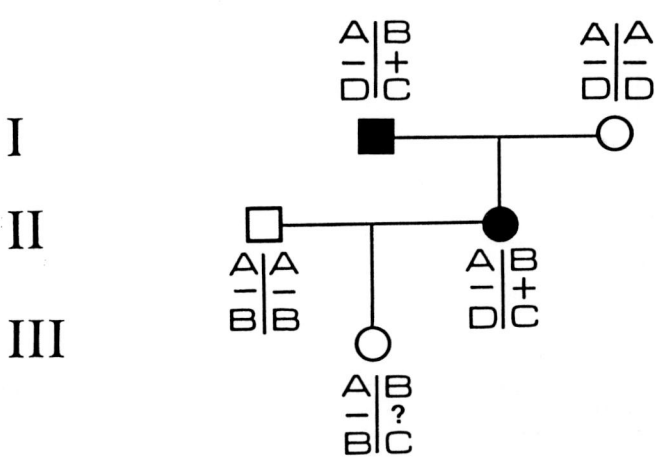

Fig. 4 Hypothetical pedigree of family informative with flanking markers. Upper letter represents D10S34 (TB14.34), lower letter represents D10S15 (MCK2) allele, and phase in indicated by the vertical divider.

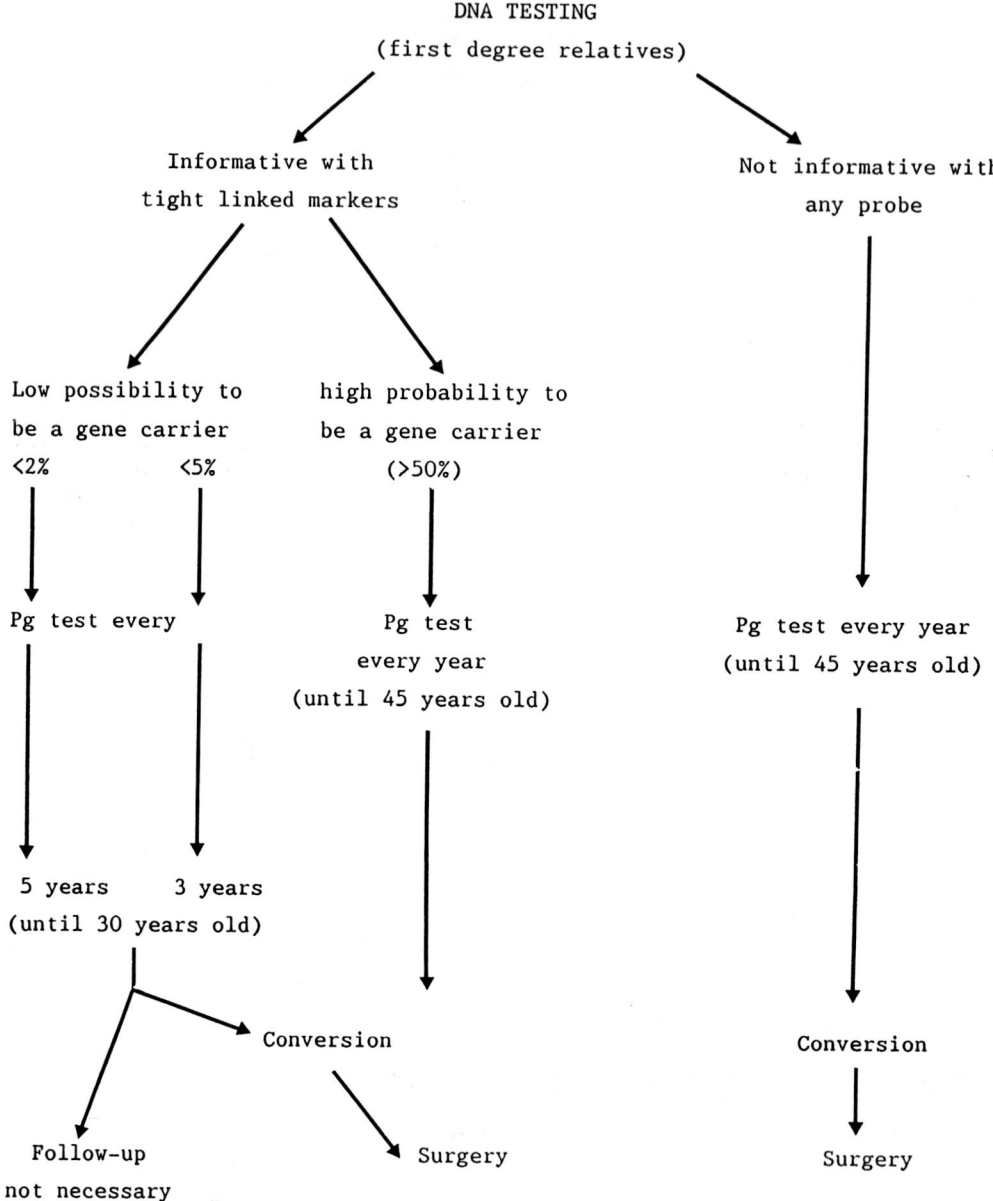

Fig. 5 Decisional tree showing the sequence of DNA test and conventional endocrine challenge. DNA test precises gene carriers who will be closely followed by PG testing; when conversion surgery can be proposed.

We shall analyse remaining multiplex MTC families with RBP3, D10S15, D10S34 and to test new probes now available: D10Z1, D10S94, MEN2.03, 48.11, FNRB (lenoir et al., 1991). This will permit to improve screening, especially in making new families informative.

Finally, genetic risk assessment will help to validate the Pg test with IRMA method by defining the significance of low CT level below 100 pg/ml (Gardet et al., 1991b). Presently, genetic screening requires familial investigations but when mutations will be characterized it will be possible to determine at the individual level who is at risk of cancer.

REFERENCES

Calmettes, C. (1984): Création d'un Groupe d'Etude des Tumeurs à Calcitonine. Bull. Cancer, 71, 3, 266-273.

Gardet, P., et al. (1991a): Screening relatives of medullary thyroid carcinoma patients. Validation of pentagastrin tests by genetic risk assessment and pathological report (submitted).

Gardet, P., et al. (1991b): Early detection of inherited MTC. London: John Libbey & Company (in this issue).

Lenoir, G.M., et al. (1991): Linkage analysis for hereditary thyroid carcinoma. London: John Libbey & Company (in this issue).

Mathew, C.G.P., et al. (1987): A linked genetic marker for multiple endocrine neoplasia type 2A on chromosome 10. Nature, 328, 527-528.

Narod, S.A., et al. (1989): Linkage analysis of hereditary MTC with and withougt pheochromocytoma. Hum. Genet., 83, 353-358.

Norum, R.A., et al. (1990): Linkage of the multiple endocrine neoplasia type 2B gene (MEN 2B) to chromosome 10 markers linked to MEN 2A. Genomics, 8, 313-317.

Sobol, H., et al. (1989a): Hereditary medullary thyroid carcinoma: genetic analysis of three related syndromes. Henry Ford Hosp. Med. J., 37, 109-111.

Sobol, H., et al. (1989b): Screening for multiple endocrine neoplasis type 2A with DNA-polymorphism analysis. New England J. Med., 321, 996-1001.

Sobol, H., (1990). Prédisposition génétique au cancer. L'exemple du cancer médullaire de la thyroïde. Localisation génique et proposition de dépistage des individus à risque. Ph D thesis, University of Lyon. pp 58bis.

VIII. Epidemiology of medullary thyroid carcinoma in Europe

VIII. *Epidémiologie du cancer médullaire de la thyroïde en Europe*

Epidemiology and genetics of medullary thyroid cancer. Preliminary results of an European concerted action

Claude Calmettes[1], Hanne Hansen[2], Eduardo Limbert[3], Pál Møller[4], Bruce Ponder[5], Friedhelm Raue[6], Hans Vasen[7] and Mischael Weissel[8]

[1] INSERM U 113, Faculté de Médecine Saint-Antoine, 75571 Paris Cedex 12, France. [2] Onkologisk afd. Rigshospitalet afsnit 5072, Blegdamsveg 9, 2100 Copenhagen, Denmark. [3] Servico de Patologia Morphologica, Instituto Portugués de Oncologia de Francisco Gentil, 1093 Lisbon Codex, Portugal. [4] Genetic Department, The Norwegian Radium Hospital 0315 Oslo, Norway. [5] Department of Pathology, University of Cambridge, CB2 1QP Cambridge, United Kingdom. [6] Department of Internal Medicine I, University of Heidelberg, 69000 Heidelberg, Germany. [7] Foundation for the Detection of Hereditary Tumours, 3501 AA Utrecht, The Netherlands. [8] Medizinische Universitätsklinik, 1090 Vienna, Austria

A research grant for a "Concerted Action", study of epidemiology and genetics of medullary thyroid cancer (MTC) was obtained from the European Communities in Bruxelles for 3 years from the beginning of 1990 ; it associates Austria, Belgium, Switzerland, Denmark, Spain, France, Germany, Italy, The Netherlands, Norway, Portugal, Sweden and United Kingdom in a common research programme.

We therefore initiated a European Study and we report, here the data that most of the different participants have been able to collect at least during the last year and our, prospective studies for the future at a European level which could be of benefit for the patients. Unfortunately, the data from Sweden are lacking, M. Telenius-Berg being absent on account of the events in Kuwait.

MOTIVATIONS AND GENERAL PURPOSE

Because of insufficient number of patients, studies in a single center are difficult in this rare disease, especially concerning MEN IIb, expression of the MEN syndrome - i.e. malignant pheochromocytoma -, prospective studies on surgical treatment - MTC reoperation, pheochromocytoma -, obtention of material, testing different technics...

Linkage studies were only initiated beginning of 1990 by G. Lenoir in LYON and B.A.J. Ponder in Cambridge. They agreed to store material, blood as well as tumors, from the patients studied in Europe and to study family members in case of the hereditary disease. Exchange of probes and training for visiting laboratories were planed.

A consensus management for early detection programme was decided; it involves a collaboration in screening of families dispersed in different countries -, establishment of national registries and collection of epidemiological data on a common form - which was established since the beginning of the action - ; it will therefore be possible to carry out an epidemiological study of the disease all over the western Europe.

Morover, one of the important goals is to inform people, specialists and non specialists, in the different countries and to invite them to participate in the study.

REGISTER OF MEDULLARY THYROID CARCINOMA IN GERMANY.

A register for medullary thyroid carcinoma was set up by the German MTC study group in 1988, (Raue F. et al. 1990) mainly focusing on the heriditary forms of MTC (multiple endocrine neoplasia = MEN types 2A and 2B). By family screening using calcitonin stimulation tests, the detection of MTC in an early curatively treatable stage is possible.

At present (December 1990), 600 patients (338 females and 262 males, ratio 1,3) with MTC have been reported by 27 cooperative centers. Mean age at diagnosis was 46,0 years ; 24,5 per cent (n = 147) had hereditary MTC, most of them MEN 2A (n = 94). 36 patients belong to the hereditary kind without other endocrinopathies (MTC only), 17 patients had MEN 2B. Mean age at diagnosis in MEN 2A patients was 36 years, in MEN 2B, 27.3 years. The number of reported patients has increased annually from 31 in 1980 to 49 patients in 1988.

A total of 452 patients were followed up over a period of .1 to 20.5 years (mean 4,6 years, median 3,7 years). The five- and ten-year survival rates were 80.5 per cent respectively 60.7 per cent for all patients, 90.7 per cent respectively 75.8 per cent in MEN 2A, 75 per cent respectively 56.3 per cent in MEN 2B and 77.5 per cent respectively 57.0 per cent in patients with the sporadic kind of MTC. Women proved to have a prognosis significantly better that men ($p < 0.001$), so has the hereditary compared with the sporadic type of MTC ($p < 0.03$) and the patients younger than 40 compared with older than 40 years ($p < 0.005$).

Total thyroidectomy is done only in 84 per cent of cases, although total thyroidectomy with central neck dissection is the therapy of choice.

A total of 353 patients is still alive, 131 of them with normal calcitonin serum levels and without localized tumor tissue. 84 live with calcitonin above the normal range but no evidence of tumor, 92 live with manifest tumor and 99 patients have died (75 of MTC, 10 of diseases other than MTC, 14 not specified).

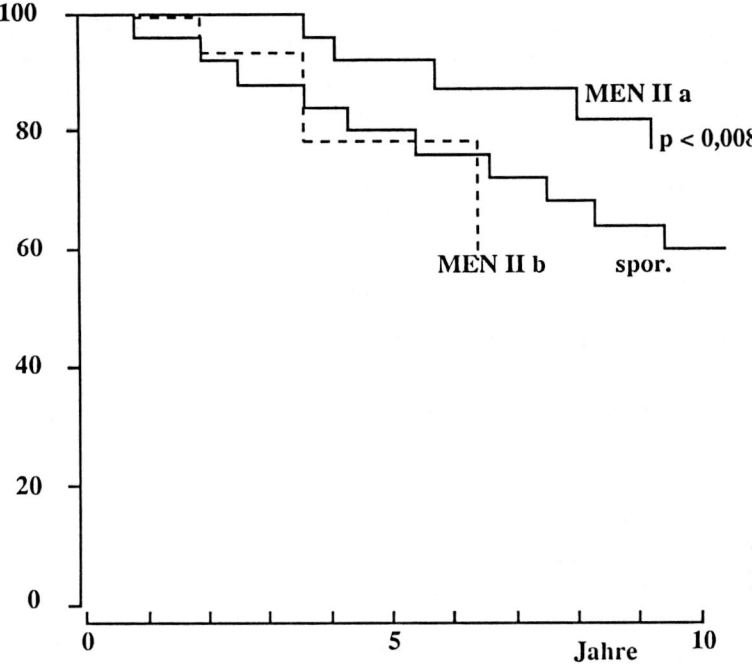

A systematic family screening with PG stimulation test is only done in 346 relatives, revealing 97 pathological tests.

This register will provide a basis for further collaborative diagnostic and therapeutic studies, e.g. systematic screening, in all relatives of MEN 2 patients and improvement of surgical treatment.

Raue F. et al. (1990) : Register für das medulläre
    schilddrüsenkarzinom in der Bundesrepublik Deutschland.
    Med Klink 85 : 113-117.

MEDULLARY CANCER IN DENMARK

Denmark is a low risk area concerning thyroid cancer ; the oncologic treatment is organized in five centers, from Alborg, Arhus to Copenhagen ; each has a catchment area of about one million people. The diagnosis is established and operation performed all over the country ; the oncologic treatment is given in these five centers, whether medical treatment, hormones and chemotherapy, as well as the follow up of the patients.

Since 1968, about 100 cases of MTC have been diagnosed (data from one center with a high load is still missing). So far, out of 21 patients with the hereditary form, 14 had MTC only, 4 had MEN 2A, 3 MEN 2B ; the biggest group was sporadic cases of MTC with an amount more than 80 patients.
The frequency of familial MTC in this period is 16 per cent, more likely more than 20 per cent.

An incidence rate of about 0.08 per cent has been calculated on the data from the danish cancer register from the sixties. In fact, MTC was not registered before 1978 but was pulled out and gives an incidence rate of 0.1 per cent for men and of 0.11 per cent for women. For all thyroid cancer, the incidence rate is of 1. for men, of 2. for women.
The number of diagnosed cases is increasing ; it varies from one to ten or more per year ; the family cases and the MEN 2 A and B can be easily recognised.

The european cooperation is welcomed as the danish MCT number is few.

MEDULLARY CANCER IN PORTUGAL

The new born MTC register began only a few months ago. It was possible to gather 51 cases but they seem to be underestimated.

The age and distribution of the population, separating sporadic cases from familial cases, have been studied. Mean age for familial cancer is 32 and for sporadic cases 57.
The evolution of the number of cases show an increase and this is probably due to a better diagnosis in the last decade and to the possibility of performing a PG test in familial cases. There are about 22.5 per cent of familial cancer. Most sporadic cases have not already beeing studied.

The distribution of all cases among the country shows that sporadic cases are distributed all over with a major prevalence in the most populated regions which stay near the coast. On the contrary, familial cases seem to be placed on nests, one in the North, one in the Center, one in the South. According to these data, mean incidence would be 0.1 and prevalence 1.2.

Geographical differences may be very interesting as they could lead to find some external causes for them and the origin of the families. Moreover, data may be compared with data from other countries.

This study was specially didactic : it was possible to transmit to other colleagues all over the country the necessity of systematic screening and standardised protocols for screening and treatment and maybe to give them experts on pathology to study difficult cases, as to obtain material for future for collaborative genetic studies.

MEDULLARY CANCER IN NORWAY

There is an excellent cancer register in Norway, a small country with about 4 million people, with a complete ascertainment of all cancer forms for long periods and that means that it is possible to do a prospective study retrospectively into the population. and analyse the data which are there.

Norway is long and is cut in two. Data from the high mountains are not yet registered ; there is a peculiar distribution of thyroid cancer in Norway : there are high prevalences in the West coast (it is not a map of inbreeding in a genetic sense); half of the population is living in the very East and South and there the frequency is low. The interesting point is that the geographic distribution is even ; it does not follow papillary carcinoma which is unevenly distributed.

Splitting out in the different forms of thyroid cancer, there is a reasonable getting to an older diagnosis of MCT because half of the patients had reached stadium 2 or 3 and if it is possible to put them down to stadium 1 or 0, it will be obviously a gain of benefit for the patients.

Looking retrospectively at the data for the last 22 years, the prevalence of medullary carcinoma in Norway is about 2.0 f or 100,000 persons living, corresponding with 3.8 per cent of all thyroid cancers. Annual incidences per 100,000 persons are 0.1 for males and 0.2 for females.

When plotting the number of new cases for each year for the last 22 years, there is a steady rate of about eight cases per year, close to twice as frequent in females as in males, with a fluctuation in small numbers : when there is a year with an additional female, there is a corresponding loss of a male, so the sums of these curves are fairly constant, about 8 persons, perhaps slighty increasing.

There are a few families in Norway and a possible new mutation. The DNA diagnostic laboratory is not made for this purpose so it is planned to ship the samples to those who are bigger in this field.

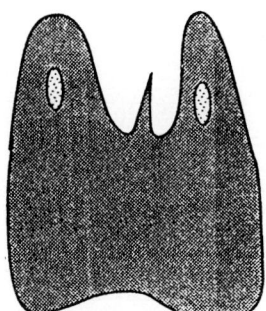

There is an age dependent logarithmic distribution which starts somewhere about 30 years of age, with an additional distribution of young patients : non genetic forms are rare and really seldom before this age. So, it could be reasonable to make a cut point of 50 years to do extensive screening studies because it would not miss any big family in confining to study that group and just skip the old group and concentrate on the young ones.

THE NETHERLANDS

There are three different registries in the Netherlands, a National Cancer Registry since 1989, Local Cancer Registries, for exemple one in Brabant, since 1975, and another in Utrecht since 1985, and a National Registry of Hereditary Cancer since 1985.
The population is 15 million.
Brabant has a population of almost 900.000 and, from 1979, 7 MTC cases have been registred ; Utrecht has a population of 1.200.000 and 7 cases have been registred since 1985.
All together, 25 families with 159 patients have been registred in the Hereditary Cancer Registry, 16 suffering from MEN 2A, 8 from MEN 2B and 1 with MTC only, with respectively 120, 11 and 28 patients, 192, 1 and 63 at risk relatives.
The cooperation looks essential for clinical and linkage studies.

AUSTRIA

The European Communities has to be thanked to have accepted the non members to participate in the concerted action on MTC. An Austrian registry is just billed up ; dr Niederle, from Vienna, had the initiative to form a group and this group had just collected the first data by telephone record organised for the meeting.
Austria has 6 million of inhabitants ; there are 215 MTC with 17 MEN 2. Most cases are in the region of Vienna.

The highest proportion - 180 - are sporadic MTC ; 18 cases are familial MTC, with 13 MEN 2A, and only from Salzburg a MEN 2B family with 4 patients.
Medullary thyroid cancer, as far we could know, is chiefly detected by chance -that means cold nodules-in 95 per cent of the cases and by the screening in 5 per cent.

SPAIN

There is no cancer registry in Spain for thyroid cancer ; so, the collection of data has been started on January 1990, so,most of the responses are lacking from most of the hospitals in the country.
The population is estimated as 30 million between Catalogna and the rest of Spain. Most cases, 76, were in Catalogna - 15 centers answered to the questionnaire- and 29 cases were collected from 6 centers In the rest of Spain.

Those cases were collected through a mean of 11,7 years for Catalogna and in a range from 5 to 20 years and for the rest of Spain the collection has been done for the last 7,8 years with a range from 4 to 10 years. This gives a number of cases per year of 6,5 in Catalogna and 3,7 for the rest of Spain and one can imagine those numbers are very 4nacurate and mainly the one for the rest of Spain. So, the approximate estimation of incidence for Catalogna is 0,069 for hundred thousand inhabitants per year which is lower that is seen for the other countries probably because there is not yet enough

information since questionnaries about the disease have not
been already returned.

The familial MCT only was diagnosed in 26 families in
Catalogna and in 2 families in the rest of Spain ; familial
MEN was found in 6 families in Catalogna and 5 in the rest of
Spain ; this discripancy could be related to the lack of
systematic screening test in all centers for the last 10
years, even if it is not the case for the last 2 years : this
collaborative study is, beside other advantages, very
important because it is making all the physicians aware that
they have really to make a screening ; it is perhaps possible
that many people still don't think so, which could explain
differences between the regions of Spain.

UNITED KINGDOM

There are about 80 cases of medullary thyroid cancer each year
in UK, of which about 20 are MEN 2 and the proportion of the
population who carries the MEN 2 gene is about 1/40 000.
The register started in about 1983 (Ponder, 1983). There are
on this register from UK of the order of 50 MEN 2A families,
which be can joined by doing genealogies, and about 25 MEN 2B
individuals and in some small families.

Conclusions can be made of some of the data in the register :
One of the first things was to calculate the age of onset
distribution of carriers MEN 2A gene and the probability that
a MEN 2A gene carrier will be detectable on a pentagastrin
stimulation test with age : half are detectable at the age of
12 and it is similar to N. Feingold's data. There is a
considerable uncertainty on a plateau between 19 and 100
because the data is based on something like 270 affected and
400 unaffected individuals : that is not still enough to
establish a probability with a high degree of confidence and
this is why it is very important to use genetic linkage to
identify gene carriers and to determine the penetrance
precisely. So, this curve has obviously an implication on how
to manage families with pentagastrin screening.
There is a similar distribution for the probability of an
individual who could carry the MEN 2A gene will presented
with clinical disease which took himself to a doctor. The
important point is that about 40 per cent of MEN 2A carriers
will not have presented clinically by the age of 70 and this
has very important implication first of all for the screening
of families. A study on the completeness of screening in the
UK found that in known families only about a third of
individual above the age of 40 had been offered screening,
probably because clinicians felt that if you had not got the
disease by the time you were 40 you had not got the gene. That
is clearly not the case. This also has implications whether to
screen the family of an apparently sporadic case. You can work
out that is a probability that somebody presenting with MTC at
any particular age will have the MEN 2A gene and it ranges
from 40 per cent for somebody aged 20 to 25 to about 10 per
cent for somebody aged 70.

B. Ponder (1983): Plasma calcitonin in medullary thyroid carcinoma. <u>Lancet 1</u>: 338

FRANCE

Among the aims of the French Medullary Study Group - Groupe d'Etude des Tumeurs à Calcitonine, GETC - were the improvement of familial screening, with the help of a network of regional coordinators, and the creation of a national register for MTC insuring medical confidence.
It was decided that a systematic and free familial screening would be made, whatever the age of the patient ; the number, age, place in the family of screened people as well as the pathological features of the proband would be taken into account in establishing the diagnosis of the sporadic form and the opportunity to stop or not the investigation.

A complete analysis of the epidemiological data is still to be made. Anyway, some conclusions can already be drawn :
The number of cases has regularly increased until about 1986, with a parallele increase in the number of familial cases and families detected ; this evolution is rather stabilized for the last 4 years : in 1987, 1988, 1989 and 1990 respectively, there was a total of 1009, 1237, 1436, 1680 cases of MTC (about 200 more patients per year). A total of 60, 77, 98 and 107 families was successively registered in the same period. The number of familial cases collected has also gone up : in the whole, 25 per cent of the cases ; anyway, it was about one third of new cases in 1989 and 1990.
In the same time, both extensive familial screening and the search for associated MEN features are associated with a decrease in apparently sporadic MEN 2A and familial MTC only (1990 : n = 43) for the benefit of familial MEN 2A (1990 : n = 58) whereas the number of MEN 2B families grows slowly (1990 : n = 6).

Genealogical studies have allowed to find common ancestors to families and to localize the main origin of familial MTC in 4 regions, 3 of them near the sea (Nord-Pas de Calais, Normandie, Bretagne), the last one not so far from the Atlantic, Charentes and West of the Massif Central. So, it is possible to inform the physicians practizing there of the occurence of the disease in their region.

Genetics studies are carried out on the responsability of G. Lenoir and H. Sobol in LYON. Blood samples have been collected from most of the familial cases and healthy relatives, and from probands in apparently sporadic cases. Results have already allowed the discrimination of people suffering or not of the hereditary form.

The main result of the French cooperative study is the extension of familial systematic screening using PG test with related improvement of the prognosis of the disease.

Calmettes C. (1984) : Création d'un Groupe d'Etude des Tumeurs à Calcitonine, <u>Bull. Cancer 71</u>: 266-273

CONCLUSIONS

From these preliminary results, and thanks to the European Communities, some conclusions can be drawn for all countries :
- the epidemiologic study was a good opportunity to stress people in doing extensive familial screening.
- the number of MTC cases has increased during the last years and there is an underestimation related to the anciennnety.
- the repartition of MCT is uneven,
- the incidence of the disase is approximatively the same, as the proportion MTC/Follicular cancers.

Moreover, members of the group offer to do screening for people belonging to families explored in other countries and to transmit research protocoles if necessary to concerned people.

So, this collaborative work can be looked as another step in the way of a progressive and deeper collaboration within Europe.

Members of the European Concerted Action

BELGIQUE
Dr Jean-Jacques BODY
    Institut Jules Bordet
    Rue Heger Bordet, 1
    B - 1000 Bruxelles
    tel (32) 2 537 3286
    fax (32) 2 537 6625

DANMARK
Dr Hanne Sand HANSEN
    Onkologist Afdeling Onk
    Rigshospitalet
    9 Blegdamsvej
    DK - 2100 KOBENHNAN O
    tel (45) 31 38 66 33

ESPANA
Dr Angeles GARCIA
    Hospital santa Cruz
    y san Pablo Avenida
    San Antonio Claret, 167
    E - 80 025 BARCELONA
    tel (34) 93 2366213
    fax (34) 93 2367633

CONFEDERATION HELVETIQUE
Dr J. FISCHER
    Klinik Balgrist
    Forchstrasse 340
    CH - 8008 ZURICH
    tel (41) 1 386 1651
    fax (41) 1 386 1652

DEUTSCHLAND
Dr Friedhelm RAUE
    Abteilung Innere Medizin I
    Endokrinologie
    und Stoffwechsel
    Medizinische
    Universitätsklinik
    FRG - 6900 HEIDELBERG
    tel (49) 6221 565671
    fax (49) 6221 565999

FRANCE
Dr Claude CALMETTES
    CHU St Antoine
    27, rue Chaligny
    F - 75 571 PARIS CEDEX 12
    tel (33) 1 40011313
    fax (33) 1 40011499

Dr Gilbert LENOIR
    International Agency for
    Research on Cancer
    150, Cours Albert Thomas
    F - 69372 LYON CEDEX 08
    tel (33) 72 73 84 85
    fax (33) 72 73 85 75

NEDERLAND
Dr Hans F.A. VASEN
    Medical School Stichting
    Opsporing Erfelijke Tumoren
    c/o University Hospital Leiden
    Rijnsburgerweg 10,
    building n°50
    ND - 2333 AA LEIDEN
    tel (31) 71 261955
    fax (31) 71 212137

OSTERREICH
Dr Mischa WEISSEL
    Universität Klinik -
    2 Medizinische
    Garnisonstrasse 13
    A - 1090 WIEN
    tel (43)   40 4 002124

SVERIGE
Dr Margareta TELENIUS BERG
    Department of Surgery
    S - 10401 STOKHOLM
    Tél (46) 87294140
    fax (46) 8336659

ITALIA
Dr Maria-Luisa BRANDI
    University of Florence,
    Dept of Pathophysiology
    Via Chiantigana 133/C
    I - 50 126 FLORENCE
    tel (39) 55 422190
    fax (39) 55 641026

NORGE
Dr Pal MOLLER
    Institute for
    Cancer Research Montebello
    N - 0310 OSLO 3
    tel (47) 2 50 60 50
    fax (47) 2 52 55 59

PORTUGAL
Dr Edward LIMBERT
    Servicio de Patologia
    Morfologica Instituto
    Portugues
    de Oncologia
    de Francisco Gentil
    Rua Prof. Lima Basto
    P - 1093 LISBOA CODEX
    Tél (98) 351 1 7264988
    fax (98) 351 1 7261529

UNITED KINGDOM
Dr Bruce A.J. PONDER
    Dept of Pathology
    Tennis Court Road
    UK - CAMBRIDGE CB2 1QP
    tel (44) 0223   333711
    fax (44) 0223 333375

<u>Other countries: physicians to be contacted</u>

HELLAS
Dr Demetrios KOUTRAS
    University of Athens -
    Dept of Clinical Therapeutics
    80, Vas. Sofias Avenue
    GR - 115 28 ATHENES
    tel (30) 1 7771 706
    fax (30) 1 7770 473

YUGOSLAVIA
Dr Marija AUERSPERG
    The Institute of Oncology
    Zaloska 2
    Y - 61 105 LJUBLIAJNA
    tel (38) 61 323 063

HUNGARIA
Dr Janos SZANTO
    Rath György u 7/9
    H - 1122 Budapest

Conclusions

Conclusions

J. Tourniaire

Clinique Endocrinologique, Hôpital de l'Antiquaille, 69321 Lyon Cedex 05, France

To sum up this fruitfull Congress would be very difficult. I prefer to focus on some important questions.

1. The first question is : where are the limits of the medullary thyroid cancer (MTC) ?

One point is clear : MTC secretes calcitonin and is often a genetic disease. But many points remain open for discussion. Geneticists are looking to the sequential defects between the primary event and the tumor revelation. Pathologists discuss about etiher ectodermic or endodermic origin of the C.cell according to the existence of mixed follicular and medullary lesions and sometimes positivity of the lesions for both thyroglobulin and calcitonin. There is perhaps more to it than mere exciting theoritical problem because of diagnosis and even prognosis implications. Biologists have developed a list of neuropeptides that can be found in these tumors. It looks like the " mille e tre" women of the Don Giovanni's list in the Mozart's opera. Each item is interesting as such, but finally wath significance is there in possessing the whole lot ?

2. The second question concerns diagnosis with two aspects : MTC and multiple endocrine neoplasia (type II).

For MTC the introduction of IRMA technic gives us a better sensitivity but there is -at the present time- an uncertain zone, when the calcitonin delta under pentagastrin (pg) is between 30 and 100 pg/ml. Some complementary markers could be of interest in such a case : for instance PAS 57 determination, or the radioreceptor assay for CGRP. They have to be tested on large series. In any cases imaging technics and venous sampling catheterization are useful only for recurrences or metastasis diagnosis. Beyond the classical technics, the unexpansive technecium D MSA seems to be both sensitive and specific enough. Cytology is of practical interest only in the diagnosis of sporadic cases before surgery.

In MEN 2, pheochromocytoma is the main association. It is generally clinically silent. It can be found before MCT and even in some patients with negative pg test. The consensus is that urinary and plasma metanephrine determination are the best tools for diagnosis." Adrenal medullary disease " can be clinically, but also biologically and radiologically asymptomatic. Its only symptom is a MIBG captation. Carefulness is required since nobody has presented adrenal biopsies in such cases. A long follow-up will be necessary before to conclude. The epidemiologist's work is fascinating : in french we call it "un travail de bénédictin " ; rather in fact a Mormon's labour! Their backward and forward inquiries give opportunities to link apparently distincts families and to discover the geographic origin of the mutation, and to reduce the number of " MTC only " families. Probably the brightest recent progress in the field comes from genetic studies. The MEN 2 gene is not identified but it is definitely situated near the centromer of chromosome 10. DNA analysis gives a precise estimation of the risk for every member of a family and it allows us to focus the screening. However everybody must know the limits of the method

It depends on the family size, on the informativeness of the probe, and on the lack of genetic heterogeneity. Finally pg test and DNA analysis are both required together in the risk determination. We have to remember that the result is but a statistic one. Clinicians know that the patients wish a yes or no answer.

3. The aim of all studies is to improve the prognosis. With the diagnosis age reduction, we can offer surgical treatment in time. It is clear thas the prognosis depends on the patient age, the tumor size, and the clinical lymph involvement. The quality of the neck dissection and lymphadenectomy is a key point and requires and experimented surgeon. Surgery remains - at the present time - our unique hope of complete cure. Unfortunately, radiotherapy and chimiotherapy are disappointing. New drugs and the use of sophisticated technics such as the radioactive antibodies have to be developed in the future.

Finally the most obvious conclusion is that cooperative studies between the different members of the scientific community are required. So this MCT Congress is only the first of a series and it is the opening of the MCT common market.

Good bye to everybody; Let's hope we shall meet again soon.

Author Index
Index des auteurs

Akwright A., 159
Allannic H., 163
Andry G., 207
Auvert B., 159

Barbosa J.A., 121
Basolo F., 81
Baulieu J.L., 125, 175, 187
Bellet D., 73, 237
Bellis G., 163
Billaud E., 115
Boiteau V., 169
Bondeson L., 101
Born W., 39
Bouillaud E., 115
Busnardo B., 229

Caillou B., 53, 159, 193, 237
Calmettes C., 9, 85, 149, 163, 169, 183, 187, 255
Caron J., 169, 187
Casanova S., 169
Chanson P., 175
Chatellier G., 115
Chauveau M.E., 175
Chaventré A., 163
Chayvialle J.A., 89
Clarke S.E.M., 111
Cola A., 81
Comoy E., 115
Corvol P., 115

Delisle M.J., 103
Delprat C.C., 221
Dor P., 207
Dupont J.L., 187
Dutrieux-Berger N., 159

Farkas D., 149, 169
Feingold N., 149, 169
Fischer J.A., 39
Floquet J., 159
Franc B., 65, 159
Fugazzola L., 81

Gardet P., 193, 213, 237
Gardner E., 137
Gay G., 175
Goslings B.M., 229
Grouzmann E., 115
Guillausseau P.J., 175, 229

Guillausseau-Scholer C., 175
Guilloteau D., 73
Guliana J.M., 19

Hansen H., 255
Henry J.F., 187
Hoefnagel C.A., 221
Holm R., 59
Houcke-Lecomte M., 159
Houdent C., 163
Hsiao R.J., 121

Jones C., 137
Jullienne A., 19
Justrabo E., 159

Krenning E.P., 85
Kvols L., 85

Labat-Moleur F., 159
Lamberts S.W.J., 85
Lange F., 159
Lasmoles F., 19
Le Bolic M.F., 159
Lenoir G., 237
Lenoir G.M., 145, 245
Limbert E., 255
Lips C.J.M., 241
Lubetzki J., 175

Marmousez T., 199
Meer A., 183
Milhaud G., 5, 19
Minvielle S., 19
Modigliani E., 85, 169, 229
Mole S.E., 137
Moller P., 255
Moore J., 137
Mornex R., 187
Moukhtar M.S., 19
Mulligan L.M., 137
Munck A., 183

Nakamura Y., 137
Narod S., 145, 245
Nesland J.M., 59
Neumann H.P.H., 121

O'Connor D.T., 121
Opocher G., 187

Pacini F., 81
Pages A., 65, 159
Papi L., 137
Parmentier C., 193, 213, 237
Parmer R.J., 121
Patey M., 159
Pinchera A., 81
Plouin P.F., 115, 187
Pluot M., 159
Ponder B., 255
Ponder B.A.J., 137
Proye C., 163, 187, 199

Raue F., 31, 187, 255
Reubi J.C., 85
Rigaud C., 159
Rosenberg-Bourgin M., 149, 169

Saint-André J.P., 159
Sambade C., 59
Sarfati E., 175
Sarrazin D., 213
Schlumberger M., 193, 213, 237
Scopsi L., 99
Segond N., 19
Sherübl H., 31
Shuffenecker I., 145, 245
Sobol H., 145, 167, 237, 245
Sobrinho-Simões M., 59

Telenius H., 137
Tourniaire J., 267
Travagli J.P., 193, 213, 237
Tubiana M., 3

Valdés Olmos R.A., 221
Vasen H.F.A., 241, 255
Vathaire (de) F., 193, 213
Viennet G., 159
Vildé F., 159

Weissel M., 229, 255
Williams E.D., 45

Zink A., 31

Colloques **INSERM**
ISSN 0768-3154

Other *Colloques* published as co-editions by John Libbey Eurotext and INSERM

153 Hormones and Cell Regulation (11th European Symposium). *Hormones et Régulation Cellulaire (11ᵉ Symposium Européen).*
Edited by J. Nunez and J.E. Dumont.
ISBN : John Libbey Eurotext 0 86196 104 8
   INSERM 2 85598 324 X

158 Biochemistry and Physiopathology of Platelet Membrane. *Biochimie et Physiopathologie de la Membrane Plaquettaire.*
Edited by G. Marguerie and R.F.A. Zwaal.
ISBN : John Libbey Eurotext 0 86196 114 5
   INSERM 2 85598 345 2

162 The Inhibitors of Hematopoiesis. *Les Inhibiteurs de l'Hématopoïèse.*
Edited by A. Najman, M. Guignon, N.C. Gorin and J.Y. Mary.
ISBN : John Libbey Eurotext 0 86196 125 0
   INSERM 2 85598 340 1

164 Liver Cells and Drugs. *Cellules Hépatiques et Médicaments.*
Edited by A. Guillouzo.
ISBN : John Libbey Eurotext 0 86196 128 5
   INSERM 2 85598 341 X

165 Hormones and Cell Regulation (12th European Symposium). *Hormones et Régulation Cellulaire (12ᵉ Symposium Européen).*
Edited by J. Nunez, J.E. Dumont and E. Carafoli.
ISBN : John Libbey Eurotext 0 86196 133 1
   INSERM 2 85598 347 9

167 Sleep Disorders and Respiration. *Les Evénements Respiratoires du Sommeil.*
Edited by P. Lévi-Valensi and D. Duron.
ISBN : John Libbey Eurotext 0 86196 127 7
   INSERM 2 85598 344 4

169 Neo-Adjuvant Chemotherapy. *Chimiothérapie Néo-Adjuvante.*
Edited by C. Jacquillat, M. Weil, D. Khayat.
ISBN : John Libbey Eurotext 0 86196 150 1
   INSERM 2 85598 349 5

171 Structure and Functions of the Cytoskeleton. *La Structure et les Fonctions du Cytosquelette.*
Edited by B.A.F. Rousset.
ISBN : John Libbey Eurotext 0 86196 149 8
   INSERM 2 85598 351 7

Colloques INSERM
ISSN 0768-3154

172 The Langerhans Cell. *La Cellule de Langerhans.*
Edited by J. Thivolet, D. Schmitt.
ISBN : John Libbey Eurotext 0 86196 181 1
INSERM 2 85598 352 5

173 Cellular and Molecular Aspects of Glucuronidation. *Aspects Cellulaires et Moléculaires de la Glucuronoconjugaison.*
Edited by G. Siest, J. Magdalou, B. Burchell
ISBN : John Libbey Eurotext 0 86196 182 X
INSERM 2 85598 353 3

174 Second Forum on Peptides. *Deuxième Forum Peptides.*
Edited by A. Aubry, M. Marraud, B. Vitoux
ISBN : John Libbey Eurotext 0 86196 151 X
INSERM 2 85598 354 1

176 Hormones and Cell Regulation (13th European Symposium). *Hormones et Régulation Cellulaire (13ᵉ Symposium Européen).*
Edited by J. Nunez, J.E. Dumont, R. Denton
ISBN : John Libbey Eurotext 0 86196 183 8
INSERM 2 85598 356 8

179 Lymphokine Receptors Interactions. *Interactions Lymphokines-récepteurs.*
Edited by D. Fradelizi, J. Bertoglio
ISBN : John Libbey Eurotext 0 86196 148 X
INSERM 2 85598 359 2

191 Anticancer Drugs (1st International Interface of Clinical and Laboratory responses to anticancer drugs). *Médicaments anticancéreux (1ʳᵉ Confrontation internationale des réponses cliniques et expérimentales aux médicaments anticancéreux).*
Edited by H. Tapiero, J. Robert, T.J. Lampidis
ISBN : John Libbey Eurotext 0 86196 223 0
INSERM 2 85598 393 2

193 Living in the Cold (2nd International Symposium). *La Vie au Froid (2ᵉ Symposium International).*
Edited by A. Malan, B. Canguilhem
ISBN : John Libbey Eurotext 0 86196 234 9
INSERM 2 85598 395 9

Colloques INSERM
ISSN 0768-3154

194 Progress in Hepatitis B Immunization. *La Vaccination contre l'épatite B.*
Edited by P. Coursaget, M.J. Tong
ISBN : John Libbey Eurotext 0 86196 249 4
INSERM 2 85598 396 7

196 Treatment Strategy in Hodgkin's Disease. *Stratégie dans la maladie de Hodgkin.*
Edited by P. Sommers, M. Henry-Amar,
J.H. Meezwaldt, P. Carde
ISBN : John Libbey Eurotext 0 86196 226 5
INSERM 2 85598 398 3

198 Hormones and Cell Regulation (14th European Symposium). *Hormones et Régulation Cellulaire (14e Symposium Européen).*
Edited by J. Nunez, J.E. Dumont
ISBN : John Libbey Eurotext 0 86196 229 X
INSERM 2 85598 400 9

199 Placental Communications : Biochemical, Morphological and Cellular Aspects. *Communications placentaires : aspects biochimique, morphologique et cellulaire.*
Edited by L. Cedard, E. Alsat, J.C. Challier,
G. Chaouat, A. Malassiné
ISBN : John Libbey Eurotext 0 86196 227 3
INSERM 2 85598 401 7

204 Pharmacologie Clinique : Actualités et Perspectives. (6e Rencontres Nationales de Pharmacologie clinique).
Edited by J.P. Boissel, C. Caulin, M. Teule
ISBN : John Libbey Eurotext 0 86196 225 7
INSERM 2 85598 454 8

205 Recent Trends in Clinical Pharmacology (6th National Meeting of Clinical Pharmacology).
Edited by J.P. Boissel, C. Caulin, M. Teule
ISBN : John Libbey Eurotext 0 86196 256 7
INSERM 2 85598 455 6

206 Platelet Immunology : Fundamental and Clinical Aspects. *Immunologie plaquettaire : aspects fondamentaux et cliniques.*
Edited by C. Kaplan-Gouet, N. Schlegel,
Ch. Salmon, J. McGregor
ISBN : John Libbey Eurotext 0 86196 285 0
INSERM 2 85598 439 4

Colloques INSERM
ISSN 0768-3154

207 Thyroperoxidase and Thyroid Autoimmunity. *Thyroperoxydase et auto-immunité thyroïdienne.*
Edited by P. Carayon, T. Ruf
ISBN : John Libbey Eurotext 0 86196 277 X
INSERM 2 85598 440 8

208 Vasopressin. *Vasopressine.*
Edited by S. Jard, R. Jamison
ISBN : John Libbey Eurotext 0 86196 288 5
INSERM 2 85598 441 6

210 Hormones and Cell Regulation (15th European Symposium). *Hormones et Régulation Cellulaire (15e Symposium Européen).*
Edited by J.E. Dumont, J. Nunez, R.J.B. King
ISBN : John Libbey Eurotext 0 86196 279 6
INSERM 2 85598 443 2

212 Cellular and Molecular Biology of the Materno-Fetal Relationship. *Biologie cellulaire et moléculaire de la relation materno-fœtale.*
Edited by G. Chaouat, J. Mowbray
ISBN : John Libbey Eurotext 0 86196 909 1
INSERM 2 85598 445 9

IMPRIMERIE LOUIS-JEAN
BP 87 — 05003 GAP Cedex
Tél. : 92.51.35.23
Dépôt légal : 366 — Mai 1991
Imprimé en France